# The Complete Idiot's Reference Card

Here is a simplified reflexology chart for the palms of the hands. T...
were holding their palms up in front of you.

There are also reflexes on the backs of the hands and all around th... ...reflexology charts
vary slightly, but most of the major reflexes are uniform. See the back of the book to order color-
coded, detailed charts for your wall or wallet.

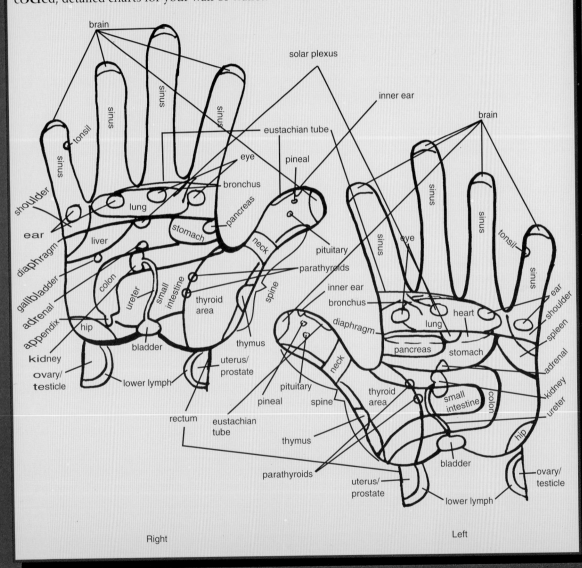

*tear here*

# Reflex Points on the Feet

Here's a simplified reflexology chart of the soles of the feet. This view shows the bottom of a pair of feet as if you were looking at someone who was lying down in front of you. This is how a reflexologist sees their subject.

Most reflexology areas are generally the same, but all charts will differ slightly. Reflexes are also found on the top side of the feet and around the ankles. See the back of the book for ordering color-coded, detailed wall charts, and/or wallet cards.

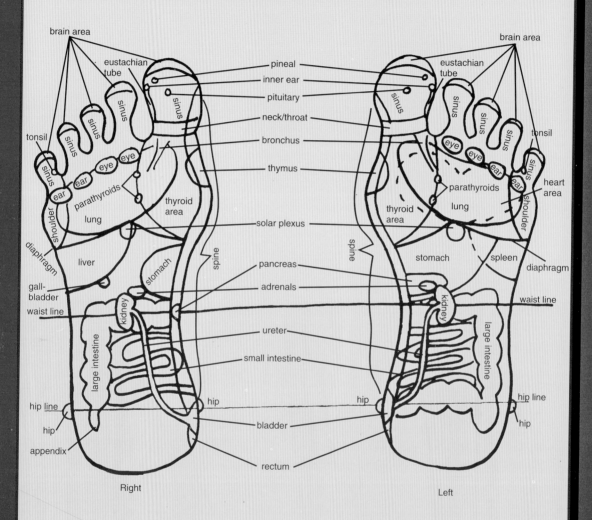

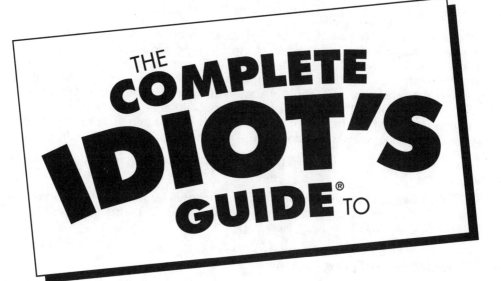

THE
# COMPLETE
# IDIOT'S
GUIDE® TO

# Reflexology

*by Frankie Avalon Wolfe*

## alpha
## books

A Division of Macmillan General Reference
A Pearson Education Macmillan Company
1633 Broadway, New York, NY 10019

Macmillan General Reference books may be purchased for business or sales promotional use. For information please write: Special Markets Department, Macmillan Publishing USA, 1633 Broadway, New York, NY 10019.

International Standard Book Number: 0-02863187-0
Library of Congress Catalog Card Number: 97-80961

01          8  7  6  5  4  3

Interpretation of the printing code: the rightmost number of the first series of numbers is the year of the book's printing; the rightmost number of the second series of numbers is the number of the book's printing. For example, a printing code of 99-1 shows that the first printing occurred in 1999.

*Printed in the United States of America*

**Note:** This publication contains information based on the research and experience of its authors and is designed to provide useful advice with regard to the subject matter covered. The authors and publisher are not engaged in rendering medical or other professional services in this publication. Circumstances vary for practitioners of the activities covered herein, and this publication should not be used without prior consultation from a competent medical professional.

# Alpha Development Team

**Publisher**
*Kathy Nebenhaus*

**Editorial Director**
*Gary M. Krebs*

**Managing Editor**
*Bob Shuman*

**Marketing Brand Manager**
*Felice Primeau*

**Acquisitions Editor**
*Jessica Faust*

**Development Editors**
*Phil Kitchel*
*Amy Zavatto*

**Assistant Editor**
*Georgette Blau*

# Production Team

**Development Editor**
*Mary Russell*

**Production Editor**
*Christy Wagner*

**Copy Editor**
*Abby Lyon Herriman*

**Cover Designer**
*Mike Freeland*

**Photo Editor**
*Richard H. Fox*

**Illustrator**
*Jody P. Schaeffer*

**Book Designers**
*Scott Cook and Amy Adams of DesignLab*

**Indexer**
*Craig Small*

**Layout/Proofreading**
*Eric Brinkman*
*Jerry Cole*
*Marie Kristine Parial-Leonardo*
*Angel Perez*
*Linda Quigley*

# Contents at a Glance

# Contents

## 11 Getting to the Heart of the Matter: The Circulatory System 141

## 12 Sexy Stuff: The Glandular System 155

## Part 3: Tools and Techniques for Feeling Good 167

## 13 Digging In: Where Do I Start? 169

## Appendices

# Foreword

Reflexology is an ancient healing art that came to us from China, Egypt, and India and was rediscovered 100 years ago. Like other ancient healing modalities, we have been able to rediscover reflexology's many benefits, and we are able to use these benefits to assist us in alleviating the stresses of the modern world.

Reflexology has the ability to bring about a state of relaxation, and because of this it is able to assist the body's own natural healing to take place. Reflexology is also able to complement other types of health care. From my own experiences I have found that reflexology is able to assist everyone, from infants right through to the elderly. It is of benefit whether our lives take active or sedentary roles, and it is able to transcend all barriers: emotional, physical, and mental.

With the increased interest in reflexology worldwide, I find it exciting that the amount of information available to the general public on this subject is increasing. It is refreshing to see a book like *The Complete Idiot's Guide to Reflexology* being published. This book explains the workings of reflexology to the layperson in easy to understand terms and still manages to contain a wealth of information for the complete novice.

It covers all the body systems and explains in simple terms the importance of each system. It covers everything the beginner needs to know and might come across when giving sessions to family and friends. It also tells you the different types of foot conditions that can occur and the importance of wearing the correct shoes.

It has been said that the foot is a reflection of our health, and reflexology gives us a means to use this reflection to improve the health of our family and friends.

No matter whether you only want to work on family or friends or you want to go further and become a professional reflexologist, you will find *The Complete Idiot's Guide to Reflexology* to be of great benefit.

—Russell McAllister

Russell McAllister is Publisher of *Reflexology World* magazine, and a Director of the International Council of Reflexologists. Mr. McAllister is a founding member of the Reflexology Association of Australia and resides in Sydney, Australia, where he has a reflexology practice.

# Introduction

When I was first asked to write this book I was delighted, then immediately anxious. I thought, "How can I write a 350-page book on the basics of reflexology and keep it entertaining?"

I thought about how over the years I have been helped by reflexology and how my clients have responded to their treatments. I thought about how reflexology is more than just a therapy involving pushing reflex points, but is also a philosophy. It shows us how our body is connected and how it reacts to stimulus and mirrors how the world is connected. This connection idea is a philosophical point of view I use in my life and my practice.

I decided to include some "fun" ideas that you might find useful, such as how to read the personality in the feet. We all have the personal power to behave correctly; however, it is entertaining to match the general personality tendencies with the shape and condition of a foot. This observance is not necessarily considered part of reflexology, but since you will be observing feet, you might be surprised how many times the foot fits the person! Utilizing this technique, you may be able to understand a little more about a person and help personalize how you deal with them.

And, if you decide to become a professional reflexologist, this book will help you to be prepared and assist you in making your practice unique and successful. It can also be used as a reference to help you remember what you learned in your classes.

I hope you have fun reading this book and that you laugh, learn, and grow.

I wish you the best of health.

## How to Use This Book

Body systems and various conditions are described in detail throughout the book. Topics are supported by sketches highlighting the relevant points. Use the tear-out card charts for reference once you are familiar with the techniques of performing effective reflexology.

The book is divided into five parts:

**Part 1, "Before You Take Your Socks Off,"** introduces you to the theory of reflexology, what it means, and what it's used for, and takes a look at its ancient history.

**Part 2, "The Body Systems: Mapping It Out,"** covers all the body systems and describes where the major reflex points are mapped on the feet and hands.

**Part 3, "Tools and Techniques for Feeling Good,"** gets into the proper techniques of reflexology to help you focus on getting results.

**Part 4, "The Practice of Reflexology,"** gives you some insight into the physical conditions of the foot. It also will help you see how your feet can tell a story about you.

**Part 5, "Reflexology in Action,"** gives some testimonials and gets into more details of how you can use reflexology to help combat certain disorders.

# Extras

In addition to all the things you'll learn in the text, this book has some special features to make your progress even more pleasant. Let me introduce you to a few extras you will see in this book.

### Tip Toe

These boxes contain little tidbits of information and highlight important facts about reflexology. Some include tips that will help you do things more easily.

### Tread Lightly

These boxes warn you about things that you will need to be cautious about. They include warnings, contraindications, and important pointers to things you need to take seriously.

### The Sole Meaning

These boxes highlight the terminology used in reflexology and will give you the language you need to understand and describe what you are doing.

### Foot Note

These boxes contain anecdotal information, personal stories, and extra bits of information about reflexology. Read them to find out a little bit more.

# Acknowledgements

I always have a great amount of gratitude to all the folks who have helped me during my times of big projects and achievements—this book is no exception.

Thanks goes first to the person I spend more time with than anyone else on the planet, my greatest helper, my gift of a husband, Townsend. (There is not enough room to thank you for everything!)

Thanks to Connie and Bob for all of your encouragement and your time in reviewing my work! Thanks to Jay Parker of Parker Portraits for your excellent photography of most of the shots in this book. And thank you Gordon a.k.a. Captain Camo for lending me your facial expressions for the funny shots in Chapter 14. (You make a great model and friend.) And to Dr. Richard Long and Dr. Zachary Brinkerhoff of the MIR for your help with some of the photographs and shared enthusiasm for the book. Thank you Werner Wirz of Canada for setting me up with your Canadian association, eh?! And a special thank you to Barbara Mosier of ARCB for the materials you supplied and your time talking with me.

The rest of the thank yous go to the friends, family members, and clients I have worked on through the years who have actually proved to ME that reflexology works! And thanks to those of you who always told me that I should write comedy. It keeps me going! Special thanks to my grandma Fran who listens to me when I doubt myself and offers encouragement and laughter. And I wish to express gratitude to all of my teachers throughout the years who inspire me to continue striving for wisdom.

Thank you Jessica Faust of Macmillan Publishing for finding me and giving me this opportunity; special thanks to Mary Russell who guided me through the process; and much appreciation is extended to my greatest reflexology teacher, Isabelle Hutton, for taking the time to do the technical editing—whew!

# Special Thanks to the Technical Reviewer

*The Complete Idiot's Guide to Reflexology* was reviewed by an expert who double-checked the accuracy of what you'll learn here, to help us ensure that this book gives you everything you need to know about reflexology. Special thanks are extended to Isabelle Hutton, R.N.

Isabelle Susanne Hutton is a Registered Nurse and a Nationally Certified Reflexologist, having practiced and taught reflexology for the past 26 years. She is responsible for teaching hundreds of students throughout the United States and Canada reflexology and other healing modalities. She is an internationally known speaker, designs and leads a variety of workshops, and is in the process of writing a book on reflexology. Isabelle has recently completed a 10-year endeavor to develop a series of Health Charts that are simple and easy to follow for anyone from the novice to the expert. She maintains a private practice and teaches at her Academy of Natural Healing in Greenwood Village, Colorado, where she celebrates her passion, reflexology, and energy work including Jin Shin Jyutsu and aromatherapy.

# Part 1
# Before You Take Your Socks Off

*Before you expose those toes to my nose there are some basics we need to cover on the concepts of reflexology! Reflexology is a natural, safe, and effective practice that helps you take responsibility for your health. Reflexology can be used in three different ways, which is one reason it is so much fun to learn.*

*First of all, reflexology is primarily used as a natural therapy to promote relaxation and healing of the body, mind, and soul. Secondly, you can use reflexology as part of a health analysis, since your feet give clues about what is going on inside your body. And finally, you can use the clues observed on your feet and hands as a tool for discovering your hidden personality traits.*

*In this section we'll take a stroll through the basics of reflexology, its history, and the fundamentals of the foot.*

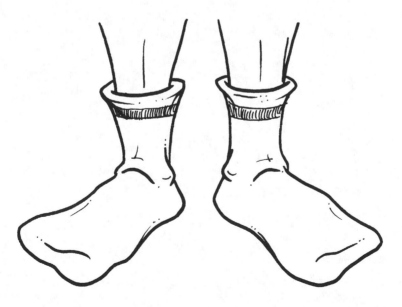

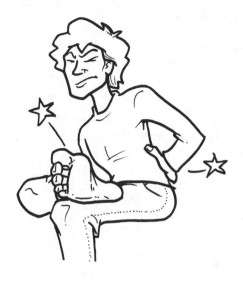

# What Is Reflexology?

When I heard that my friend, who was working as a pedicurist, was taking a class in reflexology, I immediately jumped at the chance to join her. I had no clue what reflexology was all about but I did know it had something to do with natural healing. Once we began working on each other as students I felt like my entire insides had been toned and refreshed! The cold that I was beginning to get the day before class had spontaneously disappeared and the bladder infection I felt coming on went away!

These results all came within the first four hours of my first class, and I knew that I was passionately interested in learning more about the natural, ancient, safe, and effective healing therapy known as reflexology. This chapter will lead you feet first through the philosophy behind reflexology, how it works, and how simply it can fit into your life.

## Reflexology: Go with the Flow

Let's start out by going over the basic definition of reflexology so we can get into the good stuff quickly! Broken down into its basic parts, the word *reflexology* is made up of "reflex," in this case meaning one part reflecting another part, and "ology," meaning the study of. Put together, this word means the study of how one part relates to another part. But fortunately for those of us who love to get and give reflexology sessions, there is much more to this than just the study of its parts!

Reflexology is commonly explained as the scientific theory that maps out the reflexes on the feet and hands to all the organs and the rest of the body. In other words, certain spots on the feet and hands have an energy connection to other parts of your body. By applying acupressure and massage-like techniques to the feet and hands you will positively affect all other body parts.

Although they share some similarities, acupressure, massage, and reflexology are all distinctly separate therapies from each other. A description of acupressure and acupuncture can be found in the Glossary. Also, you shouldn't confuse reflexology with massage. See the table in Chapter 21, "Healthy, Wealthy, and Wise: What You Need to Know," which contrasts the differences between reflexology and massage for further clarification.

**The Sole Meaning**

**Reflexology** literally means the study of how one part reflects or relates to another part of the body. It is a holistic therapy used for health management and maintenance and can also be used as a health and personality analysis tool.

Throughout this book I will be referring to reflexes or reflex points, areas, or spots. These will all mean the same thing. A reflex area or spot just means that it is a spot on the hands, feet, or ears that corresponds to a body part or organ elsewhere on the body. For instance, if I say, "Press on your kidney reflex," this means that I will be showing you where on your feet or hands the corresponding reflex points for the kidneys are. By applying pressure in these areas, you can positively affect your kidney(s).

## Fancy Footwork

Reflexology is more than just the study of reflex points. It is also a wonderful, natural health therapy, a health analysis tool, and sometimes it is even used to reveal the personality of the foot owner! Locating the places on the feet that correspond to different areas is great, but the true beauty of reflexology is what you can learn about yourself or your partner when you practice reflexology on them. The other beauty of reflexology is how good it makes you feel.

Reflexology can be used in three ways, including:

➤ **As a hands-on natural health body therapy.** The feet and hands and sometimes ears are worked on to create relaxation, ease pain, and stimulate the body's ability to heal itself.

➤ **A health analysis tool.** Medical doctors are the only practitioners allowed to diagnose diseases; however, as a reflexologist you will recognize many types of foot ailments, which will give you the opportunity to get proper treatment. Also, by finding tender reflex spots in your own feet or hands you just might be able to discern something about the condition of the corresponding organ. See Chapters 18, "Finding Balance: The Elemental Foot," and 20, "Podiatry Matters," for more on these subjects.

➤ **As a personality analysis tool.** Some practitioners can discern things about the personality by observing the shapes, lines, and conditions of the feet and hands. Although this isn't technically considered within the scope of reflexology, it is harmless fun and can be surprisingly accurate! See Chapter 19, "The Personality in the Feet," for more on this subject.

## The Whole Story

Since the body works as a whole unit, reflex points can actually be found many places in the body. In other words, your body is all connected; you cannot isolate any one part of the body completely without it ceasing to function. The holistic practitioner understands this "whole" concept and may utilize this knowledge to create natural therapies that apply to the whole body. There are several practices that map out reflex areas:

➤ **Foot, hand, and ear reflexology.** That's what this book is all about! However, we will be primarily concentrating on the reflexes on the feet in this book.

➤ **Bowel reflexes.** Holistic practitioners also believe that the bowel has reflex points in it. This means that an irritation or pain experienced in some part of the body may be linked to stagnation or some type of problem found in the bowel!

➤ **Iris reflexes or iridology.** This fascinating study is based on the idea that the iris of the eye (the colored part of the eye) reflects the entire body through the central nervous system, kind of like a computer screen or a TV projects an image. The iris is divided into pie-shaped pieces that map out the entire body. A trained iridologist can utilize the iris map and "read your eyes," your genetic makeup, and other information about your body.

**The Sole Meaning**

**Iridology** is the scientific analysis of the iris of the eye to determine inherent genetic weaknesses and to assess some health conditions.

➤ **Body reflexology.** Mildred Carter, famous for her foot and hand reflexology work, also has made body reflexology quite popular. Basically, the system maps out reflex points located in various areas on the body (even the tongue) that when pressed will affect a different area of the body.

Since the body is one unit, we cannot expect to isolate one area of the body and only affect that area. In fact, whatever you are exposed to or whatever you ingest has some effect on every part of you. That is why if we take very good care of at least one part of us, all other parts of us have to benefit. So in this book we will keep it simple and fun and will concentrate on taking very good care of our feet. Just keep in mind that, like everything in life, the whole is always greater than the sum of its parts.

## Putting Your Foot in Your Mouth

Reflexology is not just fancy footwork. In fact, many reflexologists are adamant that you never call their practice a foot rub, or just foot and/or hand massage. I tend to be more relaxed about semantics, but sometimes these slang terms can get you in trouble. I learned this embarrassing lesson years ago when I was taking my first reflexology class at The Colorado School of Healing Arts.

**Tread Lightly**

Most reflexologists prefer to have you call what they do **reflexology sessions**, or **hand and foot reflexology**, and not foot and hand massage, or foot rubs. And never, at least in public, ask for a hand job!

I was so excited about learning this new skill that I would practically grab any poor, innocent bystander I could just for a chance to show them how amazing reflexology can be. Of course, most people walking down the street have shoes on, so in my zealousness to practice, I began working on the hands of almost every new acquaintance.

Sharing my excitement with my younger sister one evening, I explained reflexology to her as I worked on her hands. She was impressed with how good it made her feel. Later, at a large, formal dinner party with my parents and some of their business associates, my sister and her new boyfriend were sitting across the table from me. In my overwhelming enthusiasm for my new skill, I blurted out to my sister, "Hey Brandi, have you given Tim a hand job yet?" At first I didn't understand the silence that came over the table. I have never used that term for a hand reflexology session again.

## In the Zone

To help illustrate how every part of our body is interconnected we can compare our body to the globe we live on. The globe is one whole organism just as our body is one whole organism. We affect our earth's atmosphere by what we do on the earth just as we can affect our mind by having our feet worked on. However, just as the earth requires a map to help us define where we are going, you will need a map of the reflex points of the feet and hands to understand and stimulate the areas you want to work on. Let's take a look at a couple of ways to find our bearings.

There are many ways to chart or map the feet and the whole body. Charting or dividing the body conceptually into sections helps us understand how each section works. Once we figure out all the sections, the whole makes more sense. On top of just mapping out the reflex points to corresponding organs on the soles of the feet and palms of the hands (as you can see charted on the tear card chart in the front of this book), there is another theory that reflexology encompasses: the belief that there are invisible pathways of energy that run vertically along the body. These energy flows or lines are called *zones*.

Imagine your body tattooed with pin stripes that run the length of your body from your toes on up to the top of your head, as illustrated in the following figure. These pin stripes are your zones. Working with these lines, and with points along the lines, is known as *zone therapy*.

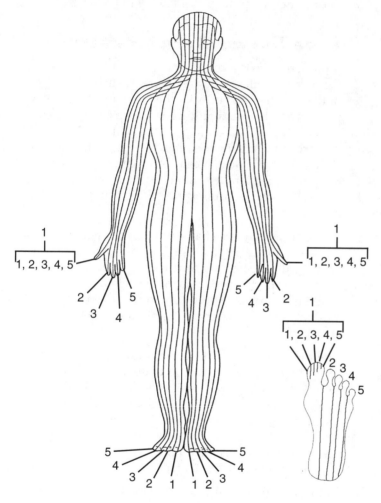

*Zone therapy divides the body into sections longitudinally. These lines of energy run through the body, affecting each organ along their path.*

It is important to understand the theory of zone therapy, because disease tends to run along these lines. For example, diabetes is a disease primarily caused by malfunctioning of the pancreas. Take a look at the zone therapy diagram. The area where the pancreas would lie is located between zones three and four. Associated complications with diabetes include problems with the kidneys, which are also located along zones three and four (on both sides), and the eyes, which are also in zones three and four.

### The Sole Meaning

**Zones** are invisible lines of energy that run longitudinally along the body. Working with these lines or sections is known as **zone therapy**, which many say is just another name for reflexology.

Each zone or section acts as a kind of link to each organ or body part along the same meridian. A break or stagnation anywhere along these lines can disrupt the flow of energy to an organ, which may cause the organ to malfunction. Breaking up these blocked energies with applied reflexology sessions or zone therapy sessions works by restoring proper energy and blood flow. This, in turn, helps restore proper energy to the organs.

## Zone Therapy Versus Reflexology

Although there is some debate about whether zone therapy and reflexology are different practices, the goal of the two therapies is really the same: to help the body balance and heal naturally, to break up congestion in corresponding organs, to improve circulation, and to help relieve pain and improve energy. So what's the difference between these two modalities? The main thing I have noticed is that I sometimes fall into a euphoric sleep when I am receiving a reflexology session. On the other hand, during my zone therapy sessions I have literally lost what felt like pounds of sweat! The difference is in the administration. You could say that the zone therapy sessions are more "active."

### Tip Toe

If a therapist is making you uncomfortable, no matter what they are calling their practice, you should let them know. If they continue to make you uncomfortable, then by all means get up and leave! Remember that you are paying someone to help you, not to help them prove a point. Don't be afraid to search for your ideal practitioner!

I have always sat in a chair for the zone therapy sessions, but we're not talking a plush, lay back and relax chair. Actually, I have had my zone therapy sessions while sitting on an old, hard, cold, orange vinyl chair. Most of the time though, shortly after the therapist began working on me, I never even noticed what I was sitting on.

The zone therapist worked deeply on my foot and lower leg using his knuckles as tools to dig into my reflex points. The therapy was applied very quickly and vigorously. The session was so vigorous that I broke a sweat in response to the healing and increased circulation that it brought to my body. The hurt-so-good feeling was so intense that I literally had to brace myself so that I didn't kick my therapist!

This is not to say that I wasn't enjoying myself. Everyone has their own level of pain tolerance, as we will discuss in more depth later. I happen to be a person who likes particularly deep work. Deep work is not for everyone though, and generally I have to search to find a reflexologist willing to go as deep as I need. If you are receiving a treatment that is too deep for you, don't be afraid to tell your therapist to back off and be more gentle.

In contrast to my zone therapy sessions, my reflexology sessions usually take place while I am lying down under warm blankets on a cushy massage table with soft music playing in the background. This situation feels much more gentle and pampering.

I enjoyed—and still enjoy—both therapies immensely. And besides, after receiving either session, I feel good, refreshed, and invigorated. So although the two therapists called their practices by different names, had different approaches, and supplied different environments for the actual session, they both still worked the same parts and the overall effects were similar for my body.

## The Toe Bone's Connected to What?

Take another look at the zone therapy model. You can see how the outside of your feet represent the outer rims of your body, such as the thighs, hips, shoulders, and each side of your head. Conversely, the insides of the feet represent the middle zones of your body, such as the bladder, spine, and digestive organs on up to the nose.

Another way to see the body mapped out on the feet is to superimpose the entire body over the sole of the foot. In the following figure you can see how the feet are associated with the parts of the body, from the head area on down to the lower bowel. The spinal column reflex area actually runs along the instep, so for some mental gymnastics try to imagine our figure superimposed sideways, too.

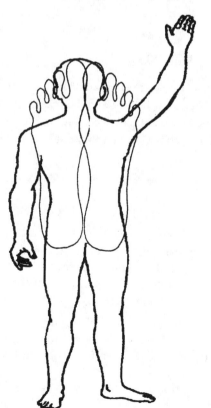

*An easy way to visualize the general reflex areas on the foot.*

Now that you've learned about zones and reflex points, you can get a general idea of how affecting energy in one place can influence another. Just think of those zones as the overall map of electricity running up and down the body on a consistent basis. We will get into the actual foot and hand maps that correspond to specific organs and how you can use them, in future chapters.

# Ooh, That Tickles!

Many people think that letting someone touch their feet will tickle. Understandable, since many of us had playful dads who held our ankles and tickled our feet unmercifully while giggling "koochey, koochey, koo!" Actually, when done properly, reflexology is anything but ticklish.

To be effective, reflexology should be a fairly firm, deep pressure applied to the feet and hands. The pressure is administered slowly to avoid discomfort. The deeper you go the slower you must apply pressure. Steady, flowing techniques are used. If anything, people feel tenderness rather than ticklishness in the feet with reflexology. The tenderness is a kind of hurts-so-good feeling, like when you press gently on a bruised area.

### Foot Note

I can't tell you how many wives have sent their reluctant husbands to me for sessions. The husbands were embarrassed because they thought they would be tickled and have to jump about and embarrass themselves! Well, I have not had one client who has felt tickled by my sessions. The only thing they were tickled about was that they felt better all over when the session was through.

# *Where Does It Hurt?*

Reflexology works by applying pressure to certain parts of the feet and hands, which stimulates the corresponding organs. Wherever you find "tender" areas, these are the clues that the corresponding organs are sluggish. The tender spots on the feet and hands are the areas that actually need the most work.

Reflexology points may be tender because at any given time we have a certain amount of toxins flowing throughout our bodies. These toxins are things like cellular waste products, uric acid, pesticide residues, and other chemicals that the body cannot or has not eliminated.

Toxic residues can linger inside us, sometimes indefinitely. Frequently, these toxins can settle along certain zones and cause interference with the energy flow to the rest of the organs along the zone pathways.

## *Walking on Pins and Needles*

Have you heard the phrase "gravity sucks"? Well, figuratively speaking, it's true. Since most of us are either on our feet or have our feet lower than our heads most of the time, these toxic waste materials can settle at the end of our nerve endings on the bottoms of our feet. These nice little deposits are what I call "crunchies."

I call them that because they usually consist of uric acid crystals, and when you apply pressure to them to break them up often you can hear them actually crunch! Once these crystals are broken up they can be carried off by the blood stream and eliminated through our natural elimination channels.

**Tread Lightly**

Toxins such as lead, mercury, aluminum, fluoride, chlorine, bacteria, and viruses have all been found in tap water. Avoid intake of these excess nasties by purchasing a water filter for your drinking water. Reverse osmosis water, in my opinion, is the cleanest, tastiest, and healthiest water for drinking, but a carbon filter is still a helpful and simple way to filter water.

You may experience a burning or even a poking sensation when these crunchies are breaking up. The good news is that the discomfort should subside almost as fast as it came. Breaking up these toxic settlements and allowing the body to eliminate them will help to restore proper energy flow to the zones and will remove excess waste from the body, leaving you feeling refreshed and more vibrant.

# Up to Your Ankles in Natural Health

Many countries have never gotten away from the use of natural health care. For some reason, though, America went for a ride, swinging from natural health care to medical science, and now we are coming back to natural health again, but with a more balanced view. Why are we going back to these ancient, healing, natural therapies?

My personal belief, which is shared by many natural health practitioners, is that health is truly a natural way of being, and it is only unnatural things that alter it. The body and its cells have an innate intelligence. Every day our heart continues to beat, we breathe, digest foods, eliminate waste, all without conscious effort! The body is an absolute miracle, and it knows what to do to be healthy and stay balanced.

How does the body get out of balance? Here's the short list:

➤ Good and bad stress

➤ Pesticides, chemicals, and fertilizers

➤ Air pollution

➤ Prescription and other drugs

➤ Environmental and electromagnetic pollution

➤ Cooked and processed foods

➤ Long work hours

These are all unnatural things that add to the imbalance of our body. Our poor bodies work so hard to keep us going in spite of all these "speed bumps" we challenge it with. If we give our body the opportunity to heal itself, then it will do a tremendous job for us to do just that.

The resurgence of natural health practices and their acceptance as normal, sensible therapies reflect our overall understanding and awareness that nature has laws and she also has cures. We should not continue to violate these simple laws, by doing things like eating processed, denatured foods, for example, and expect to have strong bodies.

**Tip Toe**

The body has a unique ability to heal and seek balance. The trick is finding out where you are out of balance and using natural therapies to even the scales. Natural balance cannot be forced because it has its own unique and temperamental formula. The opportunity for true healing must not be forced, it must be offered.

**Foot Note**

Getting in touch with nature is a good way to understand nature's laws and gain insight into the universal order. Understanding these laws helps us get in touch with our body and our health. If you study one animal or plant or bug, think of all the things that it needs to survive. Think of all the things that would fail to exist without it. See that everything on earth makes a difference, no matter how small or large. Everything in nature is connected.

## The Cure Is Underfoot

In addition to what we put in our bodies, we cannot wear shoes that insulate us from getting—and keeping—in touch with our mother planet and expect to feel grounded. Nature is a teacher. We need to stop, feel, and observe how nature works in order to understand the purpose in our lives and gain holistic insights into the world and beyond.

Reflexology is becoming a popular therapy again at least in part because we are tired of trying to drug ourselves back to health. Somehow we have finally figured out that the key to whole health cannot be found through a magic pill. We are realizing that stress-reduction skills, good relationships, exercise, organic whole foods and clean water, fresh air, sunshine, herbs, and bodywork are all part of a fine recipe for robust health and preventative maintenance.

We are changing as a people and our thoughts about old age are changing. I remember when I was little I thought that everyone lost their teeth, their hair, hearing, and eyesight when they got "old." Of course my definition of old then was 60! Now I know better, and so do most of you. With a little bit of awareness we are all changing the face of old age. We are becoming *holistic*.

My hope is that someday we will not have such a demand for nursing homes because the elderly will live stronger longer. If we can keep ourselves out of situations where we need to be cared for by someone else just by using safe, effective, natural health therapies, then *why not?* As a society, I see us really getting back into "wholism," hence the catchy phrase *holistic health*, although you'll have to supply the missing "w" for yourself.

### The Sole Meaning

**Holistic** is a term used to describe a way of living, practicing, or thinking that takes into account all factors of life. In holistic health, a practitioner will consider the physical, mental, emotional, and spiritual aspects of the person to help them back to balance.

## The Whole Philosophy on Herbs

Anyway, as I was saying before, the whole is greater than the sum of its parts. This goes for everything I can think of, including natural therapies. For instance, herbs can serve as foods and medicines. Herbs and nutrition are a part of getting well and are essential to helping reflexology maintain long-lasting effects.

All the components that make up an herb work synergistically to enhance the effect that the plant has in or on our body. For instance, many herbalists believe that rose hips, used as an herb rich in vitamin C, have a faster and better effect on a cold than a plain extracted vitamin C pill. I am an advocate of vitamin C, don't get me wrong, but my fundamental beliefs rest in wholism. Herbalists believe that the other natural components (*phytochemicals*) in the whole rose hip enhance the effectiveness of the vitamin C in our body.

Since you can't patent a plant, the pharmaceutical industry has to try to synthetically reproduce or extract some of the healing components in many plants. This extraction, coupled with specialists

### The Sole Meaning

**Phytochemicals** are natural plant substances such as hormones, bioflavonoids, or carotenoids (and thousands of others) that make up a plant and are considered nutrients for our body.

who work with diseased organs rather than the whole body, illustrates how our perceptions of health and our bodies have been distorted. We think that the parts are more valuable than the whole.

If this were truly the case, Macmillan might have tried to sign a contract only with my fingers to write this book! But the body works as a whole, and it should be treated as a whole. When dealing with reflexology we are not just working on the feet, we are influencing the entire body, mind, and spirit.

**Foot Note**

If man didn't take part in creating the universe, then I really don't believe that man can make better medicine than nature. How do we know that when we take a vitamin pill there is not some missing component that has to be synthesized by our own body in order for our body to effectively utilize the vitamin? Wouldn't you rather get the *whole* part to strengthen you instead of making your body work even harder because of what you feed it?

**Tread Lightly**

Although reflexologists are holistically oriented, don't expect them to be your holistic therapist. No one can be a specialist in everything. Usually your reflexologist will network with others in the holistic community and can refer you to other practitioners to help you with things like nutrition, herbs, psychological counseling, physical therapy, etc.

Reflexology goes hand in hand, or foot in foot, as the case may be, with other natural therapies, which makes it that much more valuable. The therapies reflexology complements include:

➤ A solid nutritional or supplement program

➤ Emotional counseling

➤ Bodywork

➤ Chiropractic care

➤ Acupuncture

➤ Aromatherapy

➤ Colonic irrigations

➤ Ear coning

All of these therapies can work together to create a holistically healthful lifestyle for you.

Reflexology is a therapeutic practice. Observing and working the reflex points can also give us some clues to our state of health. Reflexology used in this manner lets you analyze what your health issues may be and can reinforce other holistic health assessments.

Remember that medical doctors are a valuable part of our society, but they can only diagnose diseases after the symptoms manifest themselves. Reflexology may be able to lend you clues to imbalanced areas of the body and help you avoid having to be diagnosed with a full-blown disease! What a wonderful, natural, safe, noninvasive therapy tool reflexology is. It can help us prevent diseases and may even be used to detect health problems before they become serious!

# Does America Have a Foot Fetish?

What is it about the feet that's so neat? For starters, most of us have a pair of them. Many of us remember childhood rhymes such as "This Little Piggy Went to Market," which was traditionally recited by some older person speaking baby talk to us while wiggling our tootsies. But let's take a more observant look at the holistic view of the feet.

Our feet are what carry us through life. They walk us down life's path. The use of our feet is what brings us our independence. Are you walking the right path? The shape and condition of our feet can reflect if we are on the right path or not or even if we are afraid of walking this life path. Our feet give us the foundation upon which our whole body and, philosophically, our whole life rests.

In astrology, the sun sign Pisces rules the feet, and I find that many of my clients who use reflexology as their favorite form of healing are Pisces. I also know a few very good reflexologists who happen to be Pisces. So if your sun sign is the fish, take your socks off now, you're going to love this!

### The Sole Meaning

**Grounded** is a term used commonly to refer to being focused and connected to the earth or physical reality. It is used interchangeably with the phrase "having both feet on the ground." Being grounded can be used to describe a practical, down to earth, goal-oriented person.

## *Keep Your Feet on the Ground*

Our feet are the first thing that bring us back to earth and into our waking world when we get out of bed each morning. In our dreams many times we fly or float. The dream world is not where the feet are important, but in waking life they keep us in our bodies, so to speak. Did you ever hear the saying, "I was so happy I was two feet off the ground"?

**Tread Lightly**

Starting out on the right foot is taken seriously by some reflexologists. No offence to lefties, but most folks are right-handed, and it is typical for right-handed people to put their right foot forward first when taking a step. Some superstitious people make it a habit to place their right foot on the ground first when getting out of bed each morning!

We jump for joy when we hear things that make us happy. But it is important to come back down and take care of earthly matters in order to keep balance in our lives. Our feet give us independence. They help us to walk out of bad situations, run away from threatening circumstances, help us to march to the beat of a different drummer, or even tiptoe through the tulips!

Reflexology is a very grounding therapy. "One step at a time" is a helpful saying to those of us feeling overwhelmed with too many projects to do. So many of us now live our lives almost entirely in our heads! We are constantly thinking, planning, talking, and dreaming. We need time to reconnect to our roots, and one of the best ways to get grounded and become centered is concentrating on the feet.

Take a barefooted walk in the sand, and stop along the way and pick up seashells with your toes. This will exercise the muscles in the feet. Notice how it makes you feel to walk in sand. Or walk barefoot through some cold, wet grass early in the morning. These are both forms of natural reflexology and are also good therapies for the soul!

**Foot Note**

Walking barefoot in the early morning onto a nice chilly, grassy lawn filled with the morning dew is a form of reflexology. Close your eyes and feel the earth and the blades of grass between your toes. Take a nice, deep breath and experience the aroma and note how you feel. More than likely you will feel invigorated afterward. It is a great way to give your circulation a jump-start and help prepare you for a beautiful day. Need more motivation than that? Just dew it!

## The Feet, Our Earth Roots

The feet are what keep and help us stay connected to the earth. Think of our Native American peoples, or any native peoples from around the world, especially in the warmer climates, and how often they had bare feet. In the United States, many people consider the Native Americans to be the keepers of the earth. They have a deeper understanding and connection to our planet than some of our top researchers at NASA or even astronauts who view our planet from space. Some of this may have to do with their connection to the earth through their feet.

Studying with a shaman (another word for medicine man) for several years, I learned the valuable philosophy behind the words "As above, so below." I believe that the universe is all one, and if you choose any subject and study its relationship to the rest of the world, you will discover the secrets of the universe. In other words, nature has laws that are universal. There is nothing that defies this law or order. Everything has a purpose and a connection and a reason for doing what it does and being what it is. Once you can see these underlying patterns, a lot of other things will make sense to you. Since this order is inherent in anything and everything, you can discover these secrets through close observation of any subject. So, who knows, maybe if you get to know everything about your feet you will somehow get to know the rest of your body and the rest of the universe!

---

### The Least You Need to Know

➤ Reflexology is a science that maps out the connections between points on the feet and hands and the rest of the body.

➤ Using reflexology on the feet and hands positively affects all other body parts.

➤ The feet can give us clues to arising health problems and give us a chance to take preventative measures.

➤ Reflexology is a safe, natural therapy that complements all other holistic therapies.

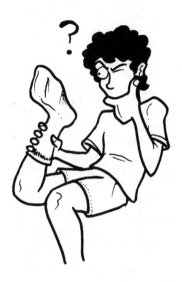

# Chapter 2

# Why Do I Want My Feet Rubbed?

## In This Chapter

➤ Discover how to balance the body with reflexology

➤ Get prepared for detoxifying

➤ Use reflexology as an anti-stress therapy

➤ Learn who can and can't use reflexology

➤ Find out how often reflexology should be used

Now that you know what reflexology is all about, I'd like to fill you in on what makes it so good. For one thing, my husband tells me it's the most fun we have together with our clothes on (but for the best benefit you will need to remove your shoes!). Reflexology stimulates the body to produce those feel-good chemicals known as *endorphins*, and so far, I have found it to be the best way to get my family members to do big favors for me!

It also ranks right up there as one of the best romantic gifts you can give your partner, especially in a pinch. Pin this thought under your cap: "Of course I didn't forget our anniversary darling. Now lay back and kick off your shoes…"

Whether you are practicing on yourself or on someone else, this chapter will help you learn about some general uses of reflexology, let you in on what you can expect, and even give you inside tips about when and how often you can use this hands-on tool for health and happiness—and why you should.

# It's a Healing Feat

Reflexology is a natural way to stimulate healing in the body, and a healthy body is a body that feels good. Many folks have been amazed at the instant relief they have had from just a few minutes of deep pressure on the feet and/or hands. Since the hands are usually accessible, you can work on yourself almost any time—in meetings, riding in a car (not if you're driving, please), watching a movie, getting your teeth cleaned— or virtually anywhere you have both hands free.

**Tread Lightly**

Just because you like reflexology doesn't mean everyone will like it. Even some of my closest friends will not let me or anyone else touch their feet! So if your offer to work on someone is declined, try not to take it personally. If you really would like to persuade them, buy them this book to show them how great reflexology can be!

The ears also have reflex points, and most of us have our ears accessible all the time. The point is that reflexology can be used almost anywhere and anytime to promote balance and give you an instant lift or quick pain relief.

A reflexologist friend of mine was on a plane recently and was fortunate enough to be sitting next to a charming young lady about seven years old. As the plane was descending, the girl began to experience excruciating pain in her ears because of sinus congestion. My friend, being the patient, healing woman that she is, instead of complaining about the little girl's cries, asked her mother for permission to work on her. The mother agreed, and my friend began to work on the girl's palms. Within minutes, the girl was drying her tears and feeling no more pain.

Now, if you are not lucky enough to be sitting next to a loving reflexologist on the plane next time your sinuses are giving you grief, have no fear! By the time you are through reading this book, you will be able to work on yourself for relief. In the meantime, check with your travel agent for specific seating arrangements or turn to Chapter 9, "Remember to Breathe! The Respiratory System," for more details about sinus reflex points on the hands and feet.

## A Delicate Balance

Spontaneous healing is great; however, most true healing takes time. Illness doesn't necessarily come about instantaneously, but is harbored and grows, sometimes long before you experience any symptoms.

My nutritional and holistic teachers over the years have all taught me the law of balance. It is only when we are imbalanced in some way, whether physically, mentally, or spiritually, that we experience ill health. We will primarily be addressing physical imbalances in this book, but keep the other two in mind for complete health.

It is great to be balanced nutritionally and maintain your health with physical therapies like reflexology, but your symptoms will continue to come back if you are in a continuing unhealthy relationship or situation. Make those changes first and then work on the physical health!

# Homeostasis: Getting It Right

Reflexology is great because it helps the body get and stay balanced. I'm not talking balanced as in walking on a balance beam. I am talking about balance as it relates to the glandular functioning of your body, or *homeostasis*. Homeostasis is really just a bio-chemical balancing act played every day of our lives by our endocrine glands. Some of the functions controlled by homeostatic mechanisms are:

➤ Heartbeat

➤ Blood production

➤ Blood pressure

➤ Body temperature

➤ Salt balance

➤ Breathing

➤ Glandular secretion

**The Sole Meaning**

**Homeostasis** is the medical term used for the body's internal balancing act. It means that our unconscious body functions such as body temperature and glandular secretions are working for us to keep us alive and functioning. Life truly is a balancing act.

Our glands all work together just like a smooth-running corporation. When one of the glands is not up to par, the whole corporation suffers. This usually means extra work for the other glands as they try to make up the work leftover by the slacker!

By using the reflex points on the soles of the feet and palms of the hands, we can stimulate those glands that are not keeping up and help the body become balanced again. For instance, symptoms of a sluggish thyroid gland could include unexplainable weight gain, lethargy, dry skin, and erratic sleeping patterns. These symptoms are signs that the body is out of balance.

More than likely, when your thyroid is out of balance and you rub your thyroid reflex point on the bottom of your foot, it will yell back at you—"ouch!" Keep on rubbing—that's just the thyroid telling you that it doesn't like getting caught sleeping on the job! (We'll get to how you can tell which areas or glands are sluggish in later chapters.)

**Tip Toe**

Kelp is a seaweed rich in organic iodine. It is used as an herbal supplement by many to nourish an underactive thyroid.

It is not just the glands that can cause imbalance in the functions of the body. The major organs can become overloaded, tired, or injured; the muscles, skin, bones, hair,

**21**

fingernails, joints, and all other parts of the body may show signs of imbalance. Bringing balance back to the body through stimulation is one goal of the reflexologist.

# Detoxing That'll Knock Your Socks Off

Most imbalances occur because of malnourishment, overuse or abuse, or too many toxins in the body causing irritations and sluggishness in certain areas. Detoxifying the body means doing some internal house cleaning. Believe it or not, our internal bodies get dusty and dirty and need to be cleansed periodically, just as our homes need a good spring cleaning.

The body has four main eliminative channels that serve as exit routes for waste products. These include:

➤ The bowel

➤ The urinary system (kidneys and bladder)

➤ The respiratory system (lungs and sinuses)

➤ The skin

When the body, or a particular organ, is sluggish due to a buildup of waste products and then we stimulate that organ to "get back to work," it will probably eliminate some toxins right away. This is called *detoxification*. When a body system is stimulated and stronger, it has the energy and ability to kick out toxins settling in it. You will know when your body is detoxifying because of the symptoms you experience.

Usually a full reflexology treatment will stimulate all the organs and therefore stir up a bunch of waste materials in the body. This is good, but you will need to know what to expect when this happens to you!

**Tread Lightly**

Although cleansing of the bowel is a good sign, you should not experience diarrhea after a reflexology treatment. A temporary cleansing due to a loosening of the bowel differs from diarrhea. Diarrhea can be caused by a parasitic or bacterial infestation that can dehydrate the body over a fairly short period of time and needs to be addressed.

## The Process of Elimination

One of the most common symptoms of detoxifying the body will be a loosening of the bowels. Many necessary, quick trips to the bathroom will prove to you that you needed cleansing. This form of detoxifying after a reflexology treatment usually lasts no longer than a day. It is also a positive sign. You should not try to stop this cleansing process by taking any medications that would constipate you—let the cleansing begin!

The urinary system will carry out waste products in the form of urine. The urine may be stronger smelling, and you may have to visit the bathroom more often for a day. This should also be encouraged. Drink plenty of pure water to help flush out the toxins.

## Sweating It Out

Sometimes when I work on someone with lung congestion, they will experience a cleansing through the lungs. This is usually in the form of a phlegmy cough. I believe the reflexology treatment loosens up old, hardened mucus, giving the lungs the opportunity to get rid of it! So, if you get copious amounts of mucus coming from your sinus passages or from your lungs in the form of a cough after reflexology, you can count on this being a cleansing process.

Do not thwart the process by taking cough medications to inhibit your lungs from expelling the mucus. This will only stop the cleansing process, which the reflexology treatment was designed to do in the first place! Instead, drink lots of water to speed up the process. Foul breath is another strange symptom that may be experienced after a deep reflexology treatment. Again, this is due to toxins in the system, usually in the lungs, that have broken free and are leaving the body.

Detoxifying through the pores of the skin can show up as any type of skin eruption, including pimples, boils, rashes, or cold sores. Sweating during a deep treatment is sometimes experienced. This is the natural way your body rids itself of waste through the skin. When a treatment is effective in detoxifying, you should not be surprised if your body odor changes for a day. In fact, after my first treatment, I smelled like maple syrup! Just before I panicked about being nicknamed Aunt Jemima, the smell subsided.

**Tip Toe**

The skin is our largest eliminative organ and we typically eliminate two pounds of waste materials (perspiration) every day, mostly through the feet.

## Stressed Out?

Reflexology promotes the production of endorphins in the body. *Endorphins* are the feel-good hormones made by the pituitary gland in the brain. The flow of endorphins in the body acts on the nervous system to help reduce pain. The effects they cause on the body are similar to the effects of morphine.

I believe that many of the painful symptoms we experience in the body are increased by stress. Stress tends to make us uptight. Literally, our muscles get tighter when we are under stress.

Just think of yourself after having a confrontational meeting at work. Are your shoulders in

**The Sole Meaning**

**Endorphins** are substances released by the pituitary gland that affect the central nervous system by reducing pain. Their effect on the body is similar to the effects of using pain-killing medications such as morphine.

your ears? Are your fists clenched? How about your jaw? Are you grinding your teeth or clenching them tight? These are all reactions to stressful situations, whether the stress is good or bad.

# Good Stress, Bad Stress, Ugly Stress

Some examples of "good" stress may be moving to a new, nicer home, starting a better job, getting married, or traveling to a new and exciting place. And of course we all experience the bad stressors, too, like accidents, conflicts with others, financial worries, and so on. When the body and mind are adjusting to anything new, the muscles tighten in response, preparing for unexpected or new challenges.

But when we are stressed all the time, the effects can eventually tire us out! We can use reflexology to help stimulate endorphins so that the body can relax, rejuvenate, and be better able to tolerate the stresses of life. By utilizing reflexology as a stress-relieving technique, the body has a chance to relax the tight muscles that can cause pain.

### Foot Note

There is something very deeply relaxing about a foot reflexology treatment. Most of my clients cannot stay conscious after a few minutes into their treatment and will doze off or enter a trance-like state of relaxation. Many businessmen and -women I have worked on say that they use their treatments with me as midafternoon catnaps that help them return to work feeling more creative and productive.

# A Balancing Act: Reducing PMS

Another form of stress is the ever-unpopular premenstrual tension. Fortunately, the stress, or tension, in the body can be released and this release can have a positive effect on symptoms of PMS. In fact, PMS symptoms are one of the most studied uses of reflexology!

Sometimes I am not sure who suffers more from PMS, women or the men who love them! But one sure thing is that reflexology has many effects on the body and can help balance the glands, reduce water retention, and promote relaxation—all of which are important factors in relieving PMS symptoms.

Besides promoting endorphin production that relieves pain and promotes relaxation, another reason reflexology seems to work on PMS is because it stimulates the glands to balance. The crankiness we feel when we are suffering from PMS is usually because our hormones are raging, our glands are going crazy, and therefore, our highs and lows are intensified. By stimulating the glands to balance through reflexology, we can help make the highs and lows less drastic.

Many times women will hold excess water (known as *edema*) and feel bloated or puffy during certain times of the month. By utilizing the reflexology points on the feet, hands, and even ears, we can encourage the urinary system to cleanse and release excess water. The effects are not only felt in the body as the swelling is reduced, but also in the brain. Excess water retention can affect certain nerves in the brain and make us ladies act very un-ladylike!

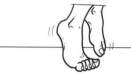

**Tip Toe**

Men, you don't need to think of PMS as an acronym for Pack My Stuff anymore! All you need to do is offer to give reflexology to your sweetheart and you can keep your suitcase in the closet!

Obviously reflexology has many uses for those of us suffering from any ailments or conditions caused by stress, tension, brain chemistry, or glandular imbalances. Relief of PMS is only one, but it is one a large percentage of the population can appreciate. We'll get into more detail in Chapters 12, "Sexy Stuff: The Glandular System," and 23, "Keeping Your Glands in Order."

# Gentle Enough for Baby, Strong Enough for a Man

Reflexology is safe and effective and only helps the body do what it was designed to do anyway. So unless you are grossly negligent (or using instruments improperly) you really can't hurt anyone with reflexology.

If you are working on yourself, you will know what hurts and what doesn't. When working on another person, you will have to utilize your people skills to stay in communication with them so that you can push deep enough to get the desired results, yet still be gentle enough that they do not become tense. Later, I will cover the specific techniques and discuss how deep to go and so on, but for now we want to talk about who can, can't, should, or shouldn't get a reflexology treatment.

Reflexology is one area in life where you should consider yourself first. Working on yourself is the best way to get started feeling the effects of reflexology. For instance, I began utilizing this therapy as a crisis management plan. When something would hurt in my body, I would go to the corresponding reflex point, and sure enough, the reflex point would be sore. I would rub the spot every chance I got. As the pain went away in my body, the tenderness would go away in my reflex point! Using the techniques on yourself will help you get in touch with your body and its functions.

**Foot Note**

Find a reflexologist and get a treatment for yourself so that you can feel firsthand what reflexology is supposed to feel like. Then you can transfer that same feel into working on yourself between treatments. See Appendix A, "Reflexology Schools, Teachers, and Associations," to help you locate a reflexologist in your area.

## Kid Stuff—Working on Baby

Babies are especially responsive to reflexology. Many mothers will instinctively rub their children's feet and hands when their child is cranky, crying, or uncomfortable. Reflexology works very well for little ones since most babies enjoy being touched. Babies' feet have undeveloped arches, and their skin and bones are usually fairly soft. You don't want to dig too deeply into a baby's feet or hands! Gentle fingertip pressure is usually enough. Short, gentle sessions are most beneficial for infants: Ten minutes is usually sufficient. It is important to not overdo when working with little ones.

**Tread Lightly**

Baby's feet should not be worked on too deeply. A gentle but firm pressure while rubbing your baby's little feet and hands is sufficient. Results for babies are usually experienced immediately and can soothe a cranky baby or help to relieve gas pains or constipation. Since the results can show up in a diaper, make sure you leave home prepared!

Many times, gas pains, nausea, and general lethargy can be relieved when you rub a baby's feet or hands for several minutes. All the babies I have ever used reflexology on have fallen asleep after a few minutes of working on them! This can be used as a trick for tired moms who need a break.

Also, babies will usually respond rather quickly to the detoxifying effects of reflexology. Therefore, this safe therapy can be used to help with gas pains due to constipation. I have found that the smaller the body, the faster the therapy works! So be aware that a child's reaction to most natural treatments can be almost instantaneous. In other words, be prepared to change a diaper if need be!

## Who Shouldn't Use It?

Men and women of any age like the feel of reflexology and can use it without problems. However, as I said earlier, pay attention to the person's pain tolerance. Someone who is generally healthy may not be very sensitive. If they already take good care of themselves and are used to other forms of bodywork such as massage, they may want or need deeper work to feel any real benefits.

Every therapy has its own set of contraindications, and reflexology is no exception. *Contraindication* means that sometimes a therapy is not recommended for someone with specific problems. We will go over a more detailed list in later chapters, but for now, here are some general things to keep in mind when using reflexology:

➤ People who are very tender to the touch can include people with degenerative conditions such as diabetes or urinary system problems, and the elderly. Do not overwork these people.

➤ When working on babies, it is important to not overwork them. Use a very gentle pressure and work no longer than 10 to 15 minutes for the entire treatment.

➤ Do not work directly on any injuries or foot conditions, and do not work an area that is painful to the touch.

➤ Do not overdo pregnant women, especially if they are prone to miscarriages.

**The Sole Meaning**

A **contraindication** is a factor that prohibits a certain treatment for a specific patient due to some condition the patient has. Although reflexology is a safe treatment for almost anyone, it has contra-indications. A complete table of the reflexology contraindications can be found in Chapter 15, "How to Touch."

## Reflexology and Pregnancy

The one serious contraindication for reflexology that I always abide by is someone who is pregnant and who has had trouble carrying a pregnancy to term in the past. This could indicate that she lacks muscle tone in the uterus, and we would not want to stimulate a cleansing, or stir up the circulation process. Personally, I will not work on anyone who has had this problem before, so as to avoid being blamed if something does go wrong.

But don't let me scare off you moms-to-be now! Typically, reflexology during pregnancy is a great way to gently relax the muscles and alleviate some of the tenderness in the feet that sometimes comes with pregnancy. Many midwives offer reflexology treatments to help their clients through labor pains!

**Tread Lightly**

Pregnant women who have had past trouble carrying their pregnancy to term should not use vigorous or deep reflexology stimulation, especially on the reproductive organ reflexes.

So, for the future moms out there, here are my recommendations:

➤ Do offer gentle reflexology treatments to yourself or to your pregnant friends.

➤ Don't overstimulate the reproductive organ reflex points.

➤ Don't use reflexology at all on someone who has had miscarriages in the past, or on anyone who is worried about miscarrying.

Although I do believe that reflexology is a wonderful therapy for pregnant ladies, the female organ reflex points should not be worked on too much. Neither should the foot be worked on too vigorously. We don't want to overstimulate the body when the body is busy building a new person!

## All Things in Time

The beauty of reflexology is that it can be used almost any time, as often as you wish, or as little as you want. (See the following Foot Note for a good rule of thumb on timing.) Since reflex points can be found on the ears, hands, and feet, there is a good chance that at least one or two of these parts will be accessible almost all the time. Reflexology can be used as a quick pick-me-up or to facilitate instantaneous relief, but it is best used as a regular therapy to promote overall balance and health.

I have found that, on occasion, the first reflexology treatment is not as effective as subsequent treatments. Sometimes this is because the person needs to get to know you a little better before they can relax totally and benefit from the stress-relieving effects. Healing through relaxation is a big part of the magic of reflexology.

For some, the first time you try reflexology you may just be breaking up some surface congestion, so you will not really notice any difference. If this is so, I suggest you try it again within a week. You may be surprised at what happens. Some of my best clients did not have anything to say after their first treatments … but when they came back for a second time, they had results, and then I couldn't keep them from coming back again and again (not that I'd want to keep them away)!

### Foot Note

If you walk barefoot each day you are giving yourself some reflexology stimulation, which is what we are naturally born to do. However, if you are getting reflexology treatments from someone, you should always allow at least 24 hours between each reflexology session to give your body time to eliminate toxins released by the previous session.

Since every body is different, each person will respond to reflexology in a different way. Sometimes the effect is more emotional than physical. I have had clients burst into tears minutes after I began working on them! This is also part of a cleansing process. When your intent as a reflexologist is to help the person you are working on heal, you will get results, however they may manifest. Do not stress yourself by attaching expectations to your reflexology results. The body will heal itself on its own time despite your ego's personal goals!

## Use It 'Til You Lose It

How often should you use reflexology? The problem you are trying to deal with will give you a clue. Although the therapy can be used as a stress reliever any time, some folks use it more seriously as a part of their health care program. If you are working on a specific ailment or chronic problem, for instance, regular treatments until healing begins are the best way to start out. I always suggest, for chronic cases, that a person use reflexology once a week for three or four weeks or until they are feeling better, then maintain with bimonthly or monthly treatments. It is important to try to get the body balanced with several treatments up front and then maintain that balance.

### Foot Note

One delightful reflexology student took my class to learn to use reflexology to help her diabetic husband. She began practicing on him every other day. At our last class together, she reported that they went to visit his doctor and the doctor asked them what they had been doing differently. She told him that she had been using reflexology. The doctor noted great improvement in her husband, including improved foot mobility, and told her, "Whatever you are doing, keep doing it!"

## Speeding Up the Healing Process

Other natural therapies used along with reflexology can complement and dramatically speed the healing process. These include:

➤ Colonic irrigations

➤ Herbs

➤ Vitamin, mineral, and enzyme therapies

➤ Proper nutrition

➤ Energy work

➤ Aromatherapy

➤ Counseling

➤ Exercise

All can make a big difference in getting healthy and then maintaining your health. Just like other natural healing therapies, using reflexology to bring your body back to health is effective, but can take some time.

We do not "catch" disease. There are a series of factors that take place over a long period of time inside our bodies before we actually experience the symptoms of imbalance. These symptoms are usually labeled as ailments or diseases. Feeling not as good as you should or having an ailment or disease is just your body's way of telling you that some things are not right. This is usually when reflexology and other forms of natural health care are sought.

By the time you are not feeling your best, there is a lot of healing that needs to take place before you can fully recover. Dr. Jack Ritchason, a well-known herbalist and nutritionist, says that it takes five to seven times the normal amount of nutrition to build and repair as it does to maintain health. I believe this holds true for using all natural therapies. One reflexology treatment will not solve all your problems, just like one magic herb pill will not. Consistency is the key to getting where you want to be.

## Hering's Law of Cure

Another good thing to remember in all natural therapies is *Hering's Law of Cure*. Hering's Law states: "All healing starts from the head down, from the inside out, and in reverse order as the symptoms have appeared." In other words, in true healing, your insides will begin healing first. The outward manifestations of healing will come last—so you may not even notice you're healing right away. Also, the symptoms that you experienced most recently will be the *last* ones to go away.

**The Sole Meaning**

**Hering's Law of Cure** is used as a standard philosophy for healing naturally. It states: "All healing starts from the head down, from the inside out, and in reverse order as the symptoms have appeared."

The body always takes care of the more chronic ailments or imbalances first. You may not be aware that your pancreas or spleen is healing, but continued effort will eventually bring the outward signs of true health. Therefore, although reflexology may work instantly to alleviate symptoms of imbalance, it will take time and continued use of reflexology to experience true healing—so be patient and enjoy the ride!

All in all, reflexology is an excellent, safe, efficient therapy that can be used on almost anyone, anytime, anywhere. Being so simple and safe, it can be integrated into anyone's lifestyle and serve as either a healing therapy or a preventative maintenance tool for health. It can even detect imbalances before you experience any symptoms. Reflexology can help the body to heal itself by detoxifying, relaxing and balancing it, and to top it off, making you feel good.

These are all good reasons to get your feet rubbed. But before we address the techniques, let's dig up a little history on reflexology in the next chapter.

---

### The Least You Need to Know

➤ Reflexology assists the body in healing by balancing glands, relaxing muscles, promoting pain-killing hormone production, and detoxifying the body.

➤ Reflexology can be used by almost anyone at any age.

➤ You can use reflexology as a natural healing therapy and as a preventative maintenance tool for health.

➤ Never work too vigorously or too deeply on a pregnant woman, a baby, or someone in a weakened state. And don't work at all on a pregnant woman who has had trouble in the past with carrying to term.

➤ Remember that natural healing takes place in the reverse order that you have experienced the problem. This means that you will need to be patient when healing naturally, as your most recent symptoms may be the last to disappear.

---

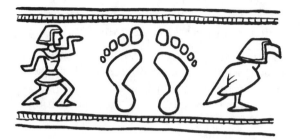

# Chapter 3

# Reflecting on History

## In This Chapter

➤ Learn the ancient roots of reflexology

➤ Compliment reflexology with other ancient natural therapies

➤ Take a firsthand look at Indian Ayurvedic practices

➤ See how the Bible refers to reflexology

➤ Meet the pioneers who modernized reflexology in the United States

> Foolish the doctor who despises the knowledge acquired by the ancients.
> —Hippocrates, *Entering the World*

It is ironic that in our modern world of computers, e-mail, technological and scientific advances, cloning, and new wonder drugs that most of us are looking back to ancient times for answers to our health concerns. Even the media has popularized the use of herbs and vitamins, and terms like "complementary medicine" are a part of everyday household vocabulary.

Reflexology, aromatherapy, meditation, and herbal medicine, although newly popular again, are not new fads. For some reason, we have lost the connection to these great natural healing therapies and are just now beginning to understand their value and bring them back into the mainstream.

In this chapter we are going to explore some ancient places where there is evidence that reflexology was used thousands of years ago. Get ready now to turn your clocks back about 5,000 years...

# Ancient Healers on the Nile

For many of us, Egypt holds a mysterious fascination. Preserved mummies, intricate gold jewelry, secret tombs and incredible structures, Egyptian gods and goddesses, and the mythological figures linked to Egypt all have an air of the exotic. Archaeologists spend years and sometimes lifetimes dedicated to uncovering ancient mysteries.

If you think about it, four to five thousand years ago there was no such thing as an "unnatural" healing therapy! People discovered what God or nature provided to take care of the body, mind, and soul. They wisely understood and applied natures' gifts to help them be strong and to help heal the ailing. Back then medicines were derived from natural substances.

**The Sole Meaning**

An **autopsy** is a medical term used to describe the dissection and examination of a dead body to determine the cause of death or the presence of disease.

The things that we do know about the ancient Egyptians are discerned by the meticulously preserved artifacts found in the secret tombs and pyramid chambers. We find that the ancient Egyptians performed surgical procedures, including brain surgery. There is evidence that they set bones, performed *autopsies*, and treated many ailments.

Most of the mummies that we observe in museums are from ancient Egyptian times. Maybe it was because of their strong belief in an afterlife that they were skillful masters in preparing the human body to be preserved after death. It is my assumption that since these people so highly regarded the body after death that they took care of the living body with a similar high regard.

## The Doctor Is In

It appears that ancient Egyptian doctors were aware of the benefits of foot and hand reflexology. One piece of evidence was revealed in a recently discovered ancient pictograph on the wall of the tomb of Ankhmahar, located at Saqqara in Egypt. The tomb was occupied by the body of an Egyptian doctor dating back to about 2500 B.C. The pictograph demonstrates two pair of Egyptians giving and receiving reflexology treatments. One of the therapists is working on a foot and the other therapist is working on a hand. The inscription is said to read, "Don't hurt me." The practitioner's reply, "I shall act so you praise me."

The fact that reflexology treatments are depicted in the tomb of a doctor lends credence to the idea that the practice was used as a healing art. I guess if we can learn how to walk like an Egyptian, we might also want to learn how to heal like the Egyptians.

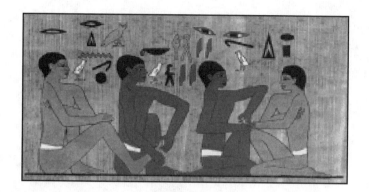

*Drawing of an Egyptian pictograph from 2500 B.C. showing the practice of reflexology.*

## *Everybody Must Get Coned*

It is interesting to note that many of the practices the ancient Egyptians used are now becoming popularized as natural health therapies and recognized as holistic medicines. How is it that we are just now catching up to this advanced civilization that existed thousands of years before us?

Another Egyptian natural therapy that is being rediscovered by the masses today is the use of *ear coning* or *ear candling*. Ear coning is used to clean out the excess wax and debris from the ear canal, and some claim it helps ease ear aches. The practice is very effective after a reflexology treatment since reflexology may help loosen stagnant mucus from the sinuses.

### Foot Note

The ancient Egyptians used hollow papyrus reeds for the practice of **ear coning**. Today, we use what are called **ear candles**. The ear candles are hollow, tube-like funnels made from sterile gauze and dipped in beeswax. One end is placed gently in the ear and the other end is lit with a flame. As the candle burns down, the smoke enters the ear and warms the wax. The flame creates a mild vacuum effect that sucks up wax and any debris into the hollow of the candle. This practice is gentle, inexpensive, and safe, but be sure to follow directions, and never do this alone. For best results, seek a practitioner to do this for you.

My clients tell me they prefer this method of cleaning out their excess wax and find it 100 percent more relaxing and gentle than the high-pressure wash used on them at some doctor's offices. With ear coning, nothing goes into the ear, you only get excess debris coming out. Ask around to find a skilled practitioner to do this for you. You should never attempt to practice ear coning alone. Thanks to the ancients, we have this gentler treatment available. If it weren't for the ancient Egyptians, I wouldn't have known I needed to clear my head occasionally!

*Irene McFee, owner of Coning Works, performing the ancient Egyptian ritual of ear coning. Irene manufactures a line of ear cones that are out of this world.*

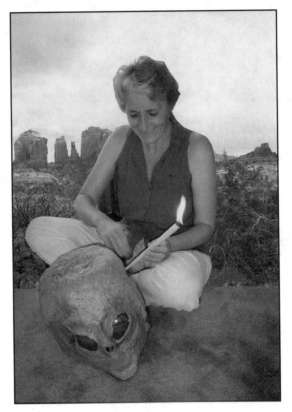

## The Sweet Smell of Feet

The ancient Egyptians also used essential oils and aromatherapy abundantly. Essential oils were commonly used as medicine. Containers of these oils have been found alongside pharaohs in their tombs, indicating that they highly regarded the pure essential oils in life and in the afterlife. Egyptians understood the uses of aromatherapy for its effects on the emotions and believed it protected their spiritual bodies as well.

They also believed that the effects of the oil essences reached beyond our physical world and could protect us from negative energies and evil spirits. Aromatherapy served many functions, including therapeutic, ritualistic, and mundane in the lives of the ancient Egyptians. It is said that Cleopatra wore sexually arousing fragrances, including ylang ylang and rose oil. Makes good scents to me!

To this day essential oils are widely used for flavoring, scenting, cleaning, and for medicinal purposes. Let's take a look at a few common oils and what some people use them for.

Here is a very short list of some commonly used essential oils of today and some of the effects they may have on us:

➤ **Peppermint oil.** Used to stimulate the senses and uplift the mind.

➤ **Lavender oil.** Used for burns and is soothing to the nervous system.

➤ **Clove oil.** Used topically to reduce pain, especially on gums for toothaches.

➤ **Oregano.** Used as a strong immune system stimulant and may help to fight bacteria and even viruses.

➤ **Tea-tree oil.** Used topically as an anti-fungal and mild antiseptic.

# Ancient Chinese Secrets

**Tip Toe**

Helichrysum oil is hard to come by, but is an excellent oil to use around the ears after a reflexology treatment and/or ear coning. The electrical properties of this oil are thought to cause the sensory hairs deep in the cochlea (part of the inner ear) to stand up, which aids hearing and can even help with ringing in the ears. Look for grade A oils when choosing essential oils.

Meanwhile, in another part of the ancient world, the Chinese were developing a sophisticated system of medicine of their own. Almost a thousand years ago, a Chinese doctor named Dr. Wang Wei was instrumental in creating a model used for teaching Chinese practitioners where the acupuncture points were on the body and the feet. Many of these points were located on the soles and the outer sides and edges of the feet and used as acupressure and acupuncture points by Chinese medical practitioners, acupuncturists, acupressure therapists, and reflexologists alike.

**Foot Note**

It isn't difficult to study ancient Chinese secrets relating to reflexology and natural health because the Chinese have not made the mistake of losing that knowledge. Instead, they have carried their knowledge of these natural therapies along with them through the ages and brought them into modern times. The Chinese holistic models of healing still hold up as well today as they did thousands of years ago. I am grateful to see so many people accepting this ancient wisdom in their lives today. We can all benefit from not just the use of reflexology, but also from the integration of the ancient Chinese holistic health philosophies into our daily lives.

Practices such as acupuncture and acupressure are directly related to reflexology and zone therapy. The Chinese meridian charts show many acupuncture points on the ears, feet, and hands that correspond to modern reflexology points. These techniques are all based on the same principals of energy lines and their corresponding body parts.

Ancient Chinese therapies are still being used worldwide today and have gained much popularity in the West. Chinese herbal medicines are widely utilized and distributed by many holistically oriented practitioners. Many natural health colleges throughout the United States base their curriculums on Chinese models and theories of health and healing.

# India Jones and the Temple of Toes

Overlooked by the West until recently, another ancient civilization that has, and still does, utilize natural therapies like reflexology is India. I traveled to India a couple of years ago, where I had the privilege of visiting with two prominent *Ayurvedic* doctors from Banaras University in Varanasi.

**The Sole Meaning**

**Ayurveda** is the ancient Indian form of healing medicine. **Ayurvedic colleges** are equivalent to Western medical schools. Ayurveda is based on the principal that illness is caused by toxin buildup in the body and/or nutritional deficiencies.

I met with the Dean of the College, Dr. B. N. Upadhyay, a biochemist, and Dr. Yamini B. Tripathi, whose grandfather was the Royal Physician to the Maharaja of Banaras. They invited me into their homes, taught me something of their philosophies, and gave me a tour of their college. Their *Ayurvedic colleges* are to them what our medical colleges are to the West. Their medical practices are grounded in natural, holistic therapies and philosophies.

Both of these respectable men expressed to me that they felt their ancient natural approach to healing, known as *Ayurveda*, has been ignored in the West in favor of the Chinese models of healing. In fact, they claim that their ancient Hindu healing practices predate even the oldest Chinese systems of healing and deserve to have more attention.

## An Indian Spa Experience

The most interesting part of my experience with Dr. Upadhyay and Dr. Tripathi was my visit to their Ayurvedic "spa." Mind you, this spa did not exactly fit the image of a pampering, upscale, hoity-toity health spot complete with bubbles and pretty people rubbing our feet. Instead, this spa came complete with rather large, intimidating monkeys that entertained themselves by trying to pee on our heads as we walked into the building.

I also noticed a striking absence of soft background music, lighted candles, and plush carpeting. I had the real feeling that once a person checked into this spa, they were motivated to get well. And in fact, Dr. Tripathi informed me that they have a better than 85 percent recovery rate. Those numbers were startling since the folks that check in are usually extremely ill already.

These doctors believe (as I do) that all sickness is caused by a nutritional deficiency and/or a build up of toxins in the system. Therefore, the first step to healing is something called *Panche Karma*. This is cleansing therapy to say the least. The entire process that takes place once you check yourself into this spa is a mixture of cleansing therapies and bodywork sure to inspire you to stay well.

## Panche Karma, Heal Me or Kill Me ... Please!

**Tread Lightly**

Although skilled Ayurvedic doctors can oversee you during strong cleansing therapies designed to heal, you should not try to administer harsh therapies yourself or unsupervised. Sometimes a building and strengthening program will work best, or even a gentle reflexology treatment will be all you need to get you back on the right track.

First you are given some *emetics*. Emetics are herbs that "push" toxins out of the body. The herbs you are given purge excess mucus from your gut and lungs through profuse vomiting. You are then given laxative herbs to prep you for the enema room. During the enema treatment you are "bled." The doctors explained to me that the blood is where the toxins circulate.

After you recover from this, they feed you some herbs with warming properties known to herbalists as *hot* or *diaphoretic herbs*. Hot herbs tend to be "yang" and help to push toxins out of the body through sweating by increasing the body temperature. Two common hot herbs include ginger and capsicum. Immediately after feeding you hot herbs they slap you into a wooden contraption with only your head sticking out. At this point you are steamed for one hour.

**Tip Toe**

Herbs that make the body warm have been used to help the body break a fever by making you sweat. This can push toxins out through the skin and fast forward cold symptoms. Some common "hot" herbs include horseradish, ginger, cayenne pepper, and cloves.

Next, they scoop your sweaty body from the sauna and lay you on a flat, wooden table, where they perform an intense, deep-tissue body massage and reflexology treatment. Scraping your flattened body from the table, you are then taken to another table where a swinging bucket of hot, herbal oil hangs over your forehead. The oil is dripped slowly onto your forehead for several hours. This is supposed to take away mental disorders, brain tumors, mental stress, and general brain malfunctions.

Now you are ready for a customized herbal and nutritional program. Voilà! Total relief from symptoms prevails, and with a nutritional program and correct living habits, health can be achieved and maintained. Now this is what I call holistic reflexology! And just a note to ease your mind: When you come see me at my holistic spa in Boise, I will be a bit more gentle on you than what I described above, and instead of monkeys, you may have elk to greet you at the entrance.

# References from the Big Book

Now let's take our history lesson a little farther west, to the lands of the Bible. I don't intend to get religious on you here. Not that I don't respect all types of religion and different depths of spirituality, quite the contrary. However, the Bible has been used by many different religious sects for centuries as a guide, as a prophecy tool, and as a reference for creating laws.

Biblical references to the feet are well known, and even the concept of reflexology can be inferred in the Bible. I think Jesus started a foot-washing fad in his day. The Bible refers to Jesus washing his disciples' feet. In a loving act, Jesus bathed his disciples' feet and told them, "You do not realize now what I am doing, but later you will understand. If you wash your feet, your whole body is clean. If you wash each other's feet, you will be blessed."

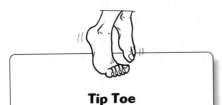

**Tip Toe**

Centipede to physician: "Doc, when my feet hurt, I hurt all over."

What was he trying to tell us here? Washing the feet for sure is a kind thing to do for another. Many reflexologists will have you bathe your feet in a foot spa before a treatment. Some even begin by washing your feet for you with a warm wet washcloth dipped in an antibacterial essential oil. I wonder if they know they are following what Jesus told his disciples to do? It doesn't matter, since it sounds like we will all be blessed for doing it anyway.

Going back to the holistic view of the feet. The feet carry us through our life journey. Romans 10:15 of the NIV Study Bible states, "How beautiful are the feet of those who bring good news." Were you ever so pleased with something someone did for you that you told them you'd kiss their feet? There are also references in the Bible that seem to indicate that the foot is seen as a sensory organ. For example, in Psalms 119:105, a nun praying to God says, "Your word is a lamp to my feet and a light for my path."

One of the most recognizable references to reflexology that I could find in the Bible begins in 1 Corinthians 12:21, "The body is a unit, though it is made up of many parts; and though all its parts are many, they form one body." And it continues:

"Now the body is not made up of one part but of many. Those parts of the body that seem to be weaker are indispensable, and the parts that we think are less honorable we treat with special honor ... so that there should be no division in the body, but that its parts should have equal concern for each other. If one part suffers, every part suffers with it; if one part is honored, every part rejoices with it."

So we go back again to the body parts all being connected. Besides this body metaphor teaching us how to treat one another and live more holistically as a community, I think the message for us here is to take care of our feet, and the rest of our body will rejoice!

# Reflexology Comes to America

I am a home-grown American citizen; however, I have been fortunate that my life has been filled with travel opportunities, too. By the time I graduated from my small Colorado mountain-town high school, I had already been to every state in the United States at least once, including Alaska and Hawaii, and had been to a couple of different countries to boot. My parents loved to travel and believed that I should be exposed to the world.

### Foot Note

If you love to travel and are looking for a mate, make sure you pick someone with high cheekbones! Dr. Bernard Jensen, in his study of personology through the facial features, says that people with high cheekbones love to travel.

I think travel, for those of us who love it, expands the mind and tends to crush any prejudices that can be harbored in a sheltered environment. Our views of how other cultures actually live and feel can be distorted when we only experience these other cultures through media coverage.

Despite my extensive traveling experience throughout the world, I am still an American and cannot help perceiving the world as an American. America is one of the youngest countries on the planet. Because of this, as Americans we all get the opportunity to be pioneers. We can relearn ancient techniques and therapies from distant lands and ancient times and bring them into our modern society in the West. We are truly fortunate to be able to be the integrators of ancient wisdom and modern knowledge and apply its practical uses to modern ailments.

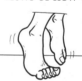

### Tip Toe

Everywhere I go folks seem to respond positively to a smile more than to anything else. A smile gives off a bright energy to those who receive it. It can make a stressed person smile back at you and help them with their day. A sincere smile is as good as medicine and seems to have a worldwide message.

# Dr. William Fitzgerald

Because of his extensive research into and application of the subject of reflexology, Dr. William Fitzgerald, an American born in 1872, is highly regarded as a pioneer of this science and art in the United States of America. Some claim that he is better known for popularizing the theory of zone therapy. Dr. Fitzgerald graduated from the University of Vermont Medical School in 1895 and traveled to Italy and the U.K. to practice medicine.

Fitzgerald discovered that deep pressure applied to the fingers of his patients had an effect similar to a local anesthetic along the zones of the body. He began using tools such as bands and clips to apply to these specific points on the fingers and toes. This simple procedure allowed Fitzgerald to actually perform minor surgeries without the use of general anesthesia or prescription drugs.

**The Sole Meaning**

Remember that **zone therapy** and **reflexology** are used interchangeably to mean the same thing. The term zone therapy was coined by a medical doctor in the late 1800s and describes the theory of energy zones that run longitudinally along the body.

Dr. Fitzgerald coined the term *zone therapy* to describe his treatments. He discovered that he could not only stop pain in certain areas of the body by applying pressure to certain "reflex" points, but that after the reflex points were released the patient was usually cured of the condition that was causing the pain in the first place!

Fitzgerald worked with a colleague, Dr. Edwin Bowers. Together they would demonstrate their theory to others in an attempt to prove the pain-relieving qualities of reflexology. To demonstrate their findings, Bowers and Fitzgerald would apply pressure to a zone reflex on their volunteer's hand and then stick a pin in the area of the face that was (hopefully) numbed by the pressure! Although not entirely embraced by the medical community, these dramatic demonstrations led to public recognition of zone therapy/reflexology in the United States.

When Fitzgerald returned to New England, he ran a hospital that used reflexology exclusively with great success. In this hospital no muscle relaxants or pain pills were prescribed. Patients were expected to take responsibility for themselves and could even administer reflexology to themselves with guidance.

Unfortunately, as time went on, people began to take less responsibility for their health and looked more and more to doctors to cure them. With the arrival of penicillin and other wonder drugs, people abused their bodies and expected a magic pill to cure them of all their ills, and reflexology fell by the wayside.

# Eunice Ingham

Another past pioneer of reflexology in the United States was a woman by the name of Eunice D. Ingham. Eunice was born in the early 1900s and spent the last part of her life in Rochester, New York, where she died in 1974. Ms. Ingham followed in

Dr. Fitzgerald's footsteps, so to speak, and utilized and taught zone therapy/reflexology to hundreds and probably thousands of people.

### Foot Note

I had the opportunity to live in Eunice's hometown of Rochester, New York, which is where she spent her last days. Unfortunately, in searching for a good reflexologist in the area I came up surprisingly short! So, if you are considering a move and want to take up reflexology, upstate New York might just be a great place to build a practice!

Eunice taught the therapeutic affects and applications of foot and hand reflexology through her classes and her books, including:

➤ *Stories the Feet Can Tell*, Ingham Publishing, 1938

➤ *Zone Therapy, Its Application to the Glands and Kindred Disorders*, Ingham Publishing, 1945 (out of print)

➤ *Stories the Feet Have Told*, Ingham Publishing, 1954

Training Centers were opened in the United States, Europe, and Great Britain to teach the Ingham Method of Reflexology. Her organization was inherited by her nephew Dwight Byers, who currently directs the International Institute of Reflexology, headquartered in St. Petersburg, Florida. (See Appendix A, "Reflexology Schools, Teachers, and Associations," for more information.)

### Foot Note

Apparently, Eunice was adamant about the importance of human touch, but from what some of her students tell me, she was not opposed to the use of tools to get the job done. One of her students told me that her approach was "Whatever works!" and she was known to use a pencil eraser to reach points hard to properly stimulate with just the fingers. Her dedication to healing the body through reflexology influenced many of today's practitioners, including many who have started their own reflexology schools.

Now that you know more history than you ever knew existed about reflexology, we have the basics covered. Congratulations! You have passed your first three prerequisites and now have a good grounding in the theory and practice of reflexology. Now it's time to get physical. In the next chapter, we'll take a closer look at feet.

---

### The Least You Need to Know

➤ Reflexology as a form of natural health care can be traced back as far as 5,000 years ago. There is evidence that doctors in ancient Egypt used reflexology as a healing practice.

➤ Ear coning and aromatherapy are other natural ancient healing practices that complement reflexology.

➤ The Bible makes references to the feet and reflexology practices. Even Jesus spoke about the importance of taking care of the feet.

➤ Indian Ayurvedic practitioners include reflexology as part of their medical healing applications.

➤ Dr. William Fitzgerald and Eunice Ingham are two famed pioneers for researching and popularizing reflexology in the United States.

---

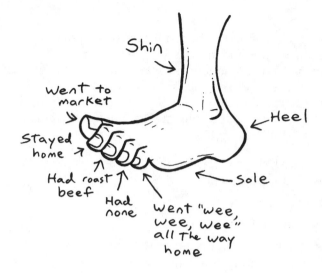

Shin

Went to market

Stayed home

Had roast beef

Had none

Went "wee, wee, wee" all the way home

Heel

Sole

# Chapter 4

# The Foot at a Glance

---

**In This Chapter**

➤ Gain insight into the function and the anatomy of the foot

➤ See how the foot serves as a sensory organ

➤ Learn about the connection between the earth and our feet

➤ Understand the four-element model and how it can help you

➤ Discover the body systems approach to health

---

There is more to the foot than meets the eye. I don't think most of us realize how much our feet really do for us. Do you know that there are people who use footbaths to cure a cold? Or that some people are so sensitive that they can actually sense color through the soles of their feet? Do you know how many bones are in your feet? Did you know that your foot can absorb substances that you apply to them? If not, kick back and we'll take a step-by-step course through the anatomy of your amazing feet.

## My, What Big Feet You Have, Grandma!

The feet are literally the foundation for the body. They help us to balance and give us a base on which to rest. The feet and toes are essential elements in body movement. They bear and propel the weight of the body during walking and running and help maintain balance when we change our body position.

**Tip Toe**

To see how much our feet adjust naturally to keep us balanced, take your shoes off and stand on one foot without holding onto anything. Notice how your weight continually shifts around to all parts of your grounded foot as you perform your balancing act.

A strong foundation for the feet means that all the bones, ligaments, and muscles are in alignment with each other and functioning as a team. You may not be aware that your whole structural system and spinal alignment relies on the correct alignment of your feet! When the spine is out of alignment you may experience any of the following problems:

➤ Headaches

➤ Lower-back pain

➤ Neck pain

➤ Pain in the hips

➤ Sciatica (a pain beginning deep in the buttock and radiating down the thigh)

Spinal adjustments can help correct these problems, and the correct alignment may be maintained by using *orthotics*. Orthotics are a type of plastic shoe insert customized to your feet by a heating and molding process. Many chiropractors and *podiatrists* (foot doctors) will offer customized orthotics to their patients to help give them a solid and stable foundation.

Orthotics can be made for each type of shoe you wear, or can just be taken out of one pair of shoes and inserted into another. You may have your feet "adjusted" by your chiropractor also. It is amazing how good it feels when you get those toes or metatarsals back into alignment.

**The Sole Meaning**

The bones of the toes are referred to as **phalanges**. The longer bones at the top of your feet are called **metatarsals**. The toes are known as the **distal part** of the foot.

## A Bone to Pick

Now let's get on with the actual physical makeup of the feet. Were you aware that the bones in the feet and hands account for about half of the bones in the entire body? The feet contain 28 bones each, and the hands contain 27 each. Twenty-six of these foot bones are very small bones, of course, unless we are talking about Michael Jordan, whose foot bones may be considered large.

The bones of the toes are referred to as *phalanges*. The longer bones you see when you look down at the top of your feet are called *metatarsals*. The toes are also referred to as the *distal part* of the foot. This is easy to remember if you think of the most distant part of your foot being the distal part. If you have an extra long foot, requiring you to make a long-distance phone call just to tie your shoes, you may easily remember this tidbit.

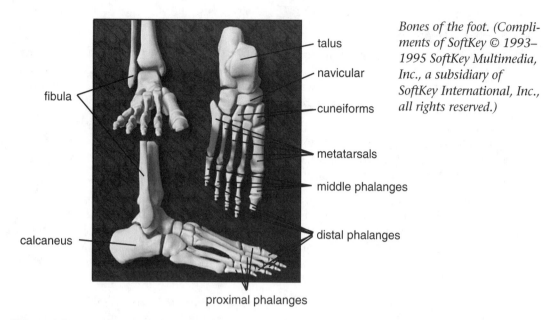

talus

navicular

cuneiforms

metatarsals

middle phalanges

distal phalanges

fibula

calcaneus

proximal phalanges

*Bones of the foot. (Compliments of SoftKey © 1993–1995 SoftKey Multimedia, Inc., a subsidiary of SoftKey International, Inc., all rights reserved.)*

## The Muscles of the Feet

Of course the foot is made up of more than just bones. In addition, each foot has about 33 muscles, which we give a real workout. While walking, it is estimated that the impact on the bottom of the foot equals about 900 pounds of pressure! Makes you really think twice about stepping on anyone's toes, doesn't it?

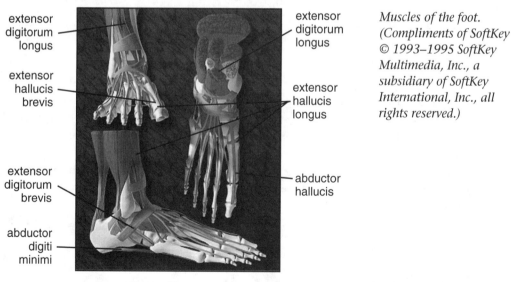

extensor digitorum longus

extensor hallucis brevis

extensor digitorum brevis

abductor digiti minimi

extensor digitorum longus

extensor hallucis longus

abductor hallucis

*Muscles of the foot. (Compliments of SoftKey © 1993–1995 SoftKey Multimedia, Inc., a subsidiary of SoftKey International, Inc., all rights reserved.)*

That bouncy spring in our step is facilitated by the arches that run lengthwise and crosswise over the foot. Some people have flat feet, which are caused by a lack of tone in the foot arches. We will discuss flat feet in more detail in Chapter 20, "Podiatry Matters."

## Foot Development

When we are babies our arches are not developed yet, so we are born with flat feet. As a baby begins to walk, the ligaments and muscles in the feet begin to form arches that help to strengthen the bones in the middle of the foot. The arches in our feet are not fully developed until we are about 16 years old.

When we are learning how to walk there are more processes going on than just the mechanics of placing one foot in front of the other. Our young brains are actually building synapses. This firing of impulses is teaching our brains how to adjust to gravity and how to balance our body weight over our legs and feet.

Not only does the baby's foot require walking for its correct formation and bone-building duties, but we adults also need to walk to exercise and maintain foot bone strength and muscle tone. Simply stated in his book *The Foot Book—Relief For Overused, Abused and Ailing Feet* (John Wiley and Sons, 1992), Glenn Copeland, D.P.M., when asked if there are any exercises that are particularly good for the feet replies, "Walking, walking, and more walking!"

Proper care of your feet is very important—after all, your feet carry you where you want to go. Many ailments of the feet, such as corns, calluses, and plantar warts, can all cause reflex problems to their corresponding body parts along the zones. Remember to take care of your feet by wearing proper shoes and getting adequate exercise like walking, and they will carry you more gently through life.

### Foot Note

One of the toughest clients I ever worked on was an ex-ballerina. She started dancing as a young girl, and her feet were literally deformed because of the years of taping her feet and wearing the ballet shoes required for her dancing. She had her shoes bronzed as an heirloom, and it struck me how similar her feet were to being cast in bronze! The poor woman was always in pain. Obviously our feet were not designed for this type of posture. But reflexology treatments helped the circulation to the feet and relieved a lot of her discomfort.

## The Foot as a Sensory Organ

The foot is a surprisingly sensitive organ that has the ability to sense subtle energy such as warmth, coolness, and other tactile sensations. All of our motor skills are coordinated through the brain. The feet have thousands of nerve endings that send pulses of information from the feet to the brain and back again in split seconds.

Feeling and sensing through the feet is a natural occurrence that we take part in every day. Do you ever notice that if your feet are cold the rest of your body feels cold? And how about when your feet are wrapped up inside a pair of hot, stifling boots on a sweltering day? What a relief it is when you can get those darn boots off and dip your feet into a crystal clear mountain stream. What a refresher! It really makes your whole body and soul feel good, doesn't it?

So you can see that we feel through our feet, and the feet affect how we feel. Let's take it to a higher level now and talk about some really sensitive tootsies. Some sensitive people are able to feel and interpret very subtle vibration changes through their feet.

**Tip Toe**

To see how the comfort of our feet changes our mental state, buy someone you know the plushest, softest, coziest pair of slippers you can find for a wintertime gift. Be there when they open them. Make them try on the slippers while you observe their facial expression. I bet they will be grinning from ear to ear when they slip their feet into the slippers.

## Colors for Healing

All matter is made up of different frequencies of vibration, and this includes color. Each color we see is just a vibration frequency pattern called light. Each color has its own "vibe," if you will. Some psychics can sense different colors with their hands or feet. Some blind people have highly refined senses through their hands and feet also.

Color vibrations have different effects on us. Of course many studies have been done on the effects of color on our psyche, and the results have been utilized widely by advertisers, merchants, and even by ourselves, unconsciously or consciously. Think of the red "power tie" that you see sported by the executive, especially when being interviewed for a high-power job. Here are some other color correlations:

➤ Blue is a cooling color and too much of it can actually make us blue or give us a chill!

➤ Green stimulates growth and is very lively and active.

➤ Yellow stimulates the mental abilities and is an attention grabber.

➤ Orange is stimulating and can be irritating if you are exposed to it for too long.

That is why yellow and orange are utilized so much in fast-food restaurants. They grab your attention to pull you in with yellow, and then they irritate you just enough with the orange so that you get out quickly! Whether we like it or not, color does have an effect on us. When was the last time you had a nice, leisurely meal at a fast-food joint?

Some holistic therapists use color therapy to help change the mood of their clients or stimulate certain organs that correlate to different colors. You can sensitize yourself to the subtleties of the different color vibrations so that someday you might be able to tell a color by walking on it barefoot! Check out the following Foot Note for a short exercise to get you started.

### Foot Note

Find some cloth in blue, yellow, and red. Cut the cloth into equal size squares. Close your eyes, and clear your mind of distractions. Rub your hands vigorously together and then hold each hand over the top of the cloth (touching or almost touching the fabric is best). Feel for any sensation. If you think you know what the color is, take a guess. If it wasn't the color you guessed, it's okay, that is part of the learning process. Make a mental note of what that color felt like to you. Test your foot sensitivity by holding your bare foot over the squares. It takes time, but these exercises will help you to become more sensitive to subtle energies.

## Watch Where You Walk

The feet are really amazing. The soles of your feet contain some of the largest pores on the body, allowing your feet to absorb whatever is applied to them. Many reflexologists use pure essential oils before or after their reflexology treatments. When the oils are applied to the feet they are absorbed almost immediately into the blood stream and go directly into the cells, creating an oxygenating effect on the whole body. Many reflexologists are also aromatherapists and will use oils that create certain therapeutic effects specifically for your needs.

### Tip Toe

Do you apply lotions to your skin and feet? Consider lotion with natural ingredients such as fruits, vegetables, and herbal products since your skin has some absorbing properties.

Another great way to take advantage of the foot's efficient absorbing properties is by applying medicinal herbs or oils to the feet. One good use of this technique is in helping a child with a parasite infection. Unfortunately, parasites are not as uncommon as you may think. I recently read a statistic that claimed an estimated 95 percent of the world's population has some type of parasitic activity going on in their body!

Many moms have asked me how to rid their toddlers of these nasty pests. I always tell them that garlic has been used for hundreds of years to rid the body of parasites. A clove can be crushed and applied to the bottom of the toddler's foot. You can even keep the clove inside the bottom of the sock if it is comfortable for the child. As he walks on this all day, the garlic's oil will be absorbed by the foot and into the blood stream. Daily application is recommended until the problem is gone.

## Footbaths—"Look, You're Soaking in It!"

Natural health experts for many years have been using therapies that treat the feet to change a body's condition. One that I use frequently on my family and myself to facilitate curing a cold or flu is a *footbath*.

Footbaths tend to work almost immediately and can be used before or after reflexology treatments, or any time you or a loved one is ill. Specifically, footbaths work because of the temperature of the water. When we submerge our sensitive feet into a tub of cold water, the blood retracts from the lower extremities and retreats to the upper body.

On the other hand, when we submerge our feet into a tub of hot water, the blood is drawn down into the lower extremities, away from the upper body. By understanding these actions, we can use footbaths to manipulate the circulation throughout the body and create certain therapeutic effects. The blood can act as a "flusher" of stagnant or congested toxins in the body or can promote healing to an area that is not getting enough blood.

If the head is congested, a cold footbath to stimulate the blood flow to the head area may help to relieve sinus congestion. Or the reverse: Using a hot footbath brings the blood to the feet and can relieve pressure-type pains that are in the upper part of the body, like a pressure headache.

Also, viruses can only survive and flourish in certain conditions and temperatures in the body, so footbaths can help create an inhospitable environment by altering the body's temperature. I have had one startling success story with a client who utilized a footbath treatment to cure a debilitating plantar wart. My client, David T. of Denver, Colorado, was a runner who ran every day. However, he had developed a plantar wart that was so

**The Sole Meaning**

A **footbath** is simply the application of water, and sometimes essential oils, to the feet and lower legs to change the condition or circulation in the body.

**Tip Toe**

In general, warts and moles seem to be extremely susceptible to suggestion, meaning that they can fall off easily if a person believes a treatment will work for them. Some claim to be able to "talk" their warts and moles into falling off!

**The Sole Meaning**

The **papovavirus hominis** is a virus that causes painful plantar warts. Footbaths may help in killing the virus.

painful he not only stopped running, but was beginning to walk with a limp.

I mentioned to him that his plantar wart was caused by a virus known as the *papovavirus hominis*, a type of virus in the body that manifests itself as plantar warts. I told him to go home, put one foot in water as cold as he could stand, and to put the foot with the plantar wart in water as hot as he could stand, and to keep his feet in the water for about 20 minutes or until the hot water cooled. The footbath worked! His plantar wart went away completely after one of these footbaths and he was happily running again!

# Introducing Your Body Systems

Now we are going to look at a way to categorize the body organs by grouping them into what we call body systems. This categorization helps you get to know your body and its functions more simply and gives us a platform to discuss the organs you will be affecting when applying reflexology techniques.

The body systems approach divides the body into general systems grouped together by their primary functions. For instance, the urinary system would consist of the kidneys, bladder, and ureter tubes, which all process uric acid waste material.

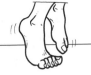

**Tip Toe**

The body systems approach has been so popular that it has been adopted by the largest, most prominent herbal company in the world, Nature's Sunshine Products, Inc., and is utilized by many of their holistic health distributors around the world, many of whom are reflexologists.

The general body systems that we will discuss are:

➤ Immune system

➤ Digestive and intestinal system

➤ Structural system

➤ Nervous system

➤ Respiratory system

➤ Urinary system

➤ Circulatory system

➤ Glandular system

In order to be able to take care of ourselves we need to have a basic understanding of how our body functions. I have found this method of categorization a fantastic tool to help people to get to know their body better and therefore enable them to take care of their health more effectively.

The next section of this book deals with these body systems and breaks each system down into its major organs and their functions. Doctors, nurses, and anatomy experts please take note: Although the information presented in the text is correct, I have had to categorize some glands and other organs in with a different system to meet the structural requirements of this book. Where an organ is not technically part of a particular system I disclose that information up front. I have also not utilized the endocrine system as a whole system, but have had to include some glands under different headings. The information presented makes the material simple to use and learn and is not meant to replace a more in-depth anatomy class. Before we proceed to the body systems, though, let's work on bringing you down to earth.

# Keeping You Grounded—The Four Elements

"Don't judge someone until you walk a mile in his moccasins" is an old saying about putting yourself in someone else's place in life and observing their actions from their point of view before you judge them. I like using moccasins in this saying rather than shoes because the reference creates an image of Native Americans, one of the peoples whose culture is most connected to the earth.

Since our feet are the parts of our bodies that touch the ground most frequently, it is understandable that our feet keep us connected to earth, or what some people call *grounded*. Walking on the earth with bare feet helps you relate to earth, reconnect to earth's rhythm, and helps to slow you down just enough to take time to remember the meaning and importance of your life.

Reflexology brings awareness to the feet. Its actual application revitalizes the circulation to the feet, and we feel the pleasure of being cared for by another person. There are numerous clichés about feet that illustrate what they really mean to us. Consider the phrase "To put your foot down." This is a grounding statement meaning to take a firm stand on something. "Dig your heels in" connotes that you are being stubborn and not budging on an issue.

**Tip Toe**

Need a new idea? Try standing up straight, hands behind your back, and stand up on your tip toes. Look straight ahead and alternate standing on your toes and coming back down until a new idea is triggered! It really works!

## *It's Elemental*

Out of the four elements that make up our world, earth, air, water, and fire, earth is the most grounding. Earth consists of things of matter and substance. Earth is thought of as dirt, density, and has some form of structure to it. In our world, physical reality is to earth as ideas are to air, emotions are to water, and willpower and passion are to fire.

These models can be used in a very broad sense to encompass types of people, colors, ideas, and general living conditions and can even be used for a general analysis of a foot. The four-element model has been used by almost all cultures around the world in some form or another, and I believe it can be used as a foundation to gain an understanding of life.

**Tip Toe**

Remember that the four-element model way of looking at things is a philosophy not a science and therefore you will see differing opinions on what things fall under what categories. It will help you if you decipher the core, baseline, most prevalent, and most typical characteristics of something before you determine what the general nature is.

I have found in all my different studies of natural health therapies, practices, and philosophies, that everything can work together using the four-element model of earth, air, fire, and water. Like the body systems model, it gives us a way to order and relate to ourselves and the universe. I not only utilize my understanding of the four elements general characteristics in my practice, but in everything I do.

## The Four-Element Model

Because the four-element model has been so helpful in my life, I'd like to introduce the basics to you so that you can apply it to reflexology. Feel free, of course, to incorporate it into other areas of your life as well. I will be referring to the four elements repeatedly, so be sure to take notes!

We all have each element in our bodies, and we can divide our body systems into these categories also. See the table later in this chapter for a breakdown of all the systems.

➤ Our structural system would belong to the earth category because it is dense and has structure.

➤ Our respiratory system would fall under the air category since the respiratory system deals mainly with breathing in and utilizing the element air.

➤ Our heart and circulatory system are associated with fire because the blood brings warmth to the rest of our body.

➤ Our urinary system falls under—guess what?—the water category.

When working with someone for the first time, you can use this four-element model to see if there is an imbalance in a certain element in their system. This will help you better to understand how to help the person. Just remember that there is no exact right or wrong way to use this model. The four elements are a philosophy and a way of looking at things. Anything in each category holds all the elements (nothing is pure in any one element). That means that the characteristics of something can change to appear more like another element. But most things have a "base personality," if you will, which can be categorized under a general element.

Let's start by getting familiar with the characteristics of each element. The following four-element model shows you their general characteristics.

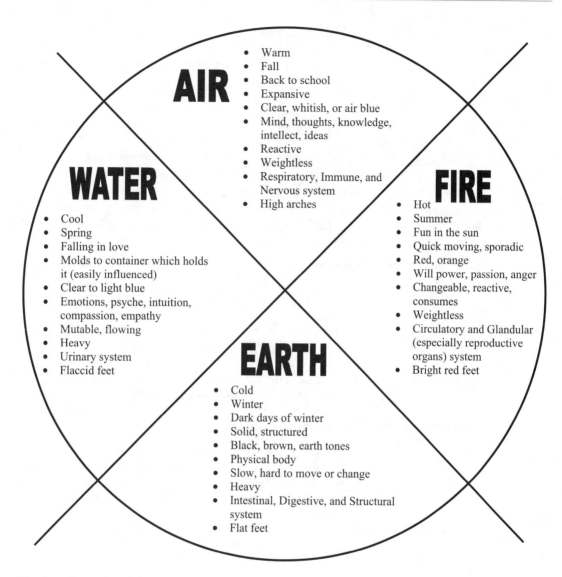

**AIR**
- Warm
- Fall
- Back to school
- Expansive
- Clear, whitish, or air blue
- Mind, thoughts, knowledge, intellect, ideas
- Reactive
- Weightless
- Respiratory, Immune, and Nervous system
- High arches

**WATER**
- Cool
- Spring
- Falling in love
- Molds to container which holds it (easily influenced)
- Clear to light blue
- Emotions, psyche, intuition, compassion, empathy
- Mutable, flowing
- Heavy
- Urinary system
- Flaccid feet

**FIRE**
- Hot
- Summer
- Fun in the sun
- Quick moving, sporadic
- Red, orange
- Will power, passion, anger
- Changeable, reactive, consumes
- Weightless
- Circulatory and Glandular (especially reproductive organs) system
- Bright red feet

**EARTH**
- Cold
- Winter
- Dark days of winter
- Solid, structured
- Black, brown, earth tones
- Physical body
- Slow, hard to move or change
- Heavy
- Intestinal, Digestive, and Structural system
- Flat feet

*The four-element model.*

Let's look at an example. On my chart, I have the emotions under water. Some may disagree with that because they think of such emotions as anger, hate, jealousy, passion, or sexual feelings. Well, in those cases, those particular emotions are display-ing fire qualities. Emotions can also appear very earthy, such as stubbornness, feeling stuck, mean, hard, cold, indifferent, etc. Similarly, when water turns to ice (because of the cold weather in the environment) it is predominately manifesting an *earth* quality. However, because our emotions *are* so changeable and seem to be influenced by our environment, they can be considered predominantly water, since water also takes on the shape of whatever container (environment) it is in.

### Foot Note

Did you ever hear someone say, he's just not "himself" anymore? This can be because a person is temporarily expressing more qualities unlike his "base element" personality qualities. For instance, a generally fiery, mobile, warm, passionate, active person becomes overwhelmed with too much earth, making him mean, stubborn, cold, analytical, and lacking in motivation. He may be taking life too seriously for whatever reason, but once the excess earth is removed he will bounce back to his fiery "self" once again, because this is his "inherent" baseline elemental personality.

### Tip Toe

If a person comes in complaining of feeling hot, her face is flushed, her feet are red, and her mouth is dry, this can be a clue for you that she is suffering from a hot condition due to too much fire in her system. You might help her by using a cooling lotion after her reflexology session. Also, offer her a cool liquid to drink.

Think of the bottom line characteristics of water. Isn't it easy to manipulate water? Freeze it, steam it, spread it out, dry it up, flavor it? You can't do all that with earth so easily. These are how our emotions work, too. We "feel" angry when someone is rude to us and become depressed, happy, passionate, and spacey based on whatever seems to be going on in our lives and environment. This is what I look for when I categorize things with the elements, and you should, too.

We all need a certain amount of fire for movement and metabolism, but too much fire can cause irritations like sore throats, heartburn, and fever. To give you a broader understanding of what I'm talking about, let's break this down to each element and its general characteristics in the following table. Can you identify yourself predominately with any one element?

## General Characteristics of the Four Elements

| Characteristic | Air | Fire | Water | Earth |
|---|---|---|---|---|
| Direction | East | South | West | North |
| Temperature | Warm | Hot | Cool | Cold |
| Colors | Transparent or light blue | Red, orange | Blue | Brown, black, earth tones |
| Part of person | Thoughts | Will | Emotion | Physical body |

| Characteristic | Air | Fire | Water | Earth |
|---|---|---|---|---|
| Associated emotions and personal characteristics | Thinker, intellectual, day dreamer, spacey | Passionate, playful, quick tempered, excitable, extrovert, generalist | Emotional, nurturing, caring, sensitive, poetic, inspiring, creative | Stable, likes order, good with numbers and facts, specific |
| Types of jobs | Writer, lecturer, journalist, philosopher, religion, lawyer, inventor, astronaut, pilot | Sales, acting, sports, motivational speaker, travel agent, party organizer | Teacher, caretaker, poet, dramatic actor, health care practitioner, musician | Construction worker, architect, CPA, sculptor, farmer, organizer, English teacher |
| Body systems | Respiratory, immune, and nervous | Circulatory and glandular | Urinary | Structural, intestinal, digestive |
| Movement | Inherently still, needs fire to move it | Fast and furious movement, mutable or sharp as in lightening | Flowing, takes the shape of its container, changeable, evaporates or freezes depending on environment | Still, slower, strong, stagnant, stable |
| Sun signs | Gemini, Aquarius, Libra | Sagittarius, Aries, Leo | Cancer, Scorpio, Pisces | Taurus, Virgo, Capricorn |
| Relation to other elements | Small amount needed to feed fire, too much can put out flame, aerates water, can move earth tiny bits at a time (wind blowing dust) | Needs air to burn, needs earth to feed it (wood), too much earth will put it out, a little water can cause steam explosion, and too much water will douse | Water needs air to keep it alive, fire to warm it, too much earth makes it muddy or freezes it | Air will move it a little, water moves it the best (mudslides), fire scorches it |

The four elements can be used to gain insight into anything, but for the purposes of this book we will focus on the analysis of the feet. Take a peek ahead to Chapter 17, "Tools of the Trade," to see a four-element chart that categorizes some common foot ailments. Knowing the elements can help you understand how they all work together to create balance. It can be really simple if we let it be.

# Foot Symbology: One Step at a Time

It is also neat to think about what the feet symbolize to you particularly. The *symbology* of the foot infiltrates your subconscious mind and has meanings that are uncovered in your dream world. Do you dream about feet? Here is an interpretation taken from Wilda B. Tanner's book *The Mystical, Magical, Marvelous World of Dreams* (Sparrow Hawk Press, 1988), which is a fantastic book I have used for years to interpret dreams:

> "Feet represent foundation, belief, understanding, your ability to stand up for your rights or to put your foot down. May also imply taking the next step, stepping in the right direction, watching your step, one step at a time."

The following is a list of foot symbolism that you can think about. See if any of these things could apply to you if you are having any of the foot conditions or if you dream about these foot conditions. I have offered this information to you so that you can take a holistic look at your problem. The list is compiled from my own teaching and integrates thoughts and symbols from Wilda Tanner's book and also Louise Hay's *Heal Your Body* (Hay House, 1994).

A holistic symbology of the feet:

**The Sole Meaning**

**Symbology** or **symbolism** describes how a symbol can represent something else. For instance, each country has a flag that symbolizes the particular country. Everyone has their own personalized set of symbolic meanings based on their life experience. This is why you can be the best interpreter of your own dream details.

➤ **Cold feet.** Symbolizes a possible lack of courage to make the decision that you know in your heart is right. Most of the time the *right* decisions are the hardest ones we can make. May imply a need to reconsider what you are getting yourself into.

➤ **Flat feet.** Symbolizes feeling a lack of support in your life. Or can symbolize that you are afraid of not being able to support yourself or that you are giving up your sense of self-reliance to take care of yourself. Or flat feet can mean that you feel a heavy responsibility in life you feel you cannot support.

➤ **Bare feet.** When you dare to go barefoot, you have the open understanding to be in touch with the earth, understand the basics of life, and are well grounded in your ideas and beliefs. If you can't bear to go bare, this may mean that you feel you are unprepared for a situation or symbolizes that you cannot tolerate or "can't stand" the situation you are in.

➤ **Problems with the heel.** Heel problems may indicate feeling susceptible to others' whims. Look closely at your relationships. Are you behaving like a heel?

➤ **Problems with the toes.** The toes represent your mobility and balance as they relate to how you are walking through life. Toes symbolize the depth or extension of your understanding as they relate to the head area in reflexology. If you have toe problems, you might want to think about how you are proceeding with your plans on your path. Is your thinking clear? If you continue to stub your toe, is there something in your life you are not willing to face and really think about? Take a good look at what your mental focus is on. The toes can give you clues as to whether you are missing something or not.

**Tip Toe**

It is fun to see how much a foot's shape can match the shape of the whole body. Some people have long, slender feet and toes and a long slender body shape to match. Others are more curvaceous and have feet to match, and some with very wide big toes have a large head.

Overall, the feet really symbolize the "earth" part of us, the down-to-earth, physical side of our being. We grow from the ground up. So, are your feet an extension of you or are you an extension of your feet?

---

## The Least You Need to Know

➤ The feet and hands contain more than half the bones in the entire body.

➤ The foot is a sensory organ that can affect the feeling of the rest of the body and will also absorb nutrients.

➤ Footbaths can be used to get immediate relief from irritating symptoms such as head colds and even plantar warts!

➤ For simplicity, the body can be categorized by organ functions into different body systems.

➤ All things can be categorized into the four-element model consisting of earth, air, fire, and water.

➤ The condition of the feet can reveal symbolic psychological factors that can help you take a look at your life situations and help you grow from them.

# Part 2
# The Body Systems: Mapping It Out

*What's the best way to your partner's heart? Instead of through the stomach, it just might be through the feet! Not only can you create goodwill by rubbing your partner's feet, but you may actually help prevent heart-related troubles!*

*Within this section lie the secrets to reflexology—how reflex points in the feet and hands affect the rest of the body. Now we get to see what those body parts correspond to on the foot map. We are going to take a body-systems approach to understanding the body's functions. Classifying major organs into basic systems is a simple way to get to know yourself from the inside out.*

*I think you will enjoy this fun look into your own body. And remember that a journey of a thousand miles begins with the first step.*

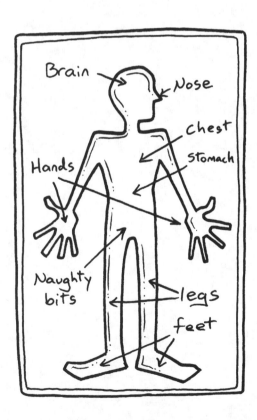

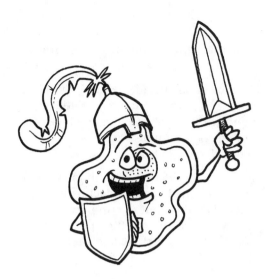

# Chapter 5

# In Your Defense: The Immune System

---

### In This Chapter

➤ Learn the importance of the immune system

➤ Understand some of its organs

➤ See how the immune system affects your health

➤ Find the immune reflex points on the feet and hands

---

There were three rabbits, the first one named Foot, the second, Foot Foot, and the third, Foot Foot Foot. One day Foot was feeling sick, so Foot Foot and Foot Foot Foot took Foot to a doctor, who told Foot Foot and Foot Foot Foot that Foot was going to die. Sure enough, Foot died. The following month, Foot Foot felt ill. So Foot Foot Foot packed Foot Foot up and took him to a different doctor. The new doctor gave Foot Foot a thorough examination and told Foot Foot Foot that Foot Foot was very ill. Foot Foot Foot became hysterical: "You've got to save him, doctor. We already have one Foot in the grave."

The moral of this corny joke is that the proper functioning of the immune system is key to your health and your life! It is like your own internal army fighting off invaders, viruses, bacteria, germs, and parasites in a battle to maintain your body's right to enjoy health. Now, get ready to be all that you can be and join me for a look at your personal armed forces.

## Granting Immunity

How do you know when your immune system is not up to par? Here are some clues: reoccurring infections, frequent colds or illness, slow-healing wounds, and frequent viral breakouts. Reflexology can play a key role in keeping your immune system strong and functioning properly.

Along with a good diet, supplements, and a positive mental attitude, reflexology is just another round of ammunition for your immune system's army of soldiers to utilize. If you are sick, or fighting off an infection or any type of disease, strengthening your immune system is the best thing you can do to help yourself.

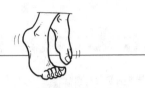

**Tip Toe**

Supplements that have been used to fight infections and build the immune system include herbs such as echinacea, goldenseal, astragalus, rose hips, and red clover, and antioxidant vitamins.

Many, many organs actually affect your immune system and are responsible for killing bugs and evicting invaders. We are going to talk only about the primary functions of each of the body systems and their principal organs for sake of the K.I.S.S. principle: Keep It Simple, Stupid (or Sweetheart, whichever you fancy).

You will find that many alternative practitioners use this simplified method to explain complicated concepts. You get all the information you need to help yourself without making your eyes glaze over from information overload, and we will take full advantage of this idea of simplicity in this book. After all, this is an introduction to your body to help you understand more about reflexology and not a prerequisite for medical school!

Before reading on you might want to glance at the following figures of the foot. This way you can get a general idea of the immune system's organs and their corresponding areas on the foot and hand. You will be seeing the same basic foot and hand charts throughout the book, filled in with different reflex locations that are discussed in each chapter. Unless otherwise indicated or made obvious to you, what you see will always be the bottom of the foot and the palm of the hand.

I have also included two lines in the diagrams. These are the hip line and the diaphragm line and are there to give you a reference point and a way to divide the feet and or hands into three sections. You can visualize anything above the diaphragm line as being reflexes to your upper body (from your diaphragm up). The middle section covers reflexes predominately in the trunk area, and the hip line is basically where your hip reflexes are. Below the hip line on the sole of the foot there are very few reflexes. Sometimes you will see the waist line through the middle of the foot; again, this is just for your orientation and happens to be the reflex area for your waist, too.

I will usually use the palm of the left hand for the diagrams. You will see this if you hold your left hand in front of you with your palm turned toward you. I primarily use a left foot also for most of the diagrams. This view would be the view of the bottom of the foot if a person was lying down and you were sitting at their feet looking at the sole of their foot.

For simplicity and clarity, I have only used this left hand or left foot throughout the pages; however, this *does not* mean that the same reflexes are not located on the same areas on the opposite foot or hand. Use the tearout card in the front of the book as a reference. For the most part, our body has a pair of everything: a pair of lungs, eyes, ears, kidneys, and so on. Just as this is true in the body, it is true for the reflex areas on the foot. Where there is only one organ on one side of the body or where the reflexes differ from one hand or foot to the other, I have included both hands or feet in the diagrams. Don't worry, I won't lose you.

Feel free to press gently on the reflex points and get familiar with these organs and reflex spots as I refer to them along the way. You can work on these immune system areas anytime you are not feeling well, and it can speed your recovery time.

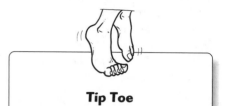

**Tip Toe**

Since your body is a whole unit, you should always work on both feet or hands to get balanced results.

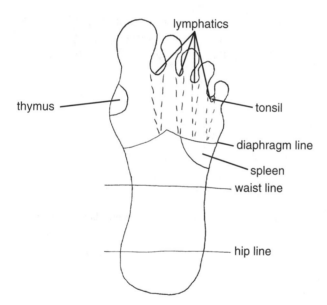

*The foot reflex points for the immune system, shown on the left foot. The lymphatic, tonsil, and thymus reflexes are also located on the right foot.*

# Your Keen Spleen

Your spleen is an organ located on the left side of the trunk of your body just under your diaphragm (or lower left rib), above the waist, to the left of the stomach, from which it is suspended. The spleen reflex on the foot is located also on the left foot, just under the ball of the foot toward the outside edge of the foot's side, as shown in the previous figure.

The main spleen reflex point on the hand is also on the left hand, below the padding of the pinky finger. Take a look at the following hand diagram to check it out.

*The left hand reflex points for the immune system. The lymphatics, tonsil, and thymus reflexes are also located in the same areas on the right hand.*

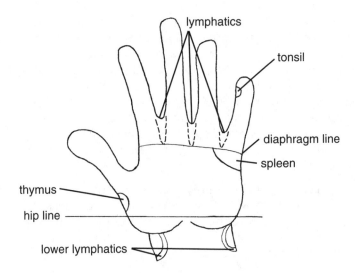

lymphatics

tonsil

diaphragm line

spleen

thymus

hip line

lower lymphatics

The spleen is responsible for storing and also filtering old and damaged blood cells, storing iron, manufacturing protective antibodies, and ridding the body of bacteria. The spleen also aids your body in producing new hemoglobin from old cells. Cool recycling program for the worn out, eh?

### Foot Note

Although our spleen is a valuable organ, some people have had severe damage to the spleen or a ruptured spleen requiring the removal of this organ (splenectomy). The body may live without the spleen as the bone marrow and liver take over the missing spleen's functions.

## Mean, Spleen, Fightin' Machine

The spleen is actually a lymphatic gland and is the largest mass of lymphatic tissue in the body. It also manufactures protective *antibodies*. Your antibodies are what go out on the battlefield and kill off offending invaders trying to stir up trouble in your system. Antibodies are therefore an important element in the functioning of your immune system.

Antibodies in general are a type of blood protein that circulates in the blood plasma to attack antigens. *Antigens* are the enemies, and can be any type of foreign invader in your body, or anything that the body does not recognize as "normal." I think of the antibodies as the equivalent of our police force here in Boise. When they see something potentially dangerous, they jump on it immediately to keep our city safe!

It's a tough neighborhood inside our bodies. It's not like the new kid in town gets welcomed with a tray of homemade cookies by his friendly neighbors! It's more like the SWAT team coming in at gunpoint to see what he's all about! "Draw guns first, ask questions later" seems to be the antibodies' basic philosophy.

## Send More Blood

Because the spleen has a big job in recycling the parts of old, worn-out cells and using their donated parts for the manufacture of new blood cells, the spleen is important to work on when there is indication of anemia in the body. *Anemia* is basically a very low blood count. Symptoms of anemia are fatigue, a pale look to the skin, and poor resistance to infection.

The spleen reflex point will be an important spot to stimulate on the foot when one has symptoms of severe fatigue or a lowered immune response. If the spleen has been removed, the liver takes over the duties of the missing spleen. The liver is the overachieving organ in the body, performing hundreds of functions. For simplicity the liver will be covered in Chapter 6, "A Lot to Swallow: The Digestive and Intestinal System," with the digestive and intestinal system.

# Lymph-ing Along

The *lymphatic system* is a network of small, transparent lymph vessels. These vessels parallel the vein and artery pathways. The lymph vessels collect fluid that seeps through the blood vessel walls and then return fluid back into the bloodstream after a filtering process.

### The Sole Meaning

**Antigens** are any type of substance foreign to our body that could be potentially dangerous. When antigens are discovered in the body, **antibodies** are created in response. Antibodies are made in the lymphoid tissue and are released into the blood stream to attack the antigen and render it less harmful.

### The Sole Meaning

**Anemia** is a reduction of the amount of hemoglobin being carried in the blood. A spleen not doing its job efficiently can cause anemia. Symptoms of anemia include fatigue, pallor, lowered immune response, and severe tiredness. Next time you're thinking "anemia boost of energy," work your spleen reflex!

The reflex areas for the lymphatic system can be found between the webbing of the toes of both feet. The webbing between the first and second toes is equivalent to the neck area lymph glands. The webbing between the second and third and third and fourth toes are the upper body and chest area in general. The webbing between the fourth and fifth toes is the reflex area for the armpits.

In the hand, the upper lymphatic areas are also located within the webbing between the fingers. The lymph system includes the tonsils and all the lymph nodes through-out the body.

### Foot Note

Although reflexologists all agree that reflexology works, not all reflexology charts are identical. You will see slight differences in almost every chart you find! This book has simplified the reflexology charts to cover the basics and focus primarily on the soles and palms. After you get the basics down, be sure to obtain a nice, detailed wall chart for yourself. It is also a good idea to carry a laminated pocket card with you for reference when you are away from home. Check out the information in the back of the book to find out where you can obtain some beautiful wall charts and pocket cards.

Most of our lymph nodes are located in the upper body around the neck and under the armpits. Since the ruler of the body is really the brain, there are numerous lymph glands in the neck to protect the brain from infection, kind of like knights guarding the king's castle.

The lymph glands are responsible for producing white blood cells that destroy infec-tion. These glands also absorb foreign invaders and kill them. You can experience the battle of your body working for you when you have a cold or sore throat and your neck glands are swollen. This is your body's defense system working hard to fight off infection locally so that the infection will not spread to the rest of the body.

## Finding Gold

Since the lymphatic system runs along the same pathways as the blood, it reminds me of a river running parallel to a highway. The highway symbolizes the arteries that are responsible for transporting the goods, like nutrients, to the places they need to go, just like the truckers bringing our groceries to the grocery stores. The lymphatic system runs alongside the roads and the lymph fluid primarily carries impurities away from the blood for filtering and reprocessing.

This analogy reminds me of a funny story told by some friends of mine who were working on constructing a bridge across the Platte River in the small mountain town of Bailey, Colorado.

The river mostly followed the highway, where truckers would haul their goods through the small valley to get back and forth between the ski towns and Denver. The river took a detour back into the woods where my friends were working. As they labored in the hot summer sun, one of my friends commented that he wondered how much gold was found in "them thar hills" and how he would use the gold that he found to buy himself a cold beer after work.

Little did he know that about a mile up river a semi-truck full of beer, specifically Coors Gold, had rolled off the highway near the river, spilling out at least half of its cargo of gold cans! When my friend looked upriver and noticed that the river looked like pure gold he thought his prayers were answered! Once the construction crew realized what was coming down the pike, they all jumped in the river and gathered as many cans of the gold stuff as they possibly could!

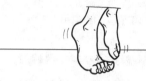

**Tip Toe**

There is power in thoughts and the spoken word, so be careful what you concentrate on and be conscious of what you say, because sometimes you get exactly what you wish for!

This story, although worth telling in and of itself, also relates directly to what we are talking about here. Think of the highway as the blood vessels in the body. The truck was the invader, which dumped its antigens into the river, representing the lymphatic system. The lymphatic system carried these invaders to the workers in the lymph glands, and they jumped on the opportunity to gather them up!

My friends, I'm sure, managed to drink all the beer and then recycle the cans so that new beer cans could be made! See how the concept "as within so without, as above so below" works in action? In the preceding story, these lymph workers were responsible for keeping the earth (our body) clean from unnatural things. Thanks guys!

## Go with the Flow

Actually though, the lymphatic system is somewhat passive, like the river is passive. The water doesn't move on its own; gravity keeps it flowing. Well, the lymphatic system does not have a pump. The lymphatic flow relies solely on the movement of the muscular system. Did you ever get swollen ankles or feet when traveling on a long road trip or even on long plane rides? This is the lymph becoming stagnant and settling in the bottom of the body.

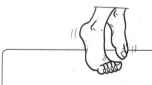

**Tip Toe**

Feeling bloated on a long plane ride? Try jumping jacks.

Jumping jacks will usually cure this edema right away. A mini tramp does wonders for moving the flow of lymph and is easier on your joints. Some vigorous stretching exercises, a large exercise ball, or anything that moves the large muscles of the body will help get the lymph flowing again. Okay, so the airlines won't let you try to squeeze your exercise ball or mini tramp in the overhead bin to take with you when you travel, what can you do? Besides general exercise, the best way to clean the lymphatic system is with reflexology! Reflexology gets the entire circulatory system moving again, which also helps the lymph flow. The essential oil of grapefruit or lemon also seems to be helpful.

## Feeding Your Army

A stagnant lymphatic system means that stagnant lymph is sitting in the lymph glands. When the lymph glands are backed up with waste products, they cannot do an efficient job of fighting off new bacteria. Stagnant lymph is equivalent to a slow-moving sewage system. It needs to get rid of waste materials to do its job effectively.

The lymph glands are composed of a considerable amount of sodium chloride and sodium carbonate. It is my belief that since each organ is predominately made of certain biochemical compounds, we can nourish the organs by feeding them foods and supplements rich in those particular compounds. A fabulous book that explains each element and the symptoms of a deficiency in the various elements, along with the foods that can correct these deficiencies, is Dr. Bernard Jensen's book, *The Chemistry of Man* (Bernard Jensen, 1983).

Sodium-rich foods that will help nourish the lymphatic system include:

➤ Apples, apricots, asparagus

➤ Barley, carrots, celery

➤ Cheeses, chick peas, collard greens

➤ Dandelion greens, egg yolks

➤ Fish, goat's milk

➤ Kelp, lentils, raw milk

➤ Mustard greens, black olives

➤ Hot red peppers, raisins

➤ Sesame seeds, strawberries, sunflower seeds

➤ Turnips, whey

Supplements rich in the following vitamins, minerals, and herbs have also been useful to the lymphatic system:

➤ **Vitamins:** A, $B_6$, C, and D

➤ **Minerals:** Magnesium and sodium copper chlorophyllin (usually added in a trace mineral supplement)

➤ **Herbs:** Bayberry, alfalfa, chamomile, echinacea, garlic, ginseng, yarrow, and parthenium

➤ **Supplements:** $CoQ_{10}$ and lecithin

A weak or stagnant lymphatic system can cause irritations such as nasal or respiratory congestion, increased mucus, lowered immune response, swollen lymph nodes, joint stiffness, over-acidity, and cysts.

# "Thymus Be Strong" Should Be a Commandment

Lymph-ing right along now, let's addresses another important component of the immune system. Many people believe that the *thymus gland* (pronounced *thigh-mus*) is really the seat of our immune system. This pinkish-gray, two-lobed organ is located in the chest cavity behind the upper sternum, below the thyroid. Basically it sits right at the base of the neck.

The location on both feet corresponding to the thymus is the medial edge of each big toe. (The medial side means the inside; it is the side of the foot that touches your other foot when you are standing with your feet together.) The point actually covers about one inch and is located almost in the middle of the joint halfway between the top of the large toe and the bottom of the large toe ball joints. On the hands, the thymus reflex area is located along the medial edge about halfway between the wrist and the tip of the thumb, and is the same for both hands.

The thymus is responsible for making cells called *T-lymphocytes*, or *T-cells*, that have a big influence on your immune system and overall strength. The lymphatic system carries white blood cells to the thymus, where they multiply and change into these special infection-fighting cells.

Although the function of the thymus is not fully understood, it is known that it plays an important part in developing immunities against various diseases. Many researchers believe the thymus produces the original lymphocytes formed in the body before birth and continues to produce them thereafter. The lymphocytes then travel from the thymus to the lymph nodes and spleen by way of the circulatory system. This shows how these organs all work together to form your immune system.

### Tread Lightly

Remember that the sodium-rich foods we are talking about are rich in the element sodium, not the table salt version. Too much table salt in the diet can only interfere with your body's delicate mineral balance and can make you retain water and raise your blood pressure. So put down that bag of salty chips and reach for the celery sticks to get the sodium your lymphatic system needs!

### Tip Toe

T-cell production is hindered in an individual with AIDS. This leaves an AIDS victim with almost no defense against any bacteria or viruses that can cause illness. Many AIDS victims die of complications associated with having no immunity, such as pneumonia. Without adequate T-cell production, illnesses that are not life-threatening to those with a healthy immune system can be deadly.

### Foot Note

When we are born our immune system is not fully developed. Actually our immune systems are not fully developed until about age 12. This is probably why children experience so many illnesses. I believe that these early illnesses are nature's way of building up or exercising our immune system, if you will. Maybe this is why our thymus is larger when we are small, because it is working hard to build our immunity. After puberty, the thymus gland begins to shrink.

## My Thymus, My Self

Some people believe our thymus is the seat of the "id," or how we identify ourselves. Just think of when someone points at you. Where does their finger usually aim? Directly at the thymus, right below your neck at the top of your chest area. Imagine that you are trying to tell someone across a crowded room "Look at me," or "I'm the one who wants to talk to you," or "Are you talking to me?" Where does your finger point? To your thymus!

This is why it is believed that the thymus is involved in more than physical immunity. This also leads to the belief that the immune system has a lot to do with how we think about ourselves and demonstrates why the thymus is so susceptible to outside forms of attack and stimulation.

My first reflexology teacher and healing woman, Isabelle Hutton, told me to tap my thymus 100 times with my fingertips daily. She believes tapping the thymus will stimulate it to produce more T-cells and therefore boost the immune system. If this is true, then maybe this is why a hug feels so good. When we hug someone, we embrace the upper chest area, which is where the thymus sits.

I tap my thymus every time I think about it, and I also try to get in as many daily hugs from my husband as I can. I figure even if it is a bunch of bologna, it still feels good and can't hurt a thing! So, go give a hug to someone you love and stimulate your immune system to boot!

### Tip Toe

When you find yourself thinking negatively or after being exposed to a negative person or situation, it won't hurt to tap your thymus several times! This may boost the immune system and protect you from getting sick or feeling down. Give it a try. After all, it worked for Tarzan.

# Laughter IS Good Medicine!

Researchers and holistic health practitioners believe that the thymus is quite susceptible to outside influences, and it has been one of the organs most studied to determine the effects of our thoughts on our immune system. The way our thoughts affect our immune system is known as *psychoneuroimmunology*.

One famous study on the impact of the mind on the immune system used two groups of volunteers. Both were normal, average, healthy adults, as similar as possible in age, health, lifestyle, and other factors. One group was asked to watch a documentary on Hitler and the evil deeds he was responsible for. The other group was asked to watch a documentary on Mother Teresa.

Afterward, a series of tests were taken on all the subjects. The most startling fact observed was that there was a significant decrease in T-cell production in the group who watched Hitler, and an equally significant increase in T-cell production in the group who watched Mother Teresa!

To me these studies were truly amazing and really made me think we should all be careful of what we expose ourselves to, especially when we are vulnerable. When we are feeling blue or doubting ourselves we are more susceptible to illness than at any other time. The moral of this story is to surround yourself with positive relationships, beautiful environments, and inspiring people. You will probably live a longer and healthier life for it!

Also, laughing stimulates your endorphins and helps your immune system gain strength. They say laughter is the best medicine, and I think this is true. Laughter is one of the best and healthiest releases for stress I know. The endorphins released by the body when you laugh help you feel better. Laughing is also good exercise! The diaphragm is stimulated, and the movement created by heavy laughter also massages the lymph glands. When you laugh, blood is forced up into your face and head area. Blood carries with it oxygen and nutrients that every cell needs to stay alive and vibrant.

> **The Sole Meaning**
>
> **Psychoneuroimmunology** is the study of how our thoughts affect our health. Broken down to its components, "psycho" means the mind, "neuro" means the nerves, "immun" stands for the immune system, and "ology" means the study of. Mind over matter is more than a cliché!

So next time you get the giggles, go all out. Laughter is contagious, and you will more than likely start a chain reaction. I believe that we all could use more laughter in our lives. You never know who you are going to help heal just because you let yourself laugh out loud in public, helping another person to laugh who was in dire need of some endorphin stimulation!

Laughter can also enhance an already jovial experience. Practicing what I preach about laughter, I like to go to comedy movies. When I think of the most enjoyable movies I have seen, it usually was because I was with a group of folks with a good sense of humor who were actively involved in laughing out loud at the funny scenes. Even if I am not with a group, but I hear a jolly fellow two rows up from me laughing hysterically at the silliest of puns, it makes me enjoy the movie that much more.

### Foot Note

When you get sleepy it is usually because there is not enough oxygen getting to the brain to keep you alert. This is why the yawn reflex is triggered. Our bodies are not dumb. Your brain invented yawning to get extra oxygen directly to the brain! Laughter also does the same thing, but it's more fun (and even more contagious than yawning!).

Think about how good you feel after a really good laugh, and make it a point to incorporate some "let-loose" time into your life. Who knows, your next reflexology treatment may be filled with laughter, and that might just be the medicine you needed.

### The Least You Need to Know

➤ The main components of the immune system are the spleen, lymph system, and thymus.

➤ The immune system can be stimulated by tapping the thymus or giving hugs to the ones we love.

➤ There is evidence that what we are exposed to mentally or verbally can affect our immune systems either positively or negatively.

➤ Laughter is good medicine!

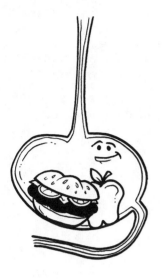

# Chapter 6

# A Lot to Swallow: The Digestive and Intestinal System

## In This Chapter

➤ Discover the importance of assimilation and elimination

➤ Learn to locate the reflex points for the digestive and intestinal organs

➤ Get to know the stomach, liver, gallbladder, and pancreas, and learn about some emotional links to your organs

➤ Meet your intestines

➤ Learn how to support your digestive health and feel better

Look through your medicine cabinet at home. What do you see? Over-the-counter medications for diarrhea, acid indigestion, heartburn, gas, constipation, and hemorrhoids? Well, well, well, these are all ailments of the intestinal and digestive tract, and the good news is that all of these things can be helped by using reflexology! Let's take a look at how these systems work together and get you working on yourself.

## Beginnings and Endings

What I refer to as the "food tube" in this chapter is an actual tube that makes up our digestive and one of the main eliminatory organs. It breaks down the foods we eat, assimilates and absorbs what we need for the body, and then eliminates what we don't need.

The top of the tube opening is the mouth. The tube takes in the food and drink we consume and sends it on its long journey from the esophagus to the stomach and on to the long, winding, scenic route through the small intestines, then down to the bowel, and its final destination.

How do you know when your intestinal and digestive systems are not working properly? Here are some clues:

➤ Heartburn, bloating, belching

➤ Sour stomach, bad breath

➤ Intestinal gas

➤ Ulcers

➤ Always feeling hungry

➤ Constipation, diarrhea

➤ Appendicitis

➤ Being overweight or being severely underweight

**The Sole Meaning**

**Rosacea** is a skin disease on the face in which the blood vessels in the cheeks and nose enlarge, causing the face to appear bright red or flushed. The cause is uncertain, but it is believed that extremes in temperature, food irritants, and too much alcohol can all play a part in aggravating the condition.

Even skin problems like acne, rashes, or *rosacea* can signal that there is improper assimilation or elimination in your system.

I believe that illness in the body many times begins in the food tube. Most of us, for starters, do not even chew our food properly. Our body relies on proper mastication of our food to start the digestive process. Our stomachs are also subject to stress and worry, and since so many of us worry or are stressed out when we are eating, our digestive functions suffer.

This is just the first half of the problem. There is an old natural health saying: "Death begins in the colon." This is probably true. Our bowels are responsible for ridding us of harmful, toxic by-products of digestion. It is the sewer system of the body. When the sewer system of a city is backed up, a health emergency is declared. When your body's sewer system is clogged up, it will also declare a health hazard, but you might not know how to interpret the signals!

This chapter will help you understand the importance of digesting, assimilating, and eliminating effectively. We will discuss all the major organs of this system, including the stomach, liver, gallbladder, pancreas, and the intestines. It is my favorite subject, and I hope you will digest and absorb the information with ease.

# Where It All Starts: The Stomach

One of my favorite lines from the *Three Stooges* television show was when Curly, Larry, and Moe were all standing on top of a building getting ready to jump to their deaths because they were downtrodden and couldn't find work. Curly had a cake in his hands and was beginning to eat it when Moe irritatingly asked him what the big idea was. Curly replied, "Mmm, so I can 'die jest' right!"

Although the first part of digestion starts when you begin chewing your food, we are going to skip right down to talking about the stomach, where lots of churning goes on to digest the foods we eat. This way, you can have your cake and digest it too!

The stomach is located high up in your abdomen about in the middle of the left side, slightly extending into the right side of the body. The stomach is somewhat protected by the left side of the rib cage. There is a reflex area for the stomach on both feet. However, it is primarily felt on the left foot, corresponding with the stomach being primarily on the left side of the body.

On the left foot, the area of the stomach is found beginning just above the midline, or waist line, section of the foot, and extends inward toward the middle of the foot about halfway across. On the right foot, it is located in the same area but does not extend as far inward across the foot.

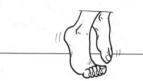

**Tip Toe**

Here's a tip to help you live or "die jest" right: Do not drink lots of liquids with your meals, especially cold liquids. This can dilute the digestive juices, contract the stomach, and interfere with proper digestion. Wait about 15 minutes before and after eating to take a drink.

The same applies to the reflex points on the hands. The stomach area is predominately found on the left hand under the pointer finger, about halfway between the thumb and pointer finger, and extends a little more than halfway across the palm. On the right hand you can find it in the same area, but it does not extend as far across the palm.

In the following two figures I have mapped out the entire digestive and intestinal system on the feet and hands so you can see the location of each reflex point.

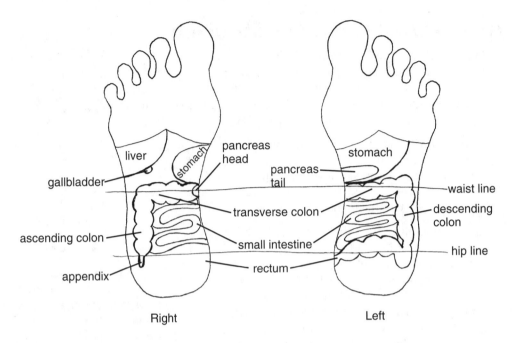

*The foot reflex points for the digestive and intestinal system.*

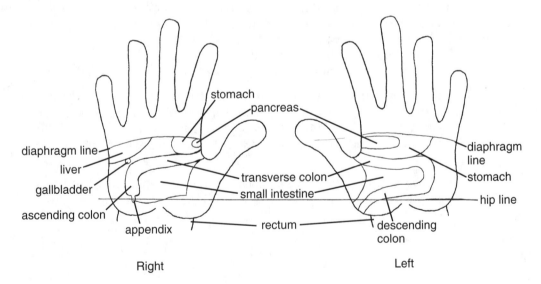

*The hand reflex points for the digestive and intestinal system.*

# Can You Stomach It?

The stomach is responsible for receiving food that has been partially digested by our saliva and chewing process. The stomach has already begun dumping digestive juices to prepare for the food coming down the tube. Once the food arrives, the stomach walls actually mash, knead, and mix the food we eat with its digestive juices and prepare the mixture to be taken to its next stop—the small intestine.

### Foot Note

One supplement that I take before every meal that has definitely changed my life is food enzymes with HCl (hydrochloric acid). Since we kill the enzymes in our foods when we cook them, these enzymes help restore the enzymes that assist digestion. My husband and I both swear that these supplements have kept us from getting ill while traveling and eating in places across the country and around the globe. We have been many places, especially third-world countries, where everyone who ate at the same restaurants suffered digestive troubles and other food poisoning symptoms, while my husband and I experienced no problems. We consider our food enzymes our insurance for a pleasurable trip!

To break down proteins in foods, your stomach produces hydrochloric acid (HCl). This acid also serves as a protective mechanism that literally "bursts" microscopic parasites and bacteria that we swallow with our food. Having a healthy amount of stomach acid is critical to keeping a strong digestive system and healthy body. If there is not enough HCl in the stomach to effectively kill off any spoiled foods or bacteria that might harm us, the stomach will trigger a reflux response to quickly eliminate these toxic substances. Many times, what we call "stomach flu" is really food poisoning.

Physically, our stomach is about 10 inches long and has a diameter that expands with the amount of food we put into it. When the stomach is empty it tends to shrink or collapse like a deflated balloon. When we overeat, the stomach stretches and proper digestion is impaired.

### Tip Toe

Peppermint is another good herb that helps stimulate digestive juices and therefore will aid digestion and may even help an upset stomach. I usually carry a small bottle of peppermint oil with me and put a dab on my tongue after meals. It not only helps my digestion but freshens my breath, too.

Think of when you overload your washer with dirty clothes. The clothes do not get as clean as they would with a proper size load since the water and soap are not able to penetrate all the tightly packed fabric. The same thing happens in the stomach when we overeat.

The perfect amount of food the stomach can handle at one time varies slightly for each person, since we all come in different sizes. However, a good rule of thumb is to limit your food portions to two handfuls of food at a time. Since we were only given two hands to eat with it makes sense that this would be the ideal amount to fill our stomach and suit our food requirements at each sitting.

## Your Stomach Can Get the Blues

It is well known that your emotions have an effect on your whole body, but many people believe that certain emotions tend to have an effect on particular organs. Emotionally speaking, the stomach is where you tend to hold worry. Worrywarts are the people who will tend to suffer stomach ailments the most.

We have all heard the phrase "you are worrying yourself sick." Many of my clients who are worriers will have indigestion and/or symptoms of a *hiatal hernia*. A hiatal hernia is a condition of the stomach in which the stomach is pushed up into the esophagus, causing symptoms such as heartburn, a lump in the throat, indigestion, and even an inability to gain weight (if underweight). Fortunately, a hiatal hernia is a correctable condition that most people get all choked up about.

### The Sole Meaning

A **hiatal hernia** is a condition of the stomach where the stomach is pushed up into the esophagus, causing pain, indigestion, heartburn, especially when lying down, a feeling of a lump in the throat, inability to gain or lose weight, anxiety attacks, and many other symptoms. Some symptoms even resemble those of a heart attack.

Speaking metaphorically, your stomach also rejects more than just spoiled foods. When you get into situations that your mind does not accept and that you are extremely worried about, you can actually loose your cookies over it! For instance, think of the barf bags on airplanes. Do you ever see anyone using them anymore? Not except in rare situations.

But when the airplane first became a real part of travel, our minds couldn't yet accept the concept. We couldn't "stomach" the idea, so to speak, of being in a huge piece of metal thousands of feet up in the air traveling at great speeds for long distances. Many folks had trouble assimilating this new idea. The worry that these new travelers experienced caused their stomachs to reject the idea completely.

## Putting Your Finger on It

Some people associate the fingers and toes with different emotions. We will talk more in depth about some beliefs about which fingers are associated with what emotions and organs in Chapter 11, "Getting to the Heart of the Matter: The Circulatory

System." But for now, realize that the body can be broken down in many different ways to be viewed symbolically and metaphorically. All can help us have more insight into our life and health.

Many believe that the finger and toe associated with worry are the thumb and large toe. When you worry about something or are listening to some important new piece of information that may affect you, you might unconsciously tuck your thumbs into your palms or curl your toes under your feet. Notice what your thumbs are doing next time you visit the dentist. Most of us worry when we are having our teeth worked on, and in my years as a dental assistant, I noticed how many people would hold their thumbs throughout an appointment!

### Foot Note

There is no real right or wrong when using finger associations, since different cultures have their different social norms. For instance, when I lived in Europe, none of the Europeans ever shook my hand. When I met a local person they would always introduce themselves and give me a light kiss on both cheeks! And as a tourist in Hawaii, my dad was driving us somewhere and a carload of young teenage Hawaiian boys passed us on the highway. They hung out their windows giving us the hand signal for "hang loose." This was a friendly gesture, we discovered later, but at the time we thought we were being told off, Hawaiian style!

When it comes to the emotions' impact on the organs, we do not necessarily know which comes first. Does a person worry because of stomach problems, or do they get stomach problems because they worry too much? Either way, there is some evidence that the two are related. So if you are experiencing troubles with your stomach, get some reflexology, and try not to worry about it. Your stomach will thank you.

## Does Liver Live Here?

Next let's talk about another major organ of the digestive system, the liver. Oh, what a great organ it is! It is truly the overachiever in the body, serving about 500 functions—and that's just those we know about so far. Your digestive system relies on the liver to manufacture bile in order to digest fats and prevent constipation and to store sugar for future use. Your liver is located on the right side of the body, just under the diaphragm. The reflex area for the liver is located on the sole of the right foot beginning just about at the waist line area and extends from the outer ridge of the foot and across the foot to about the middle.

The hand reflex area for the liver is located on the palm of the right hand just under the pad of the pinky finger and also extends across the palm toward the middle. There is also a reflex location on the top of the hand located at the point between the webbing of the thumb and first finger joint.

**Tread Lightly**

Aspartame is a chemical used as an artificial sweetener. Excess use should be avoided by people with PKU, a birth defect in which an enzyme needed to change an amino acid (phenylalanine) in the body into another substance (tyrosine) is lacking. Buildup of phenylalanine is poisonous to brain tissue. Signs include skin rashes (eczema), a mousy odor of the urine and skin, and mental retardation.

The liver has many functions, so it is appropriate that it is your largest organ, weighing an average of three pounds. It is a large, triangular, dark-colored organ that serves as a filter for all toxins that enter your bloodstream. Toxins can include most anything that isn't a natural substance. Some of the most common ones are:

➤ Over-the-counter drugs

➤ Prescription medications

➤ Alcohol

➤ Food additives

➤ Chemicals

➤ Pesticides

➤ Preservatives

We expose our bodies to these substances every day and expect the liver to take care of us. But remember, this filtering system is only one of its many functions! Most of us overburden our liver. We just can't help it because of the technologically advanced world we find ourselves in. Therefore, it is good to remember your liver and how hard it works for you so you can support it and give it a break once in a while.

## Please Deliver

The liver reminds me of the faithful, hard-working employees who labor behind the scenes of many successful corporations. It is not acknowledged when it is doing its job, making sure the accounts are in order and everything is functioning smoothly. But when a worker gets worn out and starts letting things fall through the cracks, the rest of the system suffers, and the worker is blamed for his lack of efficiency!

If you work deeply on your liver reflex area and you feel a dull ache or pain in the reflex area, it could indicate that you have a sluggish liver. If, on the contrary, your liver is overactive, you might feel more of a sharp pain when working on the liver reflex location. Working on this reflex will help your liver to rebalance. If you have either of these sensations in the liver reflex when performing reflexology, it would also be a good idea to take a break from toxins for a few days.

Symptoms of an overburdened or stressed liver may include:

➤ Diarrhea

➤ Nausea

➤ Pimples

➤ Low-grade fever

➤ Mood swings

➤ Hepatitis

➤ Gallbladder trouble

Symptoms of an underactive or sluggish liver may include:

➤ Age spots

➤ Trouble falling asleep at night and waking up feeling unrested

➤ Anemia

➤ Bruising easily

➤ Body aches

➤ Mood swings

➤ Constipation

➤ Feeling cold and tired

➤ Poor digestion

➤ Food intolerance

➤ Sensitivity to strong odors

➤ Jaundice

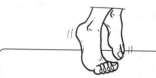

**Tip Toe**

The middle finger is associated with the liver and gallbladder and is also the finger of anger. I bet we all have learned the significance of this finger in sign language.

The liver is not only our great filter, but it also serves to lubricate the intestines with bile. It is important in forming blood cells, producing hormones, and storing and utilizing vitamins and minerals.

## Full of Bile

Our liver has been linked to the emotion anger. Repressed anger energy can be held in the liver. This is why when we cleanse the liver of its toxins, the release can have a toxic effect on our emotions! If someone is moody for no reason, you might suspect that their liver is being overburdened with toxins. This is kind of like the unappreciated worker becoming disgruntled with no time off!

When the liver works too hard for too long, it can become scarred and hardened, impairing its function. *Cirrhosis* of the liver is a potentially deadly condition of a severely damaged liver mostly experienced by alcoholics. But you don't have to be

**Tread Lightly**

Undoubtedly we all love our café lattes, but beware of becoming addicted to coffee if you already have had liver damage or a disease that affects the liver, like hepatitis.

an alcoholic to work your way into cirrhosis. You just need to continually put your body under more chemical stress than it can comfortably handle.

I have even read that regular consumption of coffee can have a hardening effect on the liver. Ironically, coffee is a stimulant that actually helps the liver to secrete bile and can therefore stimulate the bowels to move. So enjoy your coffee if you must, but be wary of overindulging.

The good news is that the liver can, and does, regenerate itself! The liver's makeup is predominately iron. It has a big influence on our own iron level that can affect the female menstrual cycle and even our blood circulation. The liver likes natural forms of iron. (This is not the same as the element iron, like construction nails are made of.) Iron from vitamin pills is hard for our body to absorb. The liver prefers food and herbal sources of iron.

Foods that are rich in iron are usually dark in color. Some of these foods include:

➤ Black cherries, black berries

➤ Spinach and other dark green, leafy vegetables

➤ Dulse, kelp

➤ Prunes, raisins

➤ Beets

➤ Red bananas

➤ Blackstrap molasses

Some herbal sources of iron include:

➤ Yellow dock

➤ Parsley

➤ Liquid chlorophyll

➤ Super blue-green algae

All of these foods and herbs nourish the blood and the liver. It is important to support your liver with the nutrients it needs to rebuild and repair itself. You can also aid your liver by using reflexology, and most important, recognize your liver and give it a break once in a while.

# You Have Some Gallbladder

The gallbladder is a pear-shaped, greenish-looking organ located on the undersurface of the right lobe of the liver. The liver and gallbladder functions are intimately linked, as demonstrated by their close proximity to one another.

The gallbladder reflex location on the foot is just about in the middle of the liver reflex area, directly below the fourth toe, midway between the waist line and the diaphragm reflex line on the right foot. The right hand also contains the gallbladder point. This point is found directly below the fourth finger, about in the middle of the liver reflex area.

### The Sole Meaning

A **gallstone** is a hard stone-like mass made up of cholesterol (blood fat), bile pigments, and calcium salts. Gallstones can cause trouble when and if they get stuck in a bile duct, where they can cause jaundice.

Basically, the gallbladder is just what its name says: a receptacle, or "bladder," that holds "gall," otherwise known as bile. The gallbladder stores the gall and releases it through the bile duct to the upper part of the small intestine to aid in the breakdown of fats and oils. This little organ can get overworked when we eat too much fat and grease. Our liver produces bile in response to fatty foods because bile emulsifies and breaks down these fats.

Loading up your diet with greasy foods can cause the gallbladder to get behind in its work. Having to deal with so much grease can sometimes lead to the formation of *gallstones* or even a gallbladder attack! The people I have known who have had these problems are convinced that reducing their fatty food intake would have been much less painful than dealing with a gallbladder attack and consequent surgery.

### Foot Note

The removal of the gallbladder may not completely do away with the painful effects of a gallbladder attack. Oddly, some people I have known who have had their gallbladders removed have had what I call "phantom" gallbladder attacks years later. They actually experienced the same painful sensations as when they had their gallbladder! Could this be the liver mourning over its missing friend? Yes, in a way. Phantom gallbladder attacks probably occur when the liver is working hard at making up for the lost gallbladder function.

In communication we use the word gall to mean nerve, as in: "You have the gall to speak to me that way?!" Having gall means having the nerve to stand up to someone or the nerve to say what is really on your mind.

If you are feeling wishy-washy and are not able to make clear decisions on what you want to do in life, where you want to go, or how to get there, you could be experiencing sluggish gallbladder energy.

We need to work on the gallbladder area to not only stimulate its function and balance in the body, but to help us take charge and have the courage to understand that we must take responsibility for ourselves to make our lives what we want them to be.

# The Pancreas: Your Sweet-Tooth Organ

The pancreas is another organ that serves many functions. It is a pinkish, semi-oblong organ about six to eight inches in length. It is located on the left side of your body midway between the diaphragm and the waist. The pancreas sits a little behind and a little below the stomach.

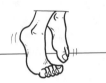

**Tip Toe**

For a swollen pancreas, known as pancreatitis, some have used a poultice made from slippery elm, marshmallow, golden seal, and fenugreek applied over the pancreas to soothe irritation. (These herbs are helpful internally also.) A poultice can be made from the dried herbs mixed with a bit of water or aloe vera juice, then applied directly to the skin.

The reflex point for the pancreas is located on the sole of each foot, but the area is larger on the left foot. It's located just under the stomach reflex point on the left foot and runs from the inside of the foot just about halfway across to the center of the foot, stopping at about the third toe. On the right foot, the spot is the same, but it does not run across as far as the left foot point and it stops under the big toe.

There are two areas of the pancreas, called the head and tail or the head and body. The pancreas head and body serve different primary functions. The head of the pancreas mainly serves our digestion and is responsible for making enzymes to help us break down our foods. These enzymes break down starches, fats, and proteins and change them to sugars and amino acids. The tail or body of the pancreas is most active in making insulin. Insulin is produced to keep our blood sugar levels adequate and regulated.

## Sugar Shock

When the pancreas is not up to par, our blood sugar level can rise dangerously high and can even lead to death. High blood sugar, or *hyperglycemia*, is known as *diabetes*. When the pancreas is overproducing insulin, the blood sugar level can become too low and the result is *hypoglycemia*. Lack of blood sugar is just as dangerous as high blood sugar, since the brain uses blood sugar, also known as *glucose*, as its constant food supply. When the brain is starved of nutrients, even for a short period of time, brain damage can occur.

The best way to help keep your blood sugar balanced is by frequently eating small meals that include lots of fibrous foods and a steady intake of protein. Sugary snacks should be avoided even if you have hypoglycemia. Sweets raise blood sugar levels only temporarily. Then blood sugar levels can drop, which makes you feel hungry for a pick-me-up snack again. This roller coaster ride over the long run can be hazardous to your health.

## Sweet Talker

Since the pancreas helps us to regulate our blood sugar levels, its function is an important part of our digestive system. The pancreas is a key gland in the *endocrine system*. The glandular system technically includes an endocrine system and an *exocrine system*. The endocrine system is a group of ductless glands that manufactures one or more hormones and secretes them directly into the bloodstream. Exocrine glands are glands that discharge their secretions to the outside via a duct.

The pancreas is an endocrine gland secreting insulin directly into the bloodstream. Another part of the pancreas serves as an exocrine gland (with ducts). The pancreatic fluid that is excreted neutralizes HCl and protects us from getting ulcers. Our pancreas has a hand in manufacturing hormones and regulating blood sugar levels, which can both affect the way we feel. I know that when my blood sugar is low I certainly get grouchy! You can see that our pancreas is important in the healthy functioning of more than just our digestive process.

Emotionally, the pancreas is related to our childlike qualities, and to the sweetness of life and how we experience it. When the pancreas points are stimulated on the feet, it will not only help you digest better and balance blood sugar levels, but it just might help you get back in touch with the child in yourself that needs to come out and play!

### The Sole Meaning

**Hyperglycemia**, better known as **diabetes**, is caused by the inability of the pancreas to produce enough insulin to keep the blood sugar balanced. Diabetes, in effect, is high blood sugar. **Hypoglycemia** is the overproduction of insulin by the pancreas, which lowers blood sugar levels, or **glucose**. Low blood sugar levels can affect brain function. If not controlled, low blood sugar can be a precursor to diabetes.

### The Sole Meaning

**Endocrine glands** are ductless glands that manufacture hormones and secrete them directly into the blood stream. Endocrine glands include the pituitary, thyroid, parathyroid, adrenals, ovaries, testes, and part of the pancreas.

**Exocrine glands** are glands that secrete through ducts. These include sweat glands and sebaceous glands just under the skin.

# Where It All Ends: The Colon

The intestinal system includes the small and large intestine (the colon), which serve similar functions and are part of the same food tube that started back at the stomach. The small intestine is a tube-like organ that has been described as an elaborate food processor! It forms a winding mass located in your trunk cavity between your waist and hips. If you could pull your small intestine out (I know, not a pretty picture) and stretch it out, it would span an amazing 20 to 26 feet! I'm just happy that it's curled up in there; I'd hate to have to be tall enough to accommodate it!

The small intestine reflex area spans the width of the entire foot from the waist line to hip line area. (As you will see, there are many overlapping areas on the feet and hands, just as our body organs are in overlapping areas.) The primary function of the small intestine is the digestion and assimilation of our nutrients, and it is where most of the nutrients from the food and supplements we eat are absorbed.

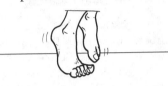

**Tip Toe**

There are no digestive enzymes in the large intestines—only an alkaline fluid that helps in the completion of digestion.

The colon, or large intestine, is also a tube-like organ that is approximately five feet long, but is wider in diameter than the small intestine. Its shape is not unlike an upside-down U. The primary function of the colon, or large intestine, is elimination of solid waste materials. The reflex area for the large intestine is broken down into three distinct areas: the ascending colon, the transverse colon, and the descending colon (known as the sigmoid), ending at the rectum reflex location.

The ascending colon begins on the lower side of the right foot, just above the heel about midway between the fourth and fifth toes, going up to about midfoot. It then takes a sharp turn toward the opposite foot and extends all the way across the foot to the instep. It picks up again on the left foot, reflecting the transverse colon starting at about the waist line. Then it spans across the foot to almost under the baby toe and takes its descent down the descending colon, making one more turn just above the heel back out toward the instep to the rectum reflex area. Whew, glad that's done, I was getting dizzy!

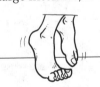

**Tip Toe**

The best way to avoid any and all diseases of the bowel is to keep your elimination channels clear. Getting reflexology treatments, drinking plenty of pure water, eating fibrous foods such as whole fruits and vegetables, taking herbal supplements like cascara sagrada and psyllium hulls, exercising, and listening to the call of nature in a timely manner will all help keep your bowel functioning properly.

The lower colon (not surprisingly) is where I seem to find most of the "crunchies" in most people's feet. The most common area of congestion in the colon may be the area where the descending colon makes its final turn before heading to the rectum (the sigmoid).

Wastes tend to accumulate at the bottom of the descending colon, so it is not surprising that this reflex area, on the left foot just below the hip line, is tender for most people. Many of us are constipated without even knowing it. The colon has an amazing ability to hold onto waste materials and harbor poisons. Like the stomach, the colon can expand as more waste is backed up into it. Portions of the bowel can even push outward, making what I call little bowel pockets. The fecal matter caught in these pockets can fester and inflame, causing a disease known as *diverticulitis*.

The role the colon plays in the body deserves a lot of attention and consideration in your health programs. The colon is your body's sewer system, and it is important to your health that you keep it moving. I have found that reflexology can be a fabulous therapy for stimulating the lower bowel into action. So those rumors about reflexologists emptying your pockets might just be true after all!

**The Sole Meaning**

**Diverticulitis** is a disease of the bowel where compacted fecal matter causes pressure in the bowel that produces small pouches, or bowel pockets, along the intestinal walls. These sacs can fester and swell, causing severe discomfort. These infected pockets can be dangerous or deadly if they burst.

---

### The Least You Need to Know

➤ Improper functioning of the digestive system can rob your body of important nutrients and lead to an array of illnesses.

➤ Your stomach is central to the digestive process.

➤ Your liver helps break down fats and serves as the major filter in the body.

➤ Your pancreas regulates your blood sugar levels, and its fluid protects you from intestinal ulcers.

➤ Your colon is your body's sewer system and must be kept clean for proper health.

➤ Reflexology, correct eating habits, and supplementation are all part of a preventative health program for your digestive and intestinal system.

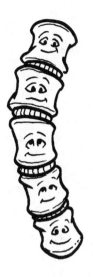

# Chapter 7

# Down to the Bone: The Structural System

## In This Chapter

➤ Learn about the structural system

➤ See how reflexology can complement chiropractic care

➤ Locate the structural reflex areas on the feet and hands

➤ Learn how reflexology can benefit your structural system

The body has three important bones: The wish bone, because everyone needs hopes, dreams and goals; the funny bone, because everything in life has to be mixed with a dose of humor; and a back bone, to give people strength to stand up for what they believe in.
—Words of Wisdom taken from a *Nampa*, Idaho, Chamber of Commerce Newsletter

Can you imagine not having any bones? Just think, the old movie *The Blob* wouldn't make any sense to us. We would have to purchase our clothes from beanbag manufacturers. Instead of rocking, we'd just have to roll. And don't even think about the Jell-O and tofu jokes we would have to endure!

### Tip Toe

The bones and teeth are made up primarily of calcium. The skin, hair, and nails are rich in silicon. Foods rich in *both* silicon and calcium include barley, beans, cauliflower, dandelion greens, millet, whole wheat, and onions.

# A Structured Environment

Our structural system is made up of more than just bones, but the bones are what give our body the structural framework on which to hang our flesh. The structural system actually encompasses the muscles, cartilage, joints, tendons, teeth, skin, and even the hair and nails. The bones give our body the ability to stand and perform intricate movements. Not to mention that it is because we have bones that our clothes don't slide off.

The body contains of a total of 206 bones. If you'll remember in Chapter 4, "The Foot at a Glance," we learned that the feet and hands contain over half the bones in the entire body. In addition to keeping us upright, the bones serve as protectors, encasing our delicate organs and keeping them from being easily exposed to damage.

There are many ailments associated with structural system imbalance, including the following:

➤ Arthritis

➤ Rheumatoid arthritis

➤ Osteoarthritis

➤ Osteoporosis

➤ Bursitis

➤ Cracking and popping of joints

➤ Muscle cramps

➤ Back pain

➤ Brittle hair and/or fingernails

➤ Tooth decay

There are several reflex points on the feet and hands that correspond to the structural system. The main ones are the spine, including the neck, the joints (knee, hip, elbow, shoulder), and the jaw and teeth. We will look at each reflex area when we talk about the particular joint, but for now you can look at the following foot and hand diagrams to see the main components of the structural system mapped out.

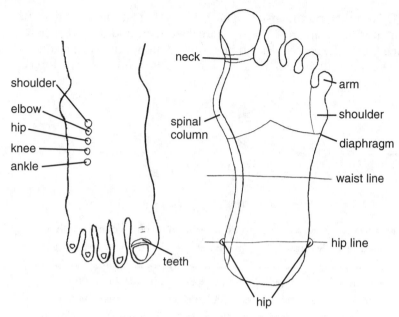

*The foot reflex areas for the structural system.*

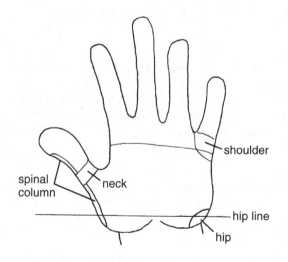

*The hand reflex areas for the structural system.*

# Having the Backbone to Get a Treatment

Have you ever been called spineless? Or felt like you have bent over backward to help someone to no avail? The spine is literally and figuratively our backbone. We use it to stand upright and to take a stand, or a bow, as the case may be.

The spine reflex can be found along the instep of each foot going all the way up to the top of the big toe, which is the head area. The neck area wraps around the entire base of the big toe. On each hand, the spine area can be found all along the outside edge of the thumb side of the hand (medial edge), running from the wrist on up to the top of the thumb.

### Foot Note

One time my husband and I were away in Mexico on a vacation when I woke up with a terrible stiff neck. The pain severely restricted my movement. We were determined not to let this problem spoil our fun, so we headed to the white, sandy beach where my helpful husband worked on my neck reflexes on my big toes as I worked on my hand reflexes. These spots were very tender and we concentrated only on the neck and spine areas for one hour. I began to feel improvement right away, and after the hour was up the kink in my neck was relieved and we were able to go scuba diving that afternoon!

Reflexology treatments will help to relax the muscles along and around the spine and back area, which can help ease back pain. I was taught to massage the reflexes to the whole spine for at least one to two minutes, although it can be "reflexed" indefinitely. This helps improve the entire circulatory system and relieve muscle tension through-out the entire body. Relaxing the muscles will also help restore the proper functioning and alignment of the spinal column.

The spine, running from the tailbone up to the base of the neck to the skull, consists of 33 bones called *vertebrae*. The spine's vertebrae are held together by ligaments and intervertebral disks, making it a flexible structure. It is a complicated structure housing an intricate network of nerves. The spine is also part of the nervous system technically, since it houses our inner wiring system of nerves.

Running through our spine is the *spinal cord*, literally the main cable to our central nervous system. All messages that are sent from the brain to the rest of the body filter through this amazing electrical network of nerves running through and along our spine. Therefore, the correct alignment of the spine is crucial for maintaining clear communication signals to the rest of the body.

## Need a Realignment?

Working the spine reflex area on the feet and hands is especially important. This is because each vertebra also affects a different organ in the body through a reflex point.

If a certain vertebra is out of alignment, meaning it is out of its normal place, the electrical impulses that run through that particular vertebra can be pinched off.

*Subluxation* (the fancy word for the misalignment of a joint) may not only cause discomfort, but it can also mean that the reflex organ will not be getting clear signals from the brain. Nor can the associated organ receive the adequate blood supply that is needed for nourishment and oxygen imperative for healthy function.

Why does a vertebra go out of alignment? Many times a muscle imbalance or spasm is the culprit. Just think of the multitudes who work on computers these days, either using a computer in their work, as their work, or even for entertainment. Because of this, many of us suffer with what my computer consultant husband calls *mouse shoulder*.

**The Sole Meaning**

**Subluxation** is the fancy word for any joint being out of alignment. If you visit a chiropractor, you will usually find that she or he will diagnose you with one or more subluxations along your spinal column. Reflexology can help chiropractic adjustments last longer by keeping the muscles relaxed. The bottom line is don't be lax about spinal care!

Mouse shoulder is when the shoulder muscles behind our shoulder blades spasm or tighten, creating a pull on the upper spine that pulls a vertebra out of its normal place. I wonder if we could come up with any other labels that we could apply to the results of our overuse of technological gizmos. Let's see, Game Boy Arm, Remote Carpal Tunnel Control Syndrome, Video Cam Paroxysm, Telephone Tic Impulse...

## Getting the Monkey Off Your Back

Sometimes an old injury like whiplash will leave a weakened area along your spine. Or damage to the ligaments could leave the vertebra vulnerable to misalignment in a particular area. Many things can cause this, including lifting something too heavy or making sudden, twisting movements like you would playing golf or softball.

**Tip Toe**

**Mouse shoulder** is a spasm of the muscles behind the shoulder blade that can pull the vertebrae in the upper neck and back out of alignment. To avoid mouse shoulder, place your mouse lower than your keyboard so that when using the mouse your wrist is not tilted back and your shoulder is relaxed and not raised toward your ear.

When working on the spine, it is always helpful to try to find the cause of the problem and eliminate it first. Then help the body to recover with natural therapies like reflexology. The following story demonstrates this.

My good friend Allison was using reflexology to ease the pain of her *sciatica* problem. The sciatica nerve is the nerve that runs from the base of your spine down your leg to the anklebone. When it is pinched off by a subluxation (misalignment) it swells and

### The Sole Meaning

**Sciatica** is a pain felt down the back and outer side of the thigh, leg, and foot, and even radiating into the heel. It is sometimes caused by a degeneration of an intervertebral disk that compresses a spinal nerve root. The onset may be sudden, brought on by awkward twisting or lifting movements.

causes a burning or deep ache that runs the length of the leg, into the buttock, and all the way to the foot.

My friend utilized chiropractic treatments and reflexology to temporarily relieve the problem. Her reflexology treatments seemed to complement her chiropractic care, helped to ease her pain, and prolonged the time between flareups. But true to her nature, Allison set out to find the cause of her ailment.

Discussing the possibilities with her chiropractor led her to question her driving position. She noticed that her condition was always worse after driving her truck. She realized that she drove with her seat too far back, causing her to overstretch her right foot in order to reach the gas pedal. This, in turn, caused her hips to rotate sideways on her spine.

This daily, awkward posture caused a muscle imbalance in her hips that misaligned one of her lower vertebrae and pinched her sciatica nerve! After having both her spine and her car seat adjusted, several reflexology treatments ended her pain, which has not come back since. Now she uses reflexology treatments for pleasure and health maintenance rather than for pain relief!

When working on yourself or another, you will usually be able to tell where the spine is out of alignment. When you are working on someone and you find a crunchy or a tender spot along the spine reflex area, this is a good indication of where the back is experiencing a subluxation. When I find a tender area on the foot, let's say on the lower spine area, I will ask the client if their lower back is sore. They always answer with a surprised "yes," and some think that I'm a fortune-teller! The analysis can be amazingly accurate! Try it on yourself and see.

# One Classy Joint

**Question:** What did one skeleton say to the other?

**Answer:** Want to meet over at my joint for a meal that will stick to your ribs?

Or maybe you'll like my grandmother Fran's joke better:

**Question:** What did the skeleton order at the bar?

**Answer:** A beer and a mop!

The joints in the body are the areas where two bones meet. The joints we will cover here are the major ones, including the shoulder, elbow, hip, knee, and jaw, which is home to the *temporal mandibular joint,* better known as *TMJ.*

Our joints offer us flexibility and help us to move in an array of amazing positions. We visualized not having bones, but what if we didn't have joints? We would all move like Barbie and Ken dolls. How would we get our socks off to get a reflexology treatment?

On the top of the foot, between the anklebone and the fourth and fifth toes, is an area where the reflex points that correspond to the joints are located. Closest to the toes is the ankle reflex. Next is the knee, hip, elbow, and shoulder.

These areas are all part of a rectangular area that encompasses all the joints for that particular side of the body. Technically these areas are not reflex points, but I want to break them down so we can talk a little bit about each. If you work this general area all along the points you see on the diagram you will be positively affecting all of your joints. Let's talk a little more about them individually.

**The Sole Meaning**

The **temporal mandibular joint**, known commonly as **TMJ**, is the hinge joint where the mandibular (lower jaw) and the temporal (upper jaw) articulate together. Discuss TMJ problems, such as popping, clicking, or pain, with your dentist for guidance.

## Lay Your Thumb on My Shoulder

Your shoulders are ball socket joints, meaning that one end of the bone is round like a ball, which fits snugly into a divot or socket-shaped bone. Ball joints offer more flexibility than a hinge joint, which can only move back and forth in one direction. The ball joint in the shoulder offers your arms a large range of movement.

On the sole of the foot, the shoulder joint reflex is located all along the base of the little toe and down toward the diaphragm line. The little toe symbolizes the arm. On the hand, the shoulder reflex area is located all along the base of the pinky finger and down toward the diaphragm line. The pinky symbolizes the arm, and the rest of the fingers represent themselves.

The shoulder gives you flexibility. My mouse shoulder always responds positively when I rub deeply on the shoulder reflex area on my hand. My husband works on the shoulder reflex area on my feet, which is always crunchy! After he is done digging his thumb into my shoulder reflex point, I thank him because my neck and shoulders feel better immediately.

**Tip Toe**

The next time your partner gives you the cold shoulder because the weight of the world is on his or her shoulders, don't fret. Instead, offer a deep shoulder reflexology treatment!

This is what I generally find with reflexology. When the discomfort in the reflex area subsides, so does the discomfort in the corresponding body part!

**Tread Lightly**

If you are experiencing tightness in your hips, a good stretch along with your reflexology sessions will help. However, a broken or fractured hip will need immediate medical attention. You can use reflexology to help alleviate some of the pain, but make sure you get yourself to a medical doctor if you have an injury.

# Reflexology Is a Hip Therapy

Your hip joints are the region of the body where the leg bones connect to your pelvis. Or as some like to say, the legs come up and make an ass of themselves! The hip-bones are located on either side of your, well, hips! The hip line on our reflex charts gives you a reference point across the heel, but the actual hip reflexes are located all around the outer ankle bones and on each side of the heel.

I also think it benefits my clients when I work from one side of the heel all along the hip reflex line. This has helped many with lower-back pain, pelvis pain, and releasing tension in the hips. The hip reflexes in the hands are located around the wrist bone on the "pinky" side of each wrist.

Here's a hip tip to see how much tension you are holding in your hips. When you lay down on your back and relax, see which way your feet fall. Do they stay basically straight up and down or do they fall inward or in opposite directions? You can suspect tension in the hips when the feet both fall to the outside of the body. This usually means that the muscles in the outer thighs and hips are tightened and are effectively pulling the feet outward. Working on the hip reflex area over a period of time should change this tension and bring the feet back to the middle.

# A Knee-Jerk Reaction

The knee joint is the joint formed by the lower end of the *femur* (the large leg bone) and the upper ends of the *tibia* and *fibula* (the shin bones) and also includes the *patella* (kneecap). Your knees are subjected to a tremendous amount of lateral stress during normal activity throughout your life. The knee is guarded by a number of ligaments to lend it support.

**The Sole Meaning**

Femur, tibia and fibula, and patella are all bones of the leg. The patella is the kneecap, the femur is the largest leg bone, and the tibia and fibula make up the shins.

Many of us participate in sporting activities such as jogging, skiing, and gymnastics, which can put much more stress on our knees than they are able to handle. Therefore, lots of us have knee problems at one time or another. Reflex areas for the knee joints are located on the top of the foot about midway between the anklebone and the webbing of the fourth and fifth toes.

The reflex to the knees is midway between the wrist and the fourth and fifth knuckles on the top (dorsal) side of each hand (not shown in the figures earlier in this chapter). Pinching the outside (pinky side) area of each hand will work the lateral sides of the body and will help loosen excess tension that might be felt in the knees.

The knee reflexes on the feet are also located on the dorsal (top) side of each foot between the ankle and the fourth and fifth toes. When the knee joints are having trouble, a gentle massage directly around the knee may prove beneficial. Usually reflexology will stimulate better circulation to the knees, which helps the knees heal.

### Foot Note

My husband is not a reflexologist, but he learned a "foot joint mobilization technique" from a reflexology video I had. Now whenever I experience pain in my knee, I ask him to use this technique in which he pulls quickly on my foot, which "snaps" my foot into alignment. The pain in my knee is immediately alleviated. See a podiatrist, chiropractor, or a reflexologist experienced in this technique, or consult the Modern Institute of Reflexology (in the back of this book) for more on foot joint mobilization.

## Go Ahead, Twist My Arm

The elbow is another joint we are all familiar with. When you come to think of it, it's really a funny-sounding word. Maybe that's why it's the place they put our funny bone! I should open up a comedy club called the Elbow Joint, where we try to stimulate your funny bone by saying the word elbow five times fast before you're allowed in!

Anyway, the elbow reflex point on the foot is located on the top part of the foot about midway between the anklebone and the webbing between the fourth and fifth toes (closer to the toes). Another area that covers the elbow, elbow, elbow, elbow (just kidding) is the little toe, which corresponds to the entire arm. The left baby toe would correspond to the left arm, and the right to the right. Similarly, the elbow reflex point on the hands is found on each pinky finger, which corresponds to the whole arm.

## Muscling In

As I mentioned earlier, the structural system is not just made of bones, but also muscles and tendons that give you the power to move your bones. Your muscles rely on magnesium and a balance of other minerals to keep them healthy.

Your muscles also like to be stretched slowly. This helps them take in a healthy blood supply and keep the circulation going so you don't get stiff and achy. Reflexology helps relax all your muscles and helps increase the circulation to your whole body, which is another reason it makes you feel so good.

### Foot Note

Sometimes I take my cues from animals. Every time my kitty wakes up, she slowly s-t-r-e-c-h-e-s her long, striped legs out behind her and then slowly stretches her front paws out in front of her before doing anything else. It is natural for an animal to stretch every time it gets up. Not so for us humans. Our kitty doesn't miss the chance to stretch. It seems to keep her calm because she sleeps all day. Stretching also helps flush out waste materials from the muscles. So stretching is good for physical and mental health!

# The Whole Tooth

Of course your teeth are not joints, but they fall under the umbrella of the structural system because the bones that support them come together at the side of your face just under your ears and make up the joint known as TMJ—temporal mandibular joint.

### Tread Lightly

One of the symptoms of a parasite infection is grinding your teeth at night. Parasites are nocturnal, so they wake up at night and begin to party, which can trigger a subconscious reaction to grind or clench your teeth. Check with your health practitioner to find out if you may have a parasite infestation. Unfortunately, it is not as uncommon as you might think.

Clicking and popping of the temporal mandibular joint can indicate TMJ problems, which can be caused by clenching or grinding your teeth. There can be other causes as well. Sometimes a filling can be too high, for example, and cause your jaw to close crookedly, which will lead to painful jaw and TMJ problems.

As always, a holistic approach to this problem is wise. Many times stress and worry will cause you to grind or clench your teeth, especially at night. In this case, a night-guard made for you by your dentist might be helpful to prevent damage to your teeth and jaw while you deal with the source of your stress.

Reflexology can help with problems of TMJ by relaxing the muscles associated with the clenching. Your teeth exert a tremendous pressure when you grind or clench them. This can damage the structure of your teeth and even trigger migraines and other headaches.

## Tracing Minerals

Tooth and jaw problems can also be a signal of a trace mineral deficiency. Your structural system holds the largest stores of calcium in the body. Proper minerals supplied by the diet or through supplementation are extremely important for myriad functions.

If your body chemistry is off due to improper digestion or irregular nutritional habits, your body may not receive the minerals it needs. When this happens, your body goes to its "stash" of minerals, located in the bones, teeth, hair, and nails. Over time, this process will weaken the overall structural system and symptoms like arthritis, osteoporosis, hip fractures, and other frequent bone breaks will begin to manifest.

Before these diseases set in, you can usually recognize a mineral or nutritional deficiency based on the condition of your fingernails, hair, and teeth. The body seems to be able to utilize the calcium found in these areas first, causing brittle hair and nails. Tooth problems may consist of cavities, tooth and gum loss, bone loss in the jaw, and teeth that fracture and crack easily. Therefore, it is important to recognize your teeth as a part of your structural system. Are you giving them everything they need?

## Pulling Out a Plumb

The jaw and teeth reflex areas are located on the top of the big toe on each foot. The teeth and jaw points run along the area just below the base of the big toe nail and up slightly on each side. The jaw and teeth reflex points on the hand run just below the base of the thumbnail on both hands.

You might remember that the thumb is also associated with worry. I think babies suck their thumbs because it pacifies them. Maybe this is also why Little Jack Horner of the nursery rhyme sat in the corner and stuck his thumb into his pie! He was probably worried that he would get caught hogging that whole plum pie!

It is understandable if you feel vulnerable when someone is working in your mouth; therefore, pressing tightly on the tooth and jaw reflex areas on the thumbs just might serve to pacify your nervousness. Later we will get more into specific techniques, but for now, hold onto those thumbs.

**Tip Toe**

It is not surprising that many people hold their thumbs when getting their teeth worked on. You can hold tightly onto the teeth reflexes on your thumbs the next time you are at your dentist to help stop discomfort. Some people have gone as far as wearing rubber bands around the base of the thumbnails to alleviate dental discomfort.

## The Least You Need to Know

➤ The structural system supports the entire body and is made up of bones, cartilage, tendons, ligaments, and muscles.

➤ The alignment of your spine is important since it affects blood supply and electrical impulse distribution to the rest of the organs. Reflexology can help to prolong your chiropractic spinal adjustments by relaxing the back muscles.

➤ The joints are where the bones come together, and, along with our muscles and tendons, they allow us to bend, twist, and move easily. Reflexology can restore circulation to the joints, which can aid healing.

➤ Stretching after a reflexology treatment will enhance the therapeutic effects of the treatment by helping to maintain flexibility and aiding the muscles to release toxins by bringing in a fresh blood supply.

➤ Reflex points below the base of the thumb correspond to the teeth and jaw and can be used to ease the discomfort of TMJ problems and help calm nerves when visiting the dentist.

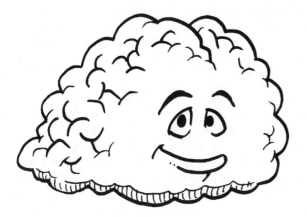

# Chapter 8

# What Nerve: The Nervous System

---

**In This Chapter**

➤ Learn about your brain

➤ Locate the nervous system reflexes on your feet and hands

➤ Get to know your pituitary and pineal glands

➤ See how your adrenals can affect your energy levels and how stress can affect your adrenals

➤ Benefit from the calming effects of reflexology

---

The nervous system is divided into two parts: the *central nervous system* and the *peripheral* or *autonomic nervous system*. The autonomic nervous system is broken down into two more parts labeled the *sympathetic* and the *parasympathetic nervous systems*.

There is now some controversy over a third type of nervous system that is believed to be activated after reading an abundance of corny jokes and puns. This system is termed the *apathetic nervous system*. Now that you are in the eighth chapter, your apathetic nervous system has probably been well exercised.

## You're Getting on My Nerves

Technically, the components of the nervous system really only consist of the brain and spinal column. But since we already talked about the spine as part of the structural

### The Sole Meaning

The **autonomic nervous system** is the part of our nervous system that is in control of our bodily functions including digestion, heartbeat, perspiration, and so on, that we do not consciously direct. The **central nervous system** includes the brain and spinal cord and controls conscious thoughts and actions like movement and talking.

system, throughout the text and in this chapter, I had to "borrow" some glands from the endocrine system and sprinkle them in with other systems where appropriate. When we discuss an endocrine gland that is not technically part of a certain body system, I will let you know as we go.

Since stress, nervousness, and tension all are connected with the hormones that the adrenals produce, we will discuss them here under the nervous system. And the pineal and pituitary are glands, but they are located *in* the brain, so we'll discuss them here as well. When you take a reflexology class, however, you will most likely be taught about the adrenals, the pituitary and pineal glands as part of the endocrine system. Now let's relax and discuss the two general parts of our nervous system, the autonomic (peripheral) and the central.

The autonomic nervous system controls the bodily functions that we do not consciously direct. Examples of these functions include our heartbeat, body temperature regulation, digestive functions, respiration, and intestinal movements. The central nervous system, including the brain and spinal cord, controls our conscious thoughts and actions like movement and talking.

I find it easier to learn new ideas and words when I use them in clever sentences. Autonomic may be used in a sentence like "I autonomically get nervous when I think that I am not in control of my intestinal movements."

Now, if you don't mind, we are going to discuss the main reflexes that affect your nervous system responses, including those for the brain, the adrenals, and two glands located in the brain: the pituitary and the pineal glands. For starters, I hope you will keep an open mind as we take a closer look at the nervous system.

Imbalances in the nervous system can go to either end of the emotional scale, meaning that disturbances can be felt as highs, known as *mania*, or lows like *depression*. Nervous system imbalances may include the following:

➤ Anxiety

➤ Depression

➤ Memory loss

➤ Alzheimer's disease

➤ ADD (Attention Deficit Disorder)

➤ Speech pattern disturbances

➤ Mental illness

➤ Premature aging

Any or all of these ailments may be linked to nervous system malfunctions due to malnutrition, something in the present or past environment, or chemical imbalances due to glandular malfunction. We will try to deal with working the reflexes here that will help stimulate your body to balance, which can be of benefit for all of these ailments.

# The Brain: Thinking on Your Feet

The brain is the primary component of the nervous system. It seems to me that studying the brain must be similar to being on the road to knowledge and enlightenment: The more you learn, the more you realize that there's a lot you don't know. Scientists, psychologists, and neuroscientists studying the brain make new discoveries only to uncover more amazing facts about how the brain actually works, leading to further experimentation.

**Foot Note**

The brain and the mind are different things. The brain is our computer, and scientists are finding out exactly how it functions. However, the mind remains a mystery. Although we know how impulses are sent to different parts of our body when we have a thought, we really don't know where the original thought is generated. Who or what is really doing the thinking? Where does inspiration come from? These are the secrets of the mind which will continue to give us thoughts to ponder.

Fortunately, we do know some physical characteristics of the brain. The brain is an organ that weighs about three pounds and is encased and protected by the bony structure called the skull. The brain represents about 97 percent of the entire central nervous system. Connected to the upper end of the spinal cord, it is responsible for issuing nerve impulses, processing nerve impulse data, and engaging in the higher order thought processes ... well, *most* of us process a higher order of thought!

The reflex points for the brain are located at the very tips of the toes. The large toe especially reflects the brain since the large toe represents the head. The same goes for the brain reflex area on the hands, located at the tip of each finger and especially the top of the thumb. The following figures show the reflex points for the brain area along with some other glands that affect the nervous system.

*The foot reflex points that affect the nervous system, along with two glands located in the brain, the pineal and pituitary. These same reflexes are located on both feet.*

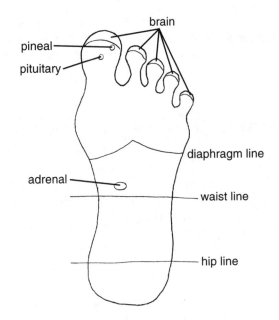

*The hand reflex points that affect the nervous system. These same reflexes are found on both hands.*

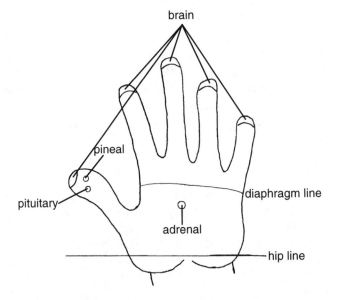

Positioned at the top of the body, literally and figuratively, the brain is the king of the hill. And it works hard for its position! The brain serves more functions than we might ever be able to discover. Along with the heart, the brain is the organ that is most vital for sustaining life.

The brain makes no bones about demanding the most attention of all the organs in the body. It uses up more nutrients, oxygen, and glucose (blood sugar) than any other organ, and it also has first dibs on these nutrients. In the internal world, the brain is the king, and the blood carries the oxygen and nutrients to it first. When the king is done feasting, the blood redistributes nutrients to the other organs in the body.

The brain is also one of the most protected organs in the body. The neck contains more lymph nodes than any other area of the body to stop viruses and infection from traveling on to the brain—like sentries around the king's castle. The brain is also the only organ that is almost entirely surrounded by a bony structure. A membrane called the *blood-brain barrier* also serves as protection around the brain. This barrier is a protective mechanism that assists us by keeping many substances that may be harmful from entering the tissue fluids surrounding the brain cells.

### The Sole Meaning

The **blood-brain barrier** is a protective mechanism made of a semi-permeable membrane that keeps solid particles and large molecules from entering the brain cells.

The body structure shows us that the brain is the most important physical part of the body and that we should take good care of it! You can be good to your brain in many different ways. Physical exercise helps bring more oxygen to the blood, a vital nutrient good for clear thinking and alertness. When you are lacking oxygen in the blood, the brain's functions are not as sharp. You get lethargic and your friends call you a "numb skull." Reflexology helps by increasing the circulation to the brain so that it can receive the oxygen and nutrients that it needs.

## Brain Food

The proper nutrients are essential in making sure that your brain is well fed and that you have enough nutrients to go around to feed the rest of your organs! Several studies done in Germany have shown the beneficial effects that the herbs ginkgo biloba and gotu kola have on improving brain function and circulation.

In Germany, ginkgo biloba is prescribed by doctors to patients with Alzheimer's disease. Studies show improvement in mental function within weeks, but the most profound effects are shown with daily use over a year or longer.

### Tip Toe

Adequate rest is an important part of recharging not only your mind, but the rest of your body. Although the brain never sleeps, your conscious mind requires time off nightly in order to keep you alert and functioning during the daytime.

Lecithin is another excellent brain food. Lecithin helps protect the brain and nerves and is also used to counteract high cholesterol. Supplements can be taken, and there is also a healthy amount found in egg yolks.

I was once told while staring off into space that I shouldn't allow my brain to wander because it was too small to be let out on its own! Another form of brain food is continuous learning. Strive to be old and wise, and your brain will defy your age.

If the brain is consistently challenged with new experiences and new things to learn, the dendrites and synapses that process the information will keep you more alert and feeling much more alive than your unproductive or inactive friends.

## Hardheadedness

As we age, we tend to slow down. Calcium deposits may form in the brain due to a lack of stimulation and lack of cerebral fluid that keeps it lubricated and soft. Can you think of folks who you would term as hardened or set in their ways, or unwilling to change their mindset?

In the elderly, this can literally mean that their brains have actually begun to calcify and therefore make them unable to be flexible in their thinking. Calcium deposits in the brain make it much more difficult for a person to change their ways, which could be literally set in stone!

### Foot Note

If we stop stimulating our brain with reflexology treatments, new challenges, and exercises, the brain can become sluggish and a calcification of the brain can begin. This calcification literally hardens parts of our brains and can make us stubborn, set in our ways, and extremely inflexible. The good news is that studies indicate that with the proper stimulation, our brains can continue to grow and we can increase our intelligence and brain function well into our 70s, 80s, and 90s! Think of senator and astronaut John Glenn as an inspiration for what you can be capable of in your 70s. The only stone that should be left unturned when you die is your tombstone!

Some people now use technology to stimulate the brain. The machines utilized for this are called *mind machines*, which use sound and light patterns to strengthen brainpower, increase memory, stimulate creativity, and accelerate learning. I purchased one in Belgium that I use on myself and in my practice. I first discovered these machines in Germany, where they are offered at health spas and even rented by hotels as a tool for stress-reduction therapy. If you are interested in learning more, see Appendix B, "Supplies and Where to Find Them," for information on where you can get a catalog.

The best way to avoid getting your brain set in stone, though, is to continue to challenge yourself regularly:

➤ See new places.

➤ Take new classes.

➤ Move about and stay flexible.

➤ Keep an open mind.

I am not advocating stopping the things that are positive and that work for you, but you can always find something new that may improve your life or that interests you. Keep your mind young by keeping it stimulated, and you will feel younger for it. Moreover, by keeping mentally youthful, you will leave good memories for the loved ones you leave behind.

**Tread Lightly**

Of course we all know that alcohol, drugs, and other toxins taken into the body kill brain cells. Use these things with discretion, if at all, to protect your brain, and fill it up with other good things to counteract the times that you do indulge!

Your thoughts, self-talk, dreams, actions, and state of mind are all controlled or influenced, by your brain. Make sure that your self-talk is positive. Mostly we find that we are harder on ourselves than anybody else will ever be. It's great to be self-regulating, but don't feed yourself negative thoughts all the time. Also, steer away from negative people. Lighten up, have some fun!

Overall, along with your regular reflexology treatments, of course, exercise, mental challenges, proper nutrients, and positive thoughts will keep you in a positive frame of mind and keep your brain and your body feeling younger and more alive!

# The Pituitary: Master Controller

The pituitary gland is a small, pea-size ball of tissue hanging from a tiny stem-like piece of flesh from the underside of the brain. Since it is located in the brain, we have categorized the pituitary under the nervous system in this book. However, this tiny gland is actually part of the endocrine system or *glandular system*. The pituitary affects myriad functions, and the messages it sends control all other glandular functions. You might consider the pituitary a little guy with a big control issue! The reflex for the pituitary gland can be found on each large toe. To locate the reflex for the pituitary

**The Sole Meaning**

The **glandular system** is a general term used to describe all the glands of the body. The glandular system is divided into two categories, the endocrine glands (without ducts) and exocrine glands (with ducts). Glands are organs or groups of cells that make and secrete fluids, such as hormones.

gland locate the bull's-eye of the swirl in your toe print. To stimulate this gland, you will have to push up and then in toward the center of the toe at the same time.

You will know when you stimulate this point because you will feel either an electric shock feeling or like someone has stuck a pin into the area! This sharp reaction is especially noticeable in people who may have calcium deposits building up in their brain!

As for the hands, the pituitary gland reflex is found on each thumb. To locate it, use the same method as for the toe. Find the middle of the swirl on the thumbprint and push up and in toward the middle of the thumb to stimulate.

## The Messenger Gland

The pituitary gland in the brain has a lot of important responsibilities. The pituitary is involved in sending messages to the rest of the glandular system and regulating growth mechanisms, skin pigmentation, blood pressure, and sexual development. This gland is responsible for the prevention of an excessive accumulation of fat. This is therefore a good point to work on if you are trying to lose weight.

Imbalances of the pituitary gland can manifest in a variety of ways, including:

➤ Obesity

➤ Growth problems

➤ Hindered or excessive body development

➤ Sexual development disturbances

➤ High or low blood pressure

➤ Feeling morose or depressed

As you can see, the pituitary gland has all kinds of responsibilities, from the physical to the emotional.

**Tread Lightly**

Feeling morose or ill-humored and depressed can be caused by an improperly functioning pituitary gland. Stimulating this gland with reflexology just might be the key to alleviating depression and lifting your spirits!

## Just a Little Bit Pregnant?

I had a coworker who began lactating although she had never had a baby and was not pregnant! She began taking black walnut hull, noted for its ability to dry up breast milk. Since the pituitary controls the sexual organs' messages, I suggested that my friend work on her pituitary reflex. Not surprisingly, her points were extremely tender!

Further medical tests revealed that she had a tumor on her pituitary gland! Her lactation stopped shortly after implementing herbs and reflexology, and the last I heard from her she was fully recovered after radiation treatment and was living happy and healthy in Hawaii! Reflexology can be complementary to medical treatments, and I think her treatments and the herbs helped speed her recovery.

## Foot Note

**Glandular body typing** is a method for analyzing a person based on their particular glandular body type. Invented by Dr. Henery Bieler, M.D., and expanded on by the Tree of Light Institute in Utah, this method identifies the dominant gland in your body, identified by your body shape and general characteristics. For instance, a pituitary type would tend to have most of their energy in their head, tending to be intellectual and idealistic. The pituitary type will look young for their age, have smallish features, and be shorter in stature. Usually these people have rounded shoulders, beautiful teeth, get baby fat all over when overweight, and women will tend to be small-breasted.

# The Pineal: Seeing the Light of Day

One of the least-understood glands in the body is the pineal gland. This gland is also part of the endocrine or glandular system, but it is located in the brain, and therefore, we will talk about it here. The pineal is located just behind and slightly above the pituitary gland.

The reflex point for the pineal is located on the upper quadrant of each big toe. In relation to the pituitary gland reflex, it is a little bit closer to the second toe and slightly above the pituitary reflex point. The stimulation of this reflex will also be felt as a sharp zing, but the zing is usually more dull than the zing of the pituitary reflex point.

On the hand, the pineal reflex point can be found on each thumb, slightly toward the pointer finger from the pituitary reflex point. See the figure earlier in this chapter to find the general location. These spots are both hard to locate when you work on yourself, but like I say, once you hit them, the "zing" will let you know you found them!

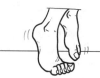

### Tip Toe

When you work the tip of the left large toe or left thumb you are effectively working the left brain, and the same goes for the right brain when you work the right thumb and toe.

## Keeping You Young

Your pineal gland is a bit of a mystery. Many believe it is responsible for dreams and even psychic abilities. We do know that the pineal gland can calcify. Usually this is found in old age, if it happens at all. Calcification of this gland has been linked to the slowing down and aging of the rest of the body and a general deterioration of health.

One dramatic study done with the pineal gland was performed on rats. Researchers switched the pineal glands of a healthy young rat with that of a much older rat showing severe signs of aging. The results were almost immediate. The young rat with the old pineal gland aged rapidly. The old rat with the young pineal gland actually gained a youthful appearance and vitality! He grew a thick, shiny coat of hair, gained back muscle tone, and his response to stimuli quickened!

## You're Getting Sleepy...

The pineal gland is responsible for producing and regulating the hormone *melatonin* in the body. Along with other functions, this hormone regulates your sleep patterns and has been linked to *Seasonal Affective Disorder*, or *SAD*. SAD is a syndrome characterized by severe depression brought on by a lack of sunshine. Many suffer from this disorder in areas where it tends to be overcast or dark during the winter months, thus its label linking it to the seasons. This condition has been improved with the use of full-spectrum light therapy.

**The Sole Meaning**

*Seasonal Affective Disorder*, otherwise known as **SAD**, is a syndrome characterized by severe depression during certain times of the year. This disorder brings on a desire to overeat, especially carbohydrates. Most notably, the depression is experienced during times when there is a lack of sunshine. Stimulating the pineal gland may help SAD people.

Melatonin is a hormone that makes us feel sleepy when nighttime comes. The pineal is stimulated by sunlight to suppress the melatonin production in the brain. This demonstrates how the pineal gland regulates our sleep/wake cycles. If you have trouble waking up in the morning, try leaving your shades open. The natural sunlight will help suppress your body's production of melatonin, and you will be able to wake refreshed. On the other hand, supplementing with melatonin might be useful when you cannot get to sleep or when you are working the night shift and are forced to sleep during the day.

The pineal gland works as the harmonizer for the rest of the glands. It is important that the pineal is working properly to keep the rest of our glands and hormones in balance. The moral of the story is that when you feel the "blahs" coming on, especially when it is an overcast day, give your pineal reflex point a few good zings and see if it doesn't help clear your mental fog!

## Adrenals: Fight or Flight

The adrenals are also glands, making them part of the glandular system, but again, we discuss them here under the nervous system because they produce chemicals that affect the nervous system and are greatly affected by stress. The adrenals are small glands that rest atop your kidneys. They are very small indeed, only about as large as the tip of your pinky finger and weighing about as much as a coin.

The adrenal reflex points are located on the soles of both feet, about midfoot, slightly above the waist line area. The adrenal reflex points on the hand are located slightly above the midpoint of the palm. The adrenals have an influence on your vigor, sense of courage, vitality, and fervor. They are linked to your ability to work hard, get excited, and even stick up for yourself!

When the adrenal reflex point is super indented, or when you work on it and it leaves a depression in the foot, you might suspect a problem with the body's ability to metabolize fats, carbohydrates, and proteins. The adrenals also serve many other functions, including:

➤ Working with insulin to maintain blood sugar balance

➤ Regulating fluid balance

➤ Improving muscle tone

➤ Promoting mineral balance in the body

Physical and mental stresses can lead to the weakening of the adrenals, as can the overuse of caffeine and other stimulants.

The adrenals produce a hormone called, appropriately, *adrenaline*. Adrenaline is known as your flight or fight response hormone. When you are under a great amount of stress, or whatever you perceive to be a great amount of stress, the adrenals pump out adrenaline and *noradrenaline*, which have an immediate and profound effect on your body, preparing you for a fight or for flight—running from danger.

The hormone raises your blood pressure, releases blood sugar to the brain, which causes acute alertness and awareness, and generally prepares the body to protect itself in any way it deems physically necessary.

**Tread Lightly**

If you find an indented adrenal reflex point, you might suspect a digestive problem. We don't diagnose with reflexology, but you might want to consider digestive disturbances or gallbladder or liver ailments that would indicate a metabolizing imbalance. You should also check the gallbladder and liver reflex areas for tenderness for more clues.

**Tip Toe**

BOO! The rush you feel when someone scares the daylights out of you is the result of adrenaline being pumped through your body. This rush can help you to move faster and fight harder than when you are in a relaxed state.

So many of us tend to overwork our adrenals through our desire to be successful. We can take on too many projects and our inner drive to meet our goals runs the body down. Too much stress keeps the adrenals on constant call, which can eventually weaken them and make us feel lethargic and even depressed.

If, in the middle of the day, you find yourself wanting for energy and looking for a candy bar or other stimulant for a boost, you might try stimulating your adrenal reflex points first. It is a healthier alternative to caffeine or a sugary snack.

---

### The Least You Need to Know

➤ Your brain needs physical as well as mental stimulation to keep you young and flexible.

➤ The pituitary is a gland located in the center of the brain. Stimulating the pituitary's reflex points may help relieve depression and also aid in weight loss.

➤ The pineal is a gland located in the brain that is associated with our sleep/wake cycles, dreaming, and even aging. Proper functioning of this gland may keep you young.

➤ The adrenals are glands that regulate your fight or flight response when you experience stress. Using reflexology may help reduce fatigue brought on by weak adrenals.

➤ Because of its overall affect on the glandular and nervous systems, reflexology is a great therapy for anxiety and depression, and may aid in balancing out the highs and lows that come from high-stress lives.

---

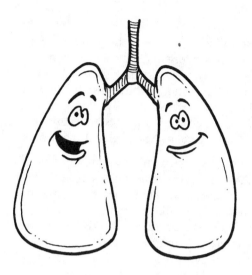

# Chapter 9

# Remember to Breathe! The Respiratory System

## In This Chapter

➤ Discover the functions of the respiratory system

➤ Learn how emotions may be linked to respiratory illness

➤ Find the respiratory system reflexes on the feet and hands

➤ Learn to breathe better with reflexology

➤ Help your eyes and ears by improving the respiratory system

Take a long, slow, deep breath and then exhale. Did your shoulders rise when you inhaled? Did you have to open your mouth to get in enough air to take that deep breath? Or did you have to exhale first? Most of us could improve our respiratory function by freeing ourselves of tension, allergies, asthma, or other respiratory problems. When we don't breathe as well as we should we can become lethargic. Let's take a look at how reflexology can ease some of these problems and get you breathing deep and feeling better!

## Divine Respiration

Starting from the nose, the major organs of the respiratory system we'll talk about here consist of the sinus cavities, bronchi, lungs, and diaphragm. The primary functions of the respiratory system include breathing, filtering dust particles, warming the body, humidifying, and exchanging oxygen with carbon dioxide.

**Tip Toe**

Hydrochloric acid (HCl) is said to break down protein complexes that can cause allergy congestion by getting into the blood stream through the liver. This may be why daily use of food enzyme tablets containing HCl have helped so many of my clients relieve long-term allergies.

In this chapter we will also talk about the eyes and ears. Although these are sensory organs, they are situated very close to the sinus cavities. When we have a respiratory ailment, like allergies for instance, the eyes itch and water and the ears feel plugged because of this proximity. I find that working the eye and ear reflex points helps my clients greatly when they have allergy-related symptoms.

The respiratory system serves many more functions than just breathing. The word *respiration* actually is used to describe all the processes associated with the release of energy into the body. By enabling our body to utilize oxygen, the respiratory system makes it possible for the body to produce energy. When the respiratory system is not up to par, the energy lags. The respiratory system also serves as a line of defense, protecting the body from harmful airborne toxins, and finally serves as an elimination channel, carrying out waste products.

Ailments of the respiratory system include:

➤ Sinusitis

➤ Allergies

➤ Asthma

➤ Bronchitis

➤ Pneumonia

➤ Emphysema

Now take a deep breath as we dive into the major components of the respiratory system.

# A Little Heavy Breathing: The Lungs

The lungs are located in the chest cavity on the left and right side of the body and are protected mostly by the rib cage. The *bronchi* are the airways to each lung and are divided into even smaller airways called *bronchioles*. The exchange of oxygen into carbon dioxide takes place in the *alveoli* (air pockets) in the terminal ends of the bronchioles.

The reflex areas for the lungs and bronchi cover almost the entire ball of the foot (the padding under the toes), and also the space between the metatarsal bones on the top and bottom of each foot. This entire area on both feet represents the chest area of the body. The bronchial tube reflexes run from the ball of the foot just under the inside edge of each large toe and up to the base of the large toe on each foot.

On the hands, the lung area covers about the whole area of the top part of the palm. Squeezing in between the webbing of the fingers on each hand will also work the chest and lung and bronchi areas. See the foot and hand illustrations to see the respiratory system mapped out, along with the eyes and ears. Notice how many of these areas overlap.

### The Sole Meaning

The **bronchi** are the airways to the lungs, and are divided into even smaller airways called **bronchioles**. The bronchioles allow the exchange of air and waste gases between the alveolar ducts and the bronchi.

**Alveoli** are small pockets that stick out along the walls of alveolar sacs in the lung. This is where carbon dioxide leaves the blood and the blood takes in oxygen.

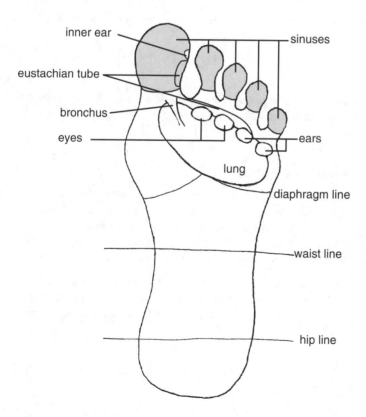

*The foot reflexes for the respiratory system, eyes, and ears. Reflexes are the same for both feet.*

*The hand reflexes for the respiratory system, eyes, and ears. Reflexes are the same for both hands.*

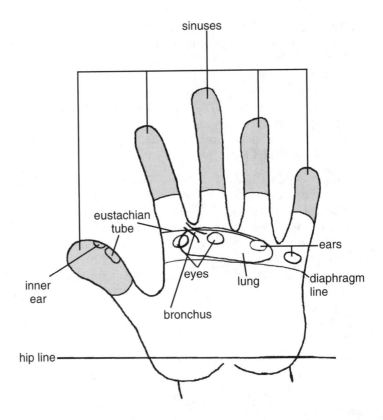

The reflexes in the left hand and foot are associated with the left lung, eye, ear, bronchi, and sinuses. The reflexes on the right hand and foot correlate to the organs on the right side of the body.

## All I Need Is the Air That I Breathe

Our lungs serve as a filter. They are the largest part of our respiratory system, and in the best conditions they are pink and clear. However, even the cleanest mountain air contains airborne dust particles and pollen that affect the condition of our lungs' filtering system. City air has an abundance of automobile exhaust, soot, and flying germs and viruses that are all mostly invisible parts of the air we breathe.

Cigarette smoke leaves the lungs with tar deposits that turn the lungs a dark black color. The fumes you work with doing home projects or even getting your nails done are all assaults on your respiratory system. Some other things that can damage your lungs include:

➤ Air pollution from vehicle and industry waste products

➤ Working with construction materials such as paints, lacquers, and insulation and airborne sawdust from grinding or sanding wood

➤ Pollution from working in industries such as mining, factory manufacturing plants employing the use of chemicals, and auto body and mechanic shops

➤ Burning wood in a wood stove or fireplace in the winter

➤ Using or working with toxic cosmetics and beauty aids such as nail polish, aerosol deodorants, and aerosol hair sprays

➤ Working with some beauty chemicals such as acrylic cosmetics (nail technicians), dental materials (dentists and assistants), and other related chemicals

**The Sole Meaning**

**Emphysema** is a disease characterized by breathlessness. Victims of this disease usually require oxygen tanks to assist their breathing. The disease occurs because the area of the lungs that is responsible for exchanging oxygen and carbon dioxide is damaged. There is no known cure for emphysema; therefore prevention is best. The disease has been linked with smoking, chronic bronchitis, and advancing age.

These toxins can fill up the passageways that are intended to filter out toxic airborne substances. This dirty filter can make it easier for other airborne toxins to enter the deeper parts of the lungs and cause asthma, bronchitis, or, even worse, lead to *emphysema*, which occurs because the areas of the lungs responsible for exchanging oxygen and carbon dioxide are damaged.

Also, when the lungs are deficient or damaged, the body is not as efficient in bringing oxygen into the blood. The blood carries oxygen to all the other organs of the body, including the brain. When the blood is not rich in oxygen the body can begin to suffocate on a cellular level.

A shortage of oxygen in the cells can cause you to feel fuzzy-headed, mentally dull, forgetful, tired, and even dizzy. When your lungs are dirty you are actually depriving your brain of the oxygen it needs to function at its best. Despite earning the label "airhead," the prognosis is quite the opposite!

## Eliminate the Negative

In addition to supplying essential oxygen to the body, the lungs carry out gaseous wastes such as carbon dioxide and cellular by-products, which makes them one of our elimination channels. The lungs can also expel tiny irritants, such as dust particles or fungi. The respiratory system coats these particles with mucus and then evicts them through coughing.

**Tip Toe**

Chinese ephedra (Ma Haung) is a controversial herb used for centuries to help asthmatics breath. It is an ingredient used in many herbal combinations designed to aid the respiratory system. Ephedra is a heart and nervous system stimulant and is not suitable for everyone, which is why it is has been banned in some states. Please ask your physician before using this effective herb.

Despite all this important activity, the lungs actually are passive, meaning that they do not move on their own. The muscle below the lungs just under the ribs is known as the *diaphragm*. It is this muscle that moves up and down, pushing air out of the lungs and allowing the lungs to fill back up. The diaphragm reflex lies just below the ball of each foot. The reference line shown as the diaphragm line in our figures is the actual diaphragm reflex area. You work this area by following the line all the way across the base of the ball of the foot with your thumb (see Chapter 14, "Let Your Fingers Do the Walking," to learn how to use finger and thumb techniques).

On each hand, the diaphragm reference line is also the same as the actual diaphragm reflex area. It spans the bottom of the padding of each hand. When you are short of breath or tense, this whole area on the feet and hands will usually be tender and feel tense also. Rub these areas until your body and lungs relax, especially if you are short of breath from nervous tension.

When the lungs are not eliminating properly, where do you think the gaseous wastes and particles go? Some continue circulating in the blood stream, keeping your immune system working overtime, leaving you even more vulnerable to illness. Some of these waste products may settle back into the tissues of the body. Settled toxins can later cause irritations such as allergies or what seems to be a cold that affects your respiratory channels.

## Breathe Deep

Try some deep-breathing exercises to help increase your lung capacity and oxygenate your cells. Keep in mind that using deep-breathing exercises may make "airheads" dizzy at first since your brain may not be used to all that oxygen! Make sure you are sitting or lying somewhere and aren't driving or doing something requiring balance the first time you attempt deep breathing.

Here's a breathing exercise to try:

➤ Breathe in through your nose for the count of 10 (or longer if you're able). Try not to move your shoulders up when you breathe in.

➤ While breathing in, concentrate on filling up the bottom of your abdomen first, then your stomach, then the bottom of your lungs, and finally the top of your lungs. Hold this breath for 20 seconds.

➤ Then, exhale slowly through your mouth for 10 seconds. Hold the exhale for 10 seconds.

➤ Repeat three more times.

Deep-breathing exercises can increase your capacity to eliminate old toxins from the body. These exercises are helpful to do during a reflexology treatment, especially when you are working on the lung areas. After the treatment, deep breathing will assist the elimination process for the lungs and upper respiratory system and will aid the whole body in its elimination and uptake of oxygen.

## Good Grief, It's Asthma

Emotionally speaking, the lungs are associated with grief. Many times, folks with chronic allergies or asthma who have not gotten well in response to reflexology and other forms of treatment are holding on to unexpressed sadness. People who have not been able to let themselves mourn over a great loss or denied themselves a grieving period can turn their tears inward, so to speak. Chronic loose coughs and other types of lung congestion may also be the result of crying on the inside.

### Foot Note

Asthma can be caused by nutritional imbalances also and can be triggered by a drop in blood sugar (hypoglycemia). Many clients of mine who have gotten their blood sugar under control have had no further problems with asthma attacks. Some nutritional supplements that have been helpful for hypoglycemics include the mineral chromium and an herbal combination of licorice root, dandelion, and horseradish.

Do you need to allow yourself some crying time? A reflexology treatment may bring this release of emotions out in you. Choose a reflexologist you feel safe with. They will understand that reflexology can trigger the release of more than just physical toxins.

Asthma can also be associated with the feeling of being suffocated mentally or emotionally by someone in your environment. Is your boss smothering your creativity? Do you feel your roommate will not allow you to speak up or express your emotions? Do you think that you are being held back because someone around you is overly protective? A holistic reflexology approach not only looks at the physical causes of illness, but takes into account other causes as well. Your lungs can give you some clues into what is going on in your emotional environment.

Breathing clean air, aerobic exercise, deep-breathing exercises, refraining from smoking, taking certain respiratory herbs like lobelia and fenugreek, and wearing protective masks when dealing with chemicals will all help protect your lungs. Reflexology can help by breaking up mucus deposits left in the lungs. Broken up, it is easier for your body to expel this old stuff, physical and emotional, leaving your lungs clear to continue doing their job for you.

# Sinus Up for Reflexology

The sinuses are the air passageways in the head located above the eyebrows, behind the eyes, and on either side of the nose. These little cavities are responsible for warming up the air we breathe before they allow it to go down into the lungs. The sinuses also have some filtering capabilities that are linked to the mucus membranes that transport mucus through small channels into the nasal cavity.

On the foot, the sinuses reflex points are represented by the soft padding on all the toes. Squeezing the toes will work these reflex points. On the hands, the finger pads represent the sinuses. You can also work on these by squeezing each finger.

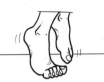

**Tip Toe**

Your sense of smell is 10,000 times more acute than your sense of taste. In fact, most food flavors are smelled, not tasted, as anyone with a heavy cold will verify. Little eddies of air are stirred up during the act of chewing and swallowing that allow the smell receptors at the roof of the nasal cavity to sense the flavors.

## *Achoo!*

When you experience a runny nose, it is usually because your nose is trying to rid itself of irritants. Your respiratory system tries to protect you by surrounding irritants with mucus to help the body eliminate the irritants (allergens) and to protect the body from absorbing the allergens. When your sinuses are overburdened, the respiratory system reacts by sneezing and coughing. If this still does not rid the system of the irritants, the sinus membranes can become irritated with mucus, which may cause the membranes to swell, creating pressure, and then you can suffer from the feeling of a stuffy head or develop a sinus headache.

Chronic sinus conditions include:

➤ Sinusitis

➤ Sinus headaches

➤ Sinus congestion

➤ Postnasal drip

All these things are irritating ailments of the sinuses. And I have personally had great success getting instantaneous sinus relief with the use of reflexology!

### Foot Note

Sneezing and coughing are powerful rejection mechanisms that your respiratory system uses to protect you from possibly harmful airborne bacteria, fungi, viruses, and tiny dust and pollen particles that have entered your system. When you sneeze, the force of the sneeze blasts germs out of your nose and mouth at an amazing rate of up to 400 miles per hour! What is the moral of the story? Make sure that you use a reliable tissue to cover up your nose and mouth next time you feel a sneeze or cough coming on!

Generally, the left sinus reflexes correspond to the left foot and hand and vice versa. However, sometimes your experiences will not necessarily reflect this division. For example, when your sinuses are clogged and you work on your left sinus reflex area, you might not feel an instant draining of the left sinus. But when you begin to work on the right hand, the left sinus may begin to drain!

I think this has to do with the buildup of pressure from increasing the circulation when working with reflexology. Or it could be that sometimes it just takes time for the work on the other side to kick in, so to speak. This has happened to me over and over, and you might experience this for yourself, too.

## Getting to Know Your Nose

Your nose contains tiny hairs in the nostrils that serve to filter airborne particles. When the smaller particles get past the nose and down into the lower airways, mucus is formed by your respiratory system in order to protect the body from the irritant. The mucus serves to coat the irritating particle and works to rid the body of the offender.

When you are exposed to irritants over and over, a buildup of mucus or an excess of mucus can be made by the nose and nasal passages. In these cases, if you take an antihistamine such as an over-the-counter drug to stop the production of mucus, the mucus can dry up and harden inside your sinus passages. This dried-up mucus is known as *catarrh*.

### The Sole Meaning

**Catarrh** rhymes with guitar and is the excessive secretion of thick phlegm or mucus by the mucus membrane of the nose or nasal cavities. The term is not used in a scientific context, but is a general term that usually refers to mucus that has been dried up or hardened in the sinus passages.

Catarrh can be built up over time in the sinus passages and be a haven for virus and fungi. The places where catarrh and mucus are settled create *anaerobic environments*, meaning that the area cannot receive oxygen efficiently. Since many parasites crave an anaerobic environment but cannot thrive in a fully oxygenated environment, it is best to keep your body free of built-up mucus and catarrh that hinders your body's potential to fully receive oxygen.

**Foot Note**

One day a little old lady went to the doctor complaining of a bad case of gas. "I have awful gas, but it doesn't bother me. You see, it's completely silent, and doesn't smell at all."

So the doctor, after examining her thoroughly, gave her some pills and told her to take one every day and come back in a week.

So the old lady went back, and when the doctor asked if her problem was any better she replied, "Well I don't know what you did to me, but now my gas smells terrible!"

The doctor replied, "Well now that we've got your sinuses cleared up, let's work on your hearing!"

# Ears to Having You Work on My Feet!

The ear reflexes are located on the padding of the ball of each foot just underneath the fourth and fifth toes. The eustachian tube is the tube that runs from the inner ear connecting it to the back of the throat. Its reflex area runs along the base of all the toes and up along the inner edge of the large toe on each foot.

The ear reflexes are on both hands and are located on the palms just below the ring and pinky fingers, and the eustachian tube reflex runs along the padding of the palm at the base of the fingers.

Clapping your hands vigorously can be considered a form of reflexology. Clapping is an easy way to affect most of the sinus areas on the hands. The fingertips are stimulated on one hand, and the eyes and ears of the other hand are stimulated simultaneously. So, you know what this means, don't you? When you see me at the next book signing I expect a standing ovation!

The inner ear is associated with your sense of balance. If you have water on your eardrum due to some type of infection or fungus growth, or have excess wax in the ear, you can become dizzy or even experience *tinnitus*, or ringing in the ears.

The ears are an excellent area to work on when you have sinus troubles. You will find that the stimulation of reflexology treatments may help relieve a congested feeling in the head. Performing an ear coning after a reflexology treatment on someone whose ears are clogged is sure to make you a hero!

I like to work on the toes vigorously on those who have ear wax buildup, or any type of sinus problem. This practice seems to break up and loosen old debris from the ear and upper sinus passages so that the body's elimination channels can easily remove it. Some people claim that they think I have changed their voice after a treatment followed by an ear coning! The only real difference is that they can hear themselves better.

One of my clients once told me that my reflexology treatments were a draining experience. I was hurt until she clarified that her sinuses drained every time I worked on her! I thought that doctors using reflexology on people in the emergency rooms to stop their asthma attacks might be a concept for a new television program. We could call it *Dr. Mucus Wellbee*. What do you think?

**The Sole Meaning**

**Tinnitus** is characterized by any noise, buzzing, or ringing in the ear. Causes of tinnitus may be excess ear wax, damage to the eardrum, Meniere's disease, or thinning blood due to overuse of aspirin or other drugs. Dr. Bernard Jensen also links tinnitus to a lack of magnesium.

# Eyes Can See Clearly Now

The eyes are wondrous, fascinating extensions of the brain that serve many functions. They deserve a whole book to themselves, but for now we will be content to tie them in with the respiratory system and reflexology.

The eyes receive information, and it is thought that they are also instruments for sending energy. And of course, the eyes provide us with the gift of sight. Since some of the sinus cavities are located close to the eyes, pressure buildup or sinus headaches can make your eyes ache or tear. When allergens are in the air, the eyes may itch and water to help reject these irritants.

**Tip Toe**

Body reflexology tip for the eyes: Gently press in with your fingertips all around your eye sockets looking for tight muscles. The pressure may create a popping sensation when the muscle releases. Loosening up these tightened muscles can bring a renewed vitality to tired eyes.

The eye reflex areas are located in the same area along the ball of each foot at the base of the toes where you found the ear reflexes. The eye points are the areas below the second and third toes. They are also found in the corresponding points on the hands. The eye reflexes are located on each palm just under the pointer and middle fingers.

Respiratory troubles are not the only things that can cause eye problems. Macular degeneration, night blindness, and glaucoma are all different diseases that have different causes, including malnutrition. Tightening of the muscles surrounding the eyes sometimes causes near- and far-sightedness, which not only distorts the shape of the eye, causing vision inadequacies, but can also slow the amount of blood circulating to the eyes.

Fluid and pressure build up behind the eye in the case of glaucoma and may be caused by tight muscles in the back of the eye squeezing off the drainage ducts, preventing them from emptying properly. Tight eyelid muscles causing friction on the eyeball may cause cataracts.

Since reflexology helps relax all muscles, this may be a wonderful way to prevent and may even reverse these muscle-related eye disorders. Whatever the cause of the eye problems, stimulating the eye reflex points on the feet and hands is a great natural and safe therapy you can use to help revitalize the eyes.

---

### The Least You Need to Know

➤ The respiratory system provides protection from airborne pollutants, makes oxygen useable to your cells, and provides energy for the body.

➤ The lungs and sinuses should be kept clear to avoid cyclical patterns of respiratory illness.

➤ The lungs are associated with grief. If you are not getting over your lung problems with natural therapies, ask yourself if you need to take the time to grieve.

➤ Working the eye reflex points on the feet and hands may help bring circulation and muscle relaxation to the eyes, which can aid vision.

➤ Squeezing the fingers and the padding of the toes can sometimes work instantaneously to relieve sinus congestion, helping to drain mucus to unclog a stuffed-up head and ears.

---

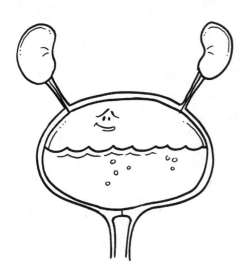

# Chapter 10

# Give Me a "P": The Urinary System

> ## In This Chapter
>
> ➤ Learn the importance of the urinary system organs
>
> ➤ Find the major urinary system reflexes on the feet and hands
>
> ➤ Understand some of the root causes of urinary troubles
>
> ➤ Learn some natural ways to correct urinary tract problems
>
> ➤ See how your emotions may affect your urinary health

My favorite radio commercial here in Boise is for a local plumbing company. Their motto is "A-1 Plumbing: We're the best place in town to take a leak."

Although you won't be calling a plumber if you have problems with your urinary system, you will still have to take care of your body's own "pipes." Your urinary system serves many more functions than just carrying off liquids from the body. Let's take a look at all that your interesting internal plumbing does for you and see how you can take better care of it with reflexology.

## Liquid Plumber

The urinary system serves as the body's plumbing system, and its organs, including the bladder, kidneys, and ureter, serve to eliminate liquid wastes from the system. The pipes also play a role in helping maintain a proper fluid balance in the body, help maintain salt balance, and keep an acid/alkaline base balance in the body fluids.

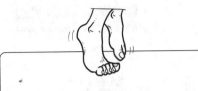

**Tip Toe**

*The recurrence of kidney stones may be prevented by adequate intake of magnesium. A few foods rich in magnesium are: yellow cornmeal, bananas, nuts, soy, and rice polishings.*

Do you have troubles with any of the following?

➤ Bladder infections

➤ Kidney infections

➤ Kidney stones

➤ Incontinence

➤ Edema

➤ Frequent urination

These are all troubles related to the urinary system. But before you call a plumber, let's try to find the cause of your troubles first!

There are many ways to support our urinary systems, and reflexology is one of them. Take a look at the illustrations of the hand and foot that follow and see where the urinary system reflexes that we are going to talk about are located.

*The foot reflexes for the urinary system. These reflexes are the same for the right foot.*

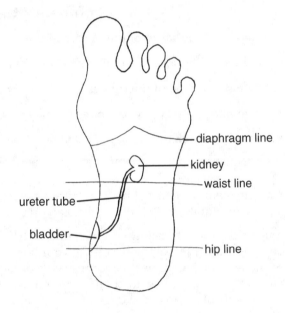

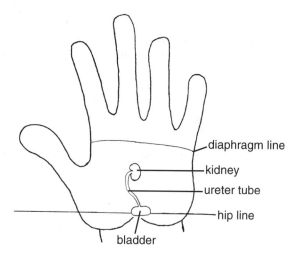

*The hand reflexes for the urinary system. These reflexes are the same for the right hand.*

diaphragm line
kidney
ureter tube
hip line
bladder

# Fill 'Er Up: The Bladder

The urinary bladder is a closed sac composed of a smooth muscle coat that stores a liquid bodily waste called urine. The bladder holds this material until it tells you by nerve impulses that it is full. When this happens, you have the urge to urinate. When you do, the bladder then flattens, and even becomes somewhat concave on the top and leans forward toward your lower abdomen. When it is full, the bladder becomes round, like a full balloon, and projects slightly upward.

The bladder reflex area is found on the sole of each foot along the medial, or inside, edge just slightly above the heel of each foot. You can find this point by using your thumb to dig around that area. You will know when you are on the bladder reflex because it will feel like a slightly hollow area. The bladder area will feel like it almost perfectly fits the tip of your thumb.

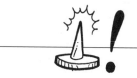

**Tread Lightly**

Ignoring your body's urge to urinate can weaken the bladder by stretching it. The stagnation may also make you more prone to bladder infections. So listen to the call of nature for bladder health.

**129**

The bladder area on the hands can be found on the lower middle palm of both hands, just above the wrist. You can tell where the bladder area in the hand is by feel also. The tip of your thumb should just naturally fit right in this little intersection of the palm. Try this tip to make it easier to find:

➤ Lay the backside of your left hand flat—palm facing up.

➤ Pretend that you are making a karate chop with your right hand directly to the base of the fingers of the left hand.

➤ Then, touch your left thumb to your right palm. If you follow the natural diagonal movement of your thumb, it will land at the bottom middle of your other hand's palm.

➤ Your thumb will be pointing to the bladder area.

## Exercise So Urine Top Condition

Bladder incontinence is a condition where urine is leaked involuntarily. This ailment is more common in women after childbirth, which can weaken the pelvic floor muscles. The good news is that since the bladder actually has a muscle surrounding it and the pelvis has muscles, they can be toned or strengthened.

**The Sole Meaning**

Kegel exercises, commonly referred to as **Kegels**, are exercises for women that involve tightening the lower pelvis muscles, simulating the same feeling as stopping urine flow. A version for men involves actually stopping urine flow, which strengthens the muscles. Talk about getting in shape.

One exercise you can use to tone your bladder area to prevent incontinence is *Kegels*. Kegels are an exercise created for women that involve voluntarily tightening the lower pelvis muscles. The exercise simulates the feeling of stopping urine flow. Contractions should be held for 6 to 10 seconds, followed by allowing the muscles to relax completely. This should be done four or five times in a row, three to four times a day.

You guys can use this exercise, too! The best way to get the effects of Kegels is to stop the flow of urine in the process of voiding your bladder. Hold it for a few seconds, then release, then hold again. The process of stopping the flow of urination will help strengthen the bladder walls and the pelvic floor muscles, and also helps your prostate gland.

## Bladder Infections: A Bad Burn

Bladder infections are a different story. Bladder infections are just that—an infection of the bladder. A pressure on the bladder to urinate even when the bladder is empty characterizes this infection. When infections are bad, blood can be passed in the urine, and urination causes a painful burning sensation. Ouch!

I can attest to the fact that bladder infections can be extremely painful. Fortunately, I am also living proof that reflexology can help speed the healing of and even prevent bladder infections!

When I first began my reflexology training, I was getting bladder infections on a regular basis. When our class was first taught about the urinary system and I found out where my bladder reflex point was, I went to town on it! I noticed that before I even started manipulation on the bladder reflex point that the area was swollen and slightly red. When I first touched my own bladder reflex point I was amazed at how crunchy and tender the spot was!

Well, to make a long story short, or a round bladder flat, every time I felt a bladder infection coming on, I would work deeply on my bladder reflex point. The area was always swollen and tender, and I would work on it until the tenderness subsided. The therapy worked! I got good at catching the beginning symptoms soon enough to work my reflex points and my full-blown, painful bladder infections never manifested. I have only had one bladder infection since that first reflexology class 10 years ago!

This latter bladder infection is one that I am convinced came on from an emotional trauma and healing crisis that I experienced. A bladder infection causes a burning pain, and I connected this to being "burnt" on an emotional level. The bladder also deals with the element water, and water is linked to our emotions!

The bladder infection happened a few weeks after I experienced a great personal betrayal in my life. Thank goodness I was already implementing good habits because the blow was devastating. Not long after the shock wore off, I became very angry about the whole situation and found myself suffering from an incredibly painful, burning bladder infection!

**Tip Toe**

Cranberry juice has been used as a safe home remedy for bladder infections for years. Cranberries change the acidity level in the bladder, which kills or prevents bacteria from irritating the bladder lining. Drink lots of fruit juice, sweetened or unsweetened cranberry juice, and lots of pure water when fighting off infection. Sugar may make your problem worse. Cranberry capsules may be taken instead.

**Tip Toe**

If you are experiencing a bladder or any type of urinary infection, ask yourself if you are feeling "pissed-off" at anyone in your life! Along with doing the right things to heal your body, try changing your perceptions and look for some good lesson that can come from such strong emotions.

I applied my knowledge of herbs and supplements and used acidophilus, cranberry, and buchu root to fight the infection while I implemented lots of reflexology treatments on myself to pull me through. Once I realized my emotional connection to the infection, I let myself cry and took another look at all the good things that were happening in my life now that that my betrayer had set me free! When I changed my perceptions, the infection cleared up. Thankfully, I learned a lot from this experience. I now see that life is most painful when you forget to see the lesson in the pain!

## Keep It Moving

Bladder infections can also be brought on by constipation. When your sewer system is backed up, the body has to deal with more toxins and fermentation than usual. The urinary system tries to deal with ridding the body of this excess and guess what? Bladder infection city! It is a good idea to also work on your colon reflex areas when you are experiencing a bladder infection. Make sure you get cleaned out so your body has a chance to heal.

Herbs can also help strengthen the bladder. Cornsilk is an herb rich in iron, silicon, and vitamin K. It also contains moderate amounts of magnesium, potassium, phosphorus, and zinc. Cornsilk has historically been used as a diuretic and has been used to help bed-wetting, bladder infections, cystitis, kidney problems, prostate health, uric acid buildup, and high blood pressure.

### Foot Note

Herbs and supplements that have been used successfully to clear up bladder infections include acidophilus supplements, cranberry, buchu root, golden seal, and cornsilk. Tea-tree oil is a natural antifungal, antibacterial oil that can be diluted with pure water and used as a douche for women suffering from reccurring bladder infections. Also, make sure the bowel is clean! Cascara sagrada has been used for hundreds of years as a natural bowel stimulant.

# Pintos or Kidneys?

> Are we really being human if we are just a human bean?
> —Author too embarrassed to take credit

The kidneys are small organs, reddish-brown in color and shaped like, guess what? a kidney bean. Except in the case of a genetic abnormality, we have two kidneys, one on each side of the body located about midback, straddling the waist line.

The kidneys are responsible for filtering toxins, wastes, ingested water, and mineral salts out of the bloodstream. Your kidneys are also responsible for regulating the acidity of the blood by excreting alkaline salts when necessary. Often, the left kidney is positioned up to an inch higher than the right kidney. Each kidney is about four to five inches long and about two inches thick, weighing four to six ounces in the average adult.

The kidneys serve important functions, including controlling water levels in the body. They also serve as filters of toxins and blood waste products contained in the liquids, foods, and air we take in.

The kidney reflex location is right in the center of the sole of the foot about the middle of the waist line. The reflex can be found on each foot, one for each side. On each hand, the kidney reflex location is on the palm just about in the center.

**Tip Toe**

The kidneys are important organs that serve many functions. The kidneys regulate body water and concentrations of electrolytes such as sodium, potassium, calcium, phosphorus, chloride, glucose, and amino acids. They aid in synthesizing vitamin D, hormones, and enzymes, and can even raise the oxygen-carrying capacity of the blood!

**Foot Note**

**Personology**, sometimes called **faceology**, is the study of the reflex areas, signs, and lines located in and on the face. In this system, the kidneys correspond to the area underneath each eye. If there are bags under the eyes, this is a sign of kidney stress or urinary system imbalance in general. When doing a holistic basic health assessment we take into account the entire person and their physical appearance as well as client complaints to discover the source of a problem.

## Drinking for Water Weight

When a person is carrying an excess amount of water weight we might be able to assume that the kidneys are not functioning effectively enough to carry off the excess waste products or that there is a mineral imbalance resulting in water retention. Kind of brings new meaning to the line in the Palmolive commercial that says, "Look, you're soaking in it!"

### The Sole Meaning

**Dehydration** is the lack of water in body tissues. Lack of sufficient water intake, vomiting, diarrhea, and sweating can all be causes of dehydration. Symptoms may include great thirst, nausea, and exhaustion. If drinking plenty of water does not immediately correct the problem, sometimes water and salts need to be administered intravenously at an emergency room.

### Tip Toe

The leaves and root of the hydrangea plant have been used by herbalists and nutritionists for years as a solvent for calculus stones and other gravel deposits in the body. Hydrangea can relieve backaches due to kidney and rheumatic problems, prevent the formation of gravel deposits, gallstones, kidney stones, and enlarged prostate glands, and help relieve the pain from each!

The body relies on a good supply of water to help it flush out waste products. Sometimes when we are not taking in enough water, the body will respond by holding onto water to protect you from *dehydration*. This is usually corrected by drinking at least eight glasses of water each day.

Along with reflexology treatments, drinking plenty of water will help your body release the water it has been hanging on to. This may take several weeks to accomplish, but once the cells of your body understand that they will be receiving enough water to keep the body balanced, they will be able to let go of their stash.

## Sticks and Stones

Kidney stones are a product of built-up mineral salts called *calculus*. Passing kidney stones through the tiny ureter canal can be severely painful. If the stone gets stuck and blocks the flow of urine, surgery may be required.

The causes of the kidney stones are generally the same as any problem with the urinary system, including the following:

➤ Too much protein in the diet

➤ Improper digestion

➤ Improper mineral intake

➤ Not drinking enough water

➤ Constipation or ignoring the call of nature

Lower-back pain may disguise itself as kidney trouble or vice versa. Take this test to see if your lower back is bothering you or if it is your kidneys giving you problems. Stand up and have someone stand beside you to brace you when you do this exercise.

➤ Stand up straight and slowly lean backward.

➤ If you get a sharp sensation of discomfort, this could indicate that your lower spine is out of alignment and pinching a nerve.

➤ If the ache is still there but leaning back does not cause a sharp pain, the kidneys could be calling for some help.

To give your kidneys the help they need, first drink plenty of water. Parsley and juniper berries are excellent herbs that help the kidneys expel toxins. Hydrangea is used in the herbal world as a stone solvent and will help break down stones naturally. Avoid caffeine-containing products that may irritate the kidneys, and see your doctor if you suspect infection or stone, and of course, work your kidney reflex areas.

If you have the feeling of a belt being cinched tightly around your waist, you could be experiencing a kidney infection. Work with the kidney reflex areas immediately, drink plenty of water, and get medical help right away! A serious kidney infection can be a life-threatening condition.

**Tread Lightly**

If you are experiencing a lot of back pain and general malaise along with a tension around your middle that feels like a belt being tightly cinched around your waist, you could be experiencing a kidney infection. In this case, drink plenty of water or parsley tea and work on your kidney reflex points on your way to the doctor's office!

## Getting in Balance

When you have high blood pressure, you should take into account the health of your kidneys also. The kidneys help keep your mineral salts in balance and therefore have a hand in regulating your blood pressure.

If you have high blood pressure, lower-back pain, bags under your eyes, and have a tendency to retain water, you have the profile of someone who might have kidney trouble. The best thing to do is eliminate acid-forming foods from your diet, including coffee and red meats, and lower your intake of cheese. Eat more raw, green vegetables and take a mineral supplement from nature such as alfalfa and liquid chlorophyll and colloidal minerals. Other supplements that may be helpful to the kidneys include vitamin D, B-complex, and l-glutamine.

See Appendix B, "Supplies and Where to Find Them," in the back of this book to locate a respectable company that will supply you with quality, natural forms of minerals. Drink much more water, cleanse the colon, and utilize reflexology every day until the blood pressure is regulated. After you are regulated, you can use reflexology less often to maintain your health.

# Urine Luck

Since we're on the subject of releasing toxins, let's talk about urine. Urine is made up of urea, creatine, uric acid, and ammonia. These are all by-products of digesting proteins. Anything that leaves an acid base in the body, such as heavy protein foods, stress, and physical exercise, can cause an over-acidic body condition. Since part of the urinary system's job is to help maintain an acid/alkaline balance in the blood stream, over-acidity can put a strain on the kidneys and the entire urinary system can be weakened.

**Tread Lightly**

Ammonia is the end product of metabolizing protein. Too much protein can cause ammonia to rise in the body and make your kidneys work harder to keep you in balance. High-protein foods to avoid while suffering from kidney problems include most meats, nuts, beans, and dairy products. Eat more greens instead.

A chemical analysis of sweat shows that it has the same components as urine. The skin serves as a "third kidney." This is why you don't urinate as much in the summer as you do in the cold months. In the summertime the skin makes up for eliminating the uric acid waste through perspiration. You also usually wear less clothing in the summertime, and therefore, the skin will evaporate wastes more easily than in the winter when you are heavily clad in long-sleeve shirts and socks.

If skin is underactive, uric acid, dead cells, and other impurities will remain in the body. The other eliminative organs, therefore, have to work harder. If skin isn't stimulated to do its job, eventually toxins will be deposited back into tissues.

Sweating and dry skin brushing are two ways to stimulate the skin to eliminate and take a load off the kidneys. You can work up a sweat in a number of interesting ways, and I'll leave that up to you. Skin-brushing might be new to you, however. Here's how to do it:

➤ Use a dry, vegetable bristle massage brush with a long handle. It is not an expensive brush. *Do not use nylon.*

➤ Use this brush first thing in the morning when you arise, before putting clothes on and before any bathing.

➤ Brush in either a circular or upward fashion always toward the heart all over the body, except the face. Use a special facial brush for this more delicate skin.

It is important for you to support the urinary system by eating lots of alkaline-forming foods with meals. Alkaline foods include most fruits and all green vegetables and leafy greens like lettuce, spinach, and parsley, as well as liquid chlorophyll.

## Ureter—Always Wanted to Meet Her

The ureter tubes are the tubes that allow urine to flow down from the kidneys into the bladder. You have two ureter tubes, one for each kidney.

The reflex area for the ureter tubes is located on the sole of each foot and runs from the kidney area down to the bladder reflex. This is actually how the area can be worked. You can work your thumb down from the kidney, down the ureter, and end at the bladder.

The reflex area for the ureter tubes is also located on each hand (palm side) and also runs from the kidney area down to the bladder reflex.

I find that this area is one of the most sensitive parts of the foot, so start gently and see what the reaction is. Sometimes uric acid buildup can settle at the bottom of the nerve endings on the feet, and when these crystals are broken up by reflexology treatments, the sensation can feel like you just stepped on a sharp rock!

Always drink plenty of water after a reflexology treatment, but especially if you find a lot of crunchies in the urinary reflexes. Your body will need extra water to help flush out the toxins.

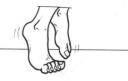

**Tip Toe**

Juicing fresh fruits and vegetables may be one of the best ways to obtain easily assimilated organic minerals, especially calcium, potassium, and silicon. Organic minerals are needed to help keep your biochemistry balanced.

# Healing and the Emotions

Your emotions have a tremendous impact on your health and should not be over-looked when you are looking for the causes of disease. The power of the mind is incredible and plays a big role in creating illness as well as health. A graphic example of this is seen in cases where people suffering from multiple-personality disorder who have full-blown diabetes or other physical illnesses in one personality have absolutely normal body chemistry with no signs of physical disease in another!

But you must take care of the physical cause of any imbalance or illness first. Your emotions cannot correct a mineral imbalance, for instance, so you always need to look at where the environmental or nutritional voids exist first and work to correct the problem from there.

For instance, if a client comes to me complaining of a pain in his finger and there is a mousetrap clinched onto his hand, I will not give him herbs to help his bones heal and perform reflexology for pain relief until we first remove the mousetrap! Otherwise he will say that my herbs did not work for him or that reflexology is worthless!

## A Model for Healing

You have to remove the environmental cause of the problem first, then correct the physical problem, and then rely on your preventative measures to keep it from occurring again. This is how all natural forms of health care should be approached.

Let's take for example chiropractic care. First, you figure out that sitting at your desk all day and working on your computer causes neck pain. Your smartest first move is to go out and get an ergonomic chair. This is fixing the environmental cause of the problem.

**Tread Lightly**

Ureteritis is an inflammation of the ureter, which is usually associated with an inflammation of the bladder. Tuberculosis in the urinary tract can also be a cause of ureteritis, which can cause the ureter tubes to become restricted and cause serious problems with the biochemical balance in the body.

Then, you get the chiropractic adjustments needed to set you straight again, which corrects the condition physically. You then implement mineral supplements and diet to keep the structural system healthy and prevent future problems.

As another form of preventative maintenance, you can use reflexology to keep the muscles relaxed and balanced. You can also use reflexology before you go in for your chiropractic adjustments to relax the muscles and make adjustments easier.

## Keeping It Simple

In searching for the root cause of your health problems, it is best to start with the most obvious causes first. After your bases are covered, then work with the more esoteric reasons that are much harder to uncover. If you remove all the obvious causes and your spine is still going out of alignment, then you need to begin to look for emotional causes.

You may need to work with a counselor to understand your underlying feelings of not being supported, or feeling like your work is "a pain in the neck." Or maybe the problem is an energy imbalance. The whole point is to cover all the obvious bases first and then work up to the more subtle levels.

**Foot Note**

Keep in mind that your thoughts and words have power. Think about the nature of your ailments and see how they could be related to the literal words you speak. Here are some examples: Hemorrhoids: How about thinking that something you do every day is a pain in the butt? Heartburn, fever, and inflammation of any kind: Do you complain that your boss "burns you up"? Urinary infections: Are you telling everyone how "pissed off" you are? Foot injuries: "I just can't stand it anymore!" If you are saying these things and subconsciously cursing yourself, try changing your situation, or change your attitude. It just may help your ailments, too!

In the case of the urinary system, we can go back to the four-element model we looked at in Chapter 4, "The Foot at a Glance," where we talked about water characterizing emotions. The releasing of liquids from your urinary system might be linked to the appropriate releasing or outflow of your emotions.

On an emotional level, I think of kidney stones as being old emotions that have not been released. Since the emotions have not been released, the toxic effects of the unexpressed or unreleased emotions have hardened and now are creating an irritation to the body.

So, for whole health, remember to think physically first and remove the possible causes of your problems. Then work on any emotional or spiritual connections and keep a positive attitude and mind-set to keep yourself healthy!

## The Least You Need to Know

➤ Your urinary system not only filters waste products, but also serves to balance and help maintain the water, sodium, and other mineral levels in the body.

➤ When the body is over-acidic due to stress, a high-protein diet, or poor digestion, the kidneys are required to work harder to filter the excess acid waste.

➤ The skin serves as a third kidney, so it is important to allow the skin to breathe and perspire by exposing it to fresh air and stimulation, such as skin brushing.

➤ If you cannot find a physical cause linked to your urinary problems, look at your emotions.

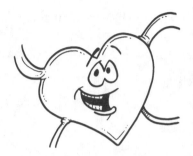

# Chapter 11

# Getting to the Heart of the Matter: The Circulatory System

## In This Chapter

➤ Learn about the main components of the circulatory system

➤ Find the heart reflexes on the foot and hand

➤ See the heart as a communicative organ

➤ Learn about your blood and how reflexology can help keep it moving

➤ See why reflexology helps in matters of the heart

Here is your chance to follow your heart and take a lighthearted look at the circulatory system. We can't live without our hearts, although some of us live with our hearts on our sleeve! Heart and soul are sometimes considered the same thing. When we give and receive reflexology, we can not only help the circulatory system, but also share good energy, which just may be a supplement the heart requires. Researchers are finding that many people live longer when they are paired up with a companion. So let's find out how we can be good to our hearts through our soles!

## Circulating Rumors and Other Things

The circulatory system is the means by which blood is pumped through the veins and arteries by the heart. The circulatory system makes it possible for all of the organs to receive nutrients, oxygen, and other substances necessary for sustaining life.

The circulatory system is not only the means of transportation to supply all these good things to the entire body, but it also takes away waste products. On a continual basis, waste by-products of oxidation and metabolism are collected by the circulatory system and carried to the correct places for elimination or recycling. It is almost like our grocery stores' delivery trucks and our garbage trucks all traveling on the same road.

The circulatory system consists of blood, the blood vessels, and the heart. Circulatory system imbalances include:

➤ High or low blood pressure

➤ High cholesterol levels

➤ Heart attacks

➤ Strokes

➤ Broken blood vessels

➤ Irregular heart beat

➤ Low or high blood count (which is also related to the liver)

➤ Mitral valve or other heart related dysfunction

Even hair loss has been linked to an imbalance in the circulatory system.

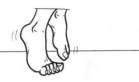

**Tip Toe**

The blood is responsible for carrying nutrients to all parts of the body. The roots of your hair require nutrients to grow and be healthy, just like all your other body parts. If you hair is falling, consider stimulating the hair roots with a massaging brush.

**Tread Lightly**

Signs of a heart attack include sudden and usually severe chest pain that may radiate through the arms and possibly the throat. If you are experiencing chest pain you could be having a heart attack. Call 911 (or your local emergency number) immediately!

## Be Still My Heart

The heart is the major organ of your circulatory system. It rests in your chest cavity slightly left of center. The heart is a muscular, cone-shaped organ about the size of a clenched fist. Mechanically, it serves as a pump. It beats normally about 70 times per minute by balanced nerve impulses and muscle contractions. Factors affecting the pulse rate include emotion, exercise, hormones, temperature, pain, and stress.

In foot and hand reflexology, the heart is really the only component of the circulatory system that is charted. Since your veins, arteries, and capillaries run throughout the body, you will be sure to stimulate the entire circulatory system when working on any parts of the feet or hands. The heart reflex area is found on the sole of the left foot and covers just about the entire ball of the foot.

On the hand, the heart area is found on the palm of the left hand and covers the area between the diaphragm line and the base of the fingers. More advanced charts may add the fourth and fifth fingers to the heart area as well. The pinky finger represents heart energy patterns, so it too can be worked as a heart reflex. See the illustrations of the left hand and foot to be sure you know where to find your heart, especially if you've been to San Francisco recently.

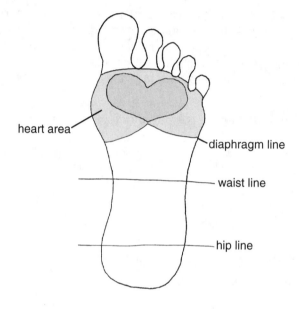

*The heart reflex on the left foot. Note: You can also work the fourth and fifth toes to stimulate cardiac reflexes.*

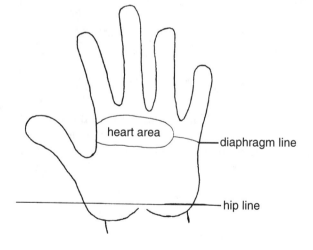

*The heart reflex on the left hand. Note: You can also work the ring and pinky fingers to stimulate the cardiac reflexes.*

# You're All Heart—and Potassium

Each organ is made up of different bio-minerals and chemicals, just as foods from the earth are made up of different minerals and chemicals. When we think of a carrot, most of us think of it as being a rich source of beta carotene (vitamin A). We also know that oranges are a rich source of vitamin C. Well, we can look at the organs of the body in this same manner.

For instance, the adrenals store vitamin C, so we can think of vitamin C as nourishment for the adrenals. The bones are made up primarily of calcium and we know that calcium nourishes the bones. The heart is predominately a potassium organ. A mineral imbalance or potassium deficiency can lead to heart fluctuations, irregularities, and sometimes high blood pressure. Foods and herbs rich in potassium feed the heart. Potassium-rich foods include:

➤ Potato peels, raisins, almonds

➤ Apples, apple cider vinegar

➤ Bananas, carrots, cucumbers

➤ Goat's milk, grapes, tomatoes

➤ Parsley, pecans, soy milk

➤ Sun-dried black olives, walnuts

Herbs rich in potassium include:

➤ Dulse, kelp, Irish moss

➤ Valerian, red clover, ginger

➤ Peppermint, parsley, licorice

➤ Horsetail, hops, garlic

➤ Hawthorn berries

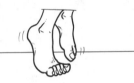

**Tip Toe**

Potassium works with sodium in all cells of the body. Potassium is stored in the muscles such as the heart. It is important in healing, aiding nerve synapses, vitality, preventing the formation of uric acid, and aiding hair growth. Without a proper potassium balance in the body, you can't have thick, long hair, great muscle tone, or a strong heart.

Potassium, sodium, calcium, and many other minerals in the body all work in a delicate balance together. Supplementing with potassium should only be done if your doctor prescribes it for you. Otherwise, take a balanced mineral supplement or try to get your minerals from raw, fresh organic fruits and vegetables. Your body knows what to do when given substances that it recognizes as real food!

## The Beat Goes On

Researchers have discovered that the heart actually has a cellular memory. Amazing observations have been made with heart transplant recipients taking on many of the characteristics of their heart donor! They also have discovered some very interesting links between our heartbeat and the earth's magnetic resonance.

The researchers have found that the human heart has a beat that resonates and actually synchronizes, or *entrains*, with the magnetic resonance of our planet, affectionately known as mother earth. Babies in the womb also resonate and rely on their own mother's heartbeat. Doesn't this give you a new way of looking at planet earth as the mother of the human race?

### The Sole Meaning

**Entrainment** is the phenomenon of self-regulated synchronization of the pulsing of two objects. For instance, clocks put together in a room and left alone can eventually synchronize and beat at exactly the same pulse. Some researchers think that our heart entrains with the beat of the earth.

# As a Man Thinketh in His Heart...

Dr. Paul Pearsall in his book *The Heart's Code* (Broadway Books, 1998) talks at length about the heart as a thinking organ. He says that to be balanced, we need to balance the intellectual messages of our brain with our subtle heart messages. The heart sends messages to us to be compassionate, cooperative, and to connect to others, whereas the brain, usually controlled by the ego, tells us to get to work and make the logical choice.

### Foot Note

Dr. Paul Pearsall stresses the importance of getting in touch with your heart's desires to balance your health and life. He suggests the following exercise: Ensure yourself a quiet environment free from interruptions. Place your hand over your heart. Ask yourself three questions, and wait for an answer before you go on to the next question. The heart will give you your answers. Ask your heart: "Am I loving fully? Am I letting go completely? Am I living totally?"

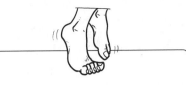

**Tip Toe**

Chinese experts in pulse diagnosis can read your pulse and give you detailed information on your body and your health. It takes decades to get good at this practice and shows the pulse is yet another way the heart communicates.

When you are in love your hearts skip a beat! When you think about the object of your desire, your heart sings and your pulse rate rises. On a more prosaic level, the foods that you eat can affect your pulse rate as well.

You can use a simple pulse rate test to determine if you might be allergic to a particular food or supplement by taking your pulse rate prior to eating the food. After ingesting a suspect food, take your pulse again. If the rate has shot up, you might be allergic to the food you tested! Wait a couple of hours and try it again to make sure. Eliminate that food from your diet and see if your symptoms improve.

## A Heart-to-Heart Talk

Dr. Pearsall also cites evidence that our hearts actually communicate with each other! Wouldn't you agree that there is a big difference between knowing something in your heart and just believing something to be true? Are you in touch with your heart's subtle communication with you? Are you putting your heart into your work, or are you letting your work damage your heart?

Many folks push themselves too much mentally and override what they know to be true in their heart. They are working jobs that are running against their natural heart's desire. They override heart energy with mental energy, and the heart physically suffers with heart attacks or other heart diseases. Wouldn't it be better if you could find your heart's desire and balance it with your intellect to make it work for you?

I am not saying that everyone needs to run out and quit their job! What I am saying is that if you are not quite fulfilled with your type of work, continue doing your best anyway. Then, every day, take some quiet time to listen to your heart's desires. You will eventually find something that warms your heart when you think about it. You should consider doing whatever that is as a hobby. You never know where this will lead you, but at least you will be giving your heart some recognition!

It could be that doing something that fills your heart will keep your heart from physically rebelling against you by ignoring it! If being with your children or your mate warms your heart more than anything, then you better figure out a way to spend more quality time with them. The ones that love you can feel your heart's connection to them. So if not for your own sake, do it for the health of your loved one's heart.

# Jin Shin Jyutsu

Jin Shin Jyutsu is an ancient art passed down from generation to generation by word of mouth until it was revived in the early 1900s by Master Jiro Murai in Japan, who used only this energy work to clear himself of a life-threatening illness. This knowledge was handed down to Mary Burmeister, who brought it to the United States in the 1950s.

Jin Shin Jyutsu is used as a self-help technique or can be applied by a trained practitioner, and also can make a nice complementary therapy before or after reflexology sessions. The practice is administered by placing the fingertips on designated "safety energy locks" located on different spots of the body to harmonize and restore energy flow.

### The Sole Meaning

In some belief systems, hurting your pinky finger means that you are trying to be someone you are not or are "trying too hard" to make something appear different than it is. In Jin Shin Jyutsu, the pinky fingers are associated with the emotion "to try, trying to, or pretense."

In Jin Shin Jyutsu, each finger represents an emotion and also two major organ energy patterns. The emotions and energy patterns associated with each finger are laid out in the following table.

| Finger | Related Emotion | Left Side Organ | Right Side Organ | Related Element |
|---|---|---|---|---|
| Thumb | Worry | Stomach | Spleen | Earth |
| Pointer finger | Fear | Bladder | Kidney | Water |
| Middle finger | Anger | Gallbladder | Liver | Earth (or wood) |
| Ring finger | Sadness | Large intestine | Lung | Air |
| Pinky finger | Try to/ pretense | Small intestine | Heart | Fire |

A good way to remember the emotion associated with your fingers is to remember a memory aid my teacher Isabelle Hutton, R.N., taught me—"Get rid of Worry F.A.S.T.!" Starting with the thumb, which is Worry, then the pointer finger Fear, middle finger Anger, ring finger Sadness, and the pinky, Trying to (or pretense).

### Foot Note

"Pretense" is usually related to a lack of self-esteem and self-worth. Acting in this manner can also become a habit for some. Some people think "Maybe they'll like me if I do one more thing for them." Pretense is doing so much for others that you drain yourself. Other "try to" or pretense behaviors include trying to prove yourself to be someone you're not just to gain approval; not living your truth; not listening to your heart; trying to obtain perfection; saying one thing and feeling another; laughing on the outside and crying on the inside.

# Keep Circulating: Veins and Arteries

The veins are the channels of transportation for blood that carry deoxygenated blood and waste products to the heart. The veins and arteries are really the same type of transportation vessels, but they are carrying their goods in different directions.

The veins and arteries are not mapped out on the foot, but a vigorous reflexology treatment brings circulation down to the feet and hands and has a warming effect on them. If your feet are not warm and your toenails look pale, you know that circulation is lacking to your extremities. Reflexology will help you restore circulation to your feet and hands.

The arteries are the blood vessels that are responsible for carrying oxygenated blood from the lungs through the heart and then away from the heart to distribute blood to the rest of the body. Our arteries should be strong but elastic. Hardening of the arteries is known as *arteriosclerosis*, a chronic disease where the arteries become thick and hard and lose their elasticity, resulting in impaired blood circulation. Symptoms may include:

➤ Cold hands and feet

➤ Blurred vision

➤ High blood pressure

➤ Difficulty thinking

➤ Difficulty breathing

### The Sole Meaning

**Arteriosclerosis** is a chronic disease where the arteries become thick, hard, and lose their elasticity, resulting in impaired blood circulation.

Causes have been linked to too much saturated fat in the diet, lack of aerobic exercise, and too much caffeine, salt, or alcohol in the diet.

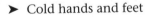

# Blood Pressure and Emotions

We used to think that high blood pressure was mostly related to arteriosclerosis or high cholesterol levels. We find this is not necessarily true. It seems that our environment and our emotions very closely influence high blood pressure. I know of a woman who is a secretary in a local high school here in Boise who had high blood pressure for years. She would check her pressure weekly and it ran very high. She tried several different methods to bring it down to no avail.

Then one day her picky, high-strung boss retired. Her blood pressure returned to normal and has not been high since! This is a classic example of how blood pressure can be affected by our environment. This effect isn't necessarily negative, though. Our blood pressure can actually lower when we think of someone we love dearly.

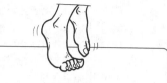

**Tip Toe**

Through strict mental discipline and deep meditation, Tibetan monks are able to control many of their own bodily functions, including body temperature, respiratory rate, heart rate, and blood pressure.

Along the same lines, connecting with a pet seems to be very beneficial for regulating blood pressure. Many hospitals have implemented a pet therapy program, which allows volunteers with trained pets to visit hospital patients on a regular basis. These animals are brought in to visit mostly with the recovering patients. The patient response is overwhelmingly positive and the recovery rates are expedited. It seems that we are positively affected by the mysterious powers of a loving animal.

# The Little Monster

I think this program is wonderful, and someday I plan to take part in this project locally. However, I believe that some pets might be able to cause high blood pressure. I had a cat once who I named Chik-a-la (pronounced *Cheek-ah-la*), which is a Lakota Sioux word for "a little." He was a stray kitten who was very little at the time I took him in, so I named him appropriately. Not long after, the sweet kitten thoughts wore off, and I decided he deserved a new name: Chik-a-la Monster!

Every morning my little monster had a new surprise for me. Some of his favorites were shredding the toilet paper rolls, diving onto hanging plants from the ceiling beams, which caused them to rip out of the ceiling and crash into a million pieces onto the floor, and climbing the drapes. Of course climbing the drapes only lasted until he was heavier, and then the entire curtain rod and drapes would tumble to the floor, serving as his cozy blanket for the afternoon.

**149**

Chik-a-la Monster was also great at finding my college papers and other homework—and shredding them—no matter how good I thought I was at hiding them between books and other papers. Oh, and we mustn't forget his obsession with clearing all windowsills of any breakable items such as ceramic potpourri holders, glass figurines, and flower vases.

Of course he waited for the flower vases to be filled with a fresh bouquet of flowers before he would destroy them. I cautiously waited for the day when I would find "REDRUM" spelled out in his litter box! Well, needless to say, I used to have a high tolerance for animals, and I even miss my little monster now, but when my cat finally passed away, so did my high blood pressure.

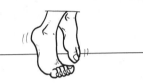

**Tip Toe**

Alcohol, food allergies, and being exposed to extremes in temperature may aggravate broken blood capillaries, especially in the face. Avoid these things and also always wear sunscreen.

## Tiny Vessels: The Capillaries

Our blood capillaries are the tiniest vessels in our circulatory system. These delicate vessels are only one single cell thick! The capillaries allow an exchange of carbon dioxide, oxygen, salts, water, and other nutrients between the blood and the tissues.

Capillaries can be easily broken, and create redness on the surface of the skin where they are broken or weakened. Some causes of broken blood vessels or capillaries include:

➤ Tight clothing

➤ Standing on your feet too much without exercise

➤ Crossing your legs

➤ Tight shoes

➤ Excessive alcohol consumption

➤ Exposure to extreme temperatures

➤ Excessive sun exposure

➤ Anything that rubs or injures the skin for a prolonged period

When working on someone whose capillaries break easily, explain to them that they might find some bruising on their lower legs after your treatments. Try not to work too deeply on them, and give them some tips on how to strengthen their capillary walls nutritionally.

A component in grape seed extract and pine bark has been found to be a powerful antioxidant and has been shown to strengthen capillary walls. Citrus bioflavonoids and vitamin K have also worked well for strengthening the capillaries. Any of these supplements would also be good for someone who suspects a risk of stroke or who bruises easily.

# Blood, Sweat, and Tears

Our blood is made up of cells carried in a liquid substance called *blood plasma*. The average adult male has about five liters of blood in his body. The liver, spleen, and bone marrow all take part in the production and recycling of blood. Some problems with blood include:

➤ A low blood count

➤ Hemophilia

➤ High blood pressure

➤ Blood clots

➤ Leukemia

➤ AIDS

**Tread Lightly**

Beware of working too deeply on a client with a blood clot. The increased circulation may dislodge the clot and could cause a stroke! Of course the same thing could happen to them if they were to walk barefoot through their front yard, but just be aware of the dangers when you are working with anyone with life-threatening illnesses, and make sure the one you are working on also understands the risks.

Blood not only carries nutrients and oxygen to other parts of the body, but it will also carry toxins, especially when our sewer system (lower bowel) is backed up. Since the skin is the closest eliminatory organ to the blood when it is overloaded with toxins, it will throw toxins out through the skin.

# Bad Blood

This is when we get zits, rashes, boils, and itching on our skin! If you are slapping zit cream on your face day and night to tame those pus pockets from hell, remember that most skin ailments are coming from the dirty condition of your blood, not necessarily your skin! So when rashes and other skin ailments pop up, look for reasons why the blood is toxic. Look first at the bowel.

When you have skin ailments, work on your bowel and liver reflex areas to help stimulate those organs. You will be amazed what a good bowel and liver cleansing will do for your skin! An herbal cleansing won't hurt either. You might want to try herbalist Ivy Bridge's daily colon cleansing drink (see the following Foot Note).

### Foot Note

Ivy Bridge's daily cleansing drink: Blend half a glass of apple juice, two tablespoons each whole leaf aloe vera juice and liquid chlorophyll, and one teaspoon or eight capsules of psyllium hulls. Drink immediately with two capsules of cascara sagrada. Follow up with eight ounces of water. Take it first thing in the morning for 60 days, then take every other day for two months, and one to two times a week indefinitely. It also helps to normalize over-acid conditions and lower cholesterol. Ivy stresses adding a daily food enzyme supplement to this cleanser to break up undigested proteins left in the digestive tract. And be sure to drink two to three quarts of water daily to flush toxins from the body.

## Warm Hands, Cold Heart?

It is more of a challenge to send good circulation to the extremities such as the feet and hands, since these areas are the farthest away from the trunk of the body where the heart "pump" is located. The body knows that the most important organs to keep nourished and warm are contained in the head and trunk areas. Since the blood warms your body, the blood tends to stay mostly in the center of your body, and your limbs are more subjected to outside temperatures than your core.

### Tip Toe

Reflexology actually stimulates the heart and all body parts through reflex action. It is believed that reflexology helps the body to dissolve blood clots—working remotely, helping directly.

When the outside temperatures are cold, the blood tends to retract toward the middle of the body. This is where the saying "cold hands and warm heart" comes from! This is a natural body function. It is only unnatural when someone has cold hands and feet all the time. This could mean that their circulation is not strong enough to get the warm blood out to the ends of the extremities. It could mean that they have low blood pressure or that they have a low blood count.

Reflexology really comes in handy in these cases because outside stimulation of the feet and hands will naturally bring blood to those areas, warming them up, nourishing the tissues, and flushing out accumulated toxins. Improved circulation through reflexology, therefore, can aid in healing the body.

And if our hearts really do communicate with each other, then you just might be able to help mend a broken heart when you give a reflexology treatment to someone you care about. I give you my heartfelt thanks for letting me share the secrets of the heart with you. Give your heartthrob a reflexology treatment, and they will quickly become your sweetheart.

---

### The Least You Need to Know

➤ The heart is the main organ of the circulatory system. Some researchers believe it can actually communicate to us and to others' hearts.

➤ Giving reflexology to someone you love will benefit their circulation and might just help mend a broken heart.

➤ High blood pressure can be caused by environmental or emotional factors. Reflexology can help balance blood pressure by creating time to relax in a stress-free environment during treatments.

➤ Skin ailments usually come from toxic blood, which comes from a toxic colon and liver. When dealing with skin problems, work the bowel and liver reflex points to stimulate cleansing.

---

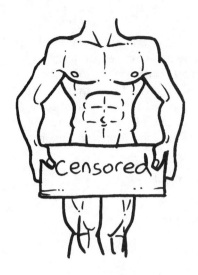

# Chapter 12

# Sexy Stuff: The Glandular System

## In This Chapter

➤ Get to know your thyroid gland and its role in your life

➤ Note key symptoms that could signal glandular imbalance

➤ Consider the role of the gonads

➤ See how your hormones affect how you feel

➤ Locate the reproductive system and thyroid reflex areas

Sex sells doesn't it? I thought sex was best to talk about last since you already got through the rest of this section (foreplay). Are you impressed with my strategic planning skills? Good. (And yes, as a matter of fact I *am* the gal who told all the retail clothing outlets to advertise sales and then put the sale stuff in the back of the store so that you have to pass the full-priced items first! That's strategy!)

Have you ever heard the question "Is it hot in here or is it me?" Well, if it is you, it just might be your glandular system in overdrive! The glandular system, as you know, encompasses many glands serving many functions. This chapter will sum up the glands that we have not talked about elsewhere, which are the reproductive organs and the thyroid gland.

## Sex and the Glands

This being the last chapter in this part, we are going to discuss the reproductive organs, glands, and the thyroid, too. But first, I am going to clarify one more time how all the glands work together so you don't forget the endocrine system.

The endocrine glands all work together as a team to keep your body in harmony. When the ovaries are surgically removed, for example, the adrenals and thyroid take over. You remember that we discussed the adrenals in the nervous system chapter since they are related to stress hormones, but they are actually a part of the endocrine system and are intimately linked to the other glands in that system.

The endocrine system consists of:

➤ The adrenals

➤ The ovaries/testes

➤ Thyroid

➤ Pancreas (part of it)

➤ Pituitary

➤ Parathyroids

➤ Thymus

➤ Pineal

Symptoms of glandular imbalance range as wide as the plains of Montana and run high and low depending on the over- or underactivity of a particular gland. Usually, glandular imbalances will involve conditions such as the following:

➤ Irregular menstrual cycles

➤ PMS or irritability

➤ Infertility

➤ Unexplained weight gain or loss

➤ Adult acne

➤ Insomnia

➤ Lethargy

➤ Racing heart

➤ Facial hair (in women)

➤ Hot flashes or feeling cold all the time

Well, now you know the worst, so let's get on with it. Take a look at the following figures to see the hand and foot reflexes for the reproductive glands, the thyroid, and the parathyroids.

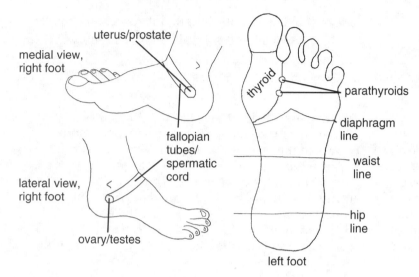

*The foot reflexes for the reproductive organs, thyroid, and parathyroids. The same reflexes are located on both feet.*

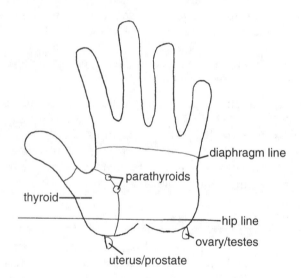

*The hand reflexes for the reproductive organs, thyroid, and parathyroids. These same reflexes are repeated on the palm of both hands.*

# The Thyroid—Metabolism Regulator

The thyroid is a small, pinkish gland that straddles the windpipe just below the Adam's apple in the throat. It is shaped kind of like a butterfly or a bat. Imagine a pink, fleshy butterfly wrapping its wings around your windpipe, and you can visualize your thyroid gland.

The hormone-secreting thyroid is mostly responsible for your metabolism. The thyroid area can be found on both feet and includes the area all around the base of the big toe (neck area) and the ball of the foot just below the big toe. You can press all around the

**The Sole Meaning**

The **parathyroids** are two pair of flat, disk-shaped glands on each side of the thyroid gland. Think of them as the spots on the ends of the wings of the pink butterfly that represents the thyroid. The parathyroids help regulate the calcium and phosphorus balance in the body. They are good reflex points to work on when dealing with arthritis and kidney stones.

base of your big toe with your thumb to work the tender spots. This therapy will also help loosen up your neck.

The thyroid area on the hands is found on both hands all along the padding of the palm at the base of the thumb.

The thyroid includes the *parathyroid glands*, which have a lot to do with keeping the calcium and phosphorus balance in the body. Their proper function is also important in poise and composure. The parathyroids are two pair of flattened tiny pieces of tissue that are on either side of the larynx on the thyroid gland. They are probably named parathyroids because there are two "pair a thyroids" on the thyroid! You can remember them as the spots on the ends of the wings of our pink thyroid butterfly.

The reflex areas for the parathyroids are two spots located together (one above the other) on the thyroid area between the webbing of the large toe and the second toe. I find these spots tender on many people.

Press in on these tender spots, hold for three seconds, and repeat two more times. These areas are also located on both feet and hands.

On the hands, these parathyroid reflexes are found on the area of the padding of the thumb about in the middle edge of where the thyroid reflex runs through the palm. The thyroid area is easy to find on the hand since most of us have lines in the palm that correspond closely to this area. Look at your palm and see if you have a curved line that outlines the padded area of your thumb. If you do, you can use it as your landmark for where the thyroid and parathyroid areas are located.

**The Sole Meaning**

**Goiter** is an enlargement of the thyroid gland usually caused by a lack of iodine. The thyroid is actually working hard to attract the nutrient **iodine** (its main source of food) and enlarges in the process.

## Iodine: Thyroid Food

There are many problems associated with a dysfunctional thyroid gland. When the gland is overactive due to an iodine deficiency it may enlarge, resulting in a condition known as *goiter*. The thyroid is actually working hard to attract the nutrient *iodine* (its main source of food) and enlarges in the process. Iodine is needed for the production of thyroid hormone. In severe cases, the swollen goiter can appear as if the person swallowed a large grapefruit that got stuck in his throat!

Iodine-rich foods nourish the thyroid gland. Some of the best sources of iodine from foods are seafood, kelp, and dulse. Other iodine-rich foods and herbs include:

➤ Artichokes, asparagus

➤ Blueberries, Brussels sprouts

➤ Carrots, cucumbers

➤ Liquid chlorophyll

➤ Peanuts, spinach

➤ Summer squash, strawberries

➤ Garlic, tofu

Reflexology cannot change an iodine deficiency. It can, however, utilize the pores on the soles of the feet, which are some of the largest pores on the body. Although nutritional sources of iodine are recommended, organic or biochemical iodine applied to the soles of the feet have been used to correct an iodine deficiency. The pores are not only good for eliminating wastes from the body, but they also absorb whatever is applied to them.

## Seesaw or Balance Beam?

It is important to keep our thyroid in balance. The thyroid can become under- or overactive, and either extreme has its own symptoms. An over-active thyroid is known as *hyperthyroidism*, and a deficient or underactive thyroid is known as *hypothyroidism*. Both can be caused by a lack of iodine. Simply speaking, the hyperthyroid is working hard to find iodine, and the hypothyroid is exhausted because it hasn't found any.

Symptoms associated with an overactive thyroid include hyperactivity, a ferocious appetite, being underweight, nervousness, irritability, emotionally imbalanced, and having a racing heart. Eyes that appear as if they are popping out of the head could also be an indication of hyperthyroidism. Say, could it be that Popeye got his name from having a pop-eyed look from a thyroid problem and that's why he craved all that spinach?

**The Sole Meaning**

A **hyperthyroid** is an overactive thyroid. The hyperthyroid uses up iodine rapidly. A **hypothyroid** is a thyroid that is worn out and under-active. It usually is too weak to produce the correct thyroid hormones.

An underactive thyroid can slow you down. There are many indications that a person has low thyroid activity. Some of the typical things I look for when assessing a client who thinks they have an underactive thyroid are given in the following list. If you think your thyroid is low, work those thyroid points every day!

See your physician to have a blood test to see if a thyroid problem can be confirmed, but remember that blood tests only show a problem when the thyroid is already half incapacitated. Eat foods and herbs rich in natural iodine. If you catch these problems early enough, most thyroids can be saved without the use of drugs or surgery. And, it is

**159**

*always* easier to prevent problems in your body than to work to correct them. Think preventatively!

Hypothyroidism signs to look for:

➤ Coarse hair, brittle nails, cold sensation

➤ Constipation, deafness, depression

➤ Difficult breathing, dry skin, emotional instability

➤ Enlarged heart, excessive and painful menstruation, hair loss

➤ Headaches

➤ Hoarseness, impaired memory, lack of sweating

➤ Lethargy, loss of appetite, low body temperature

➤ Lowered tone in voice, muscle weakness, pain over heart

➤ Pale lips, pallor of skin, palpitations

➤ Poor vision, puffy face

➤ Retarded growth in children and retarded mental development

➤ Slow movement, slow speech, slowing of mental activity

➤ Swelling of the eyelids, swollen feet and hands, thick tongue

➤ Weakness, unexplained weight gain or loss

**Foot Note**

Hypothyroidism can be caused by continued exposure to low dose radiation such as X-rays or mammograms, environmental pollution that depletes the body of vitamin A, and overuse of diet pills and other drugs. Women are eight times more likely to experience hypothyroidism than men.

A hypothyroid condition, a cold condition of the body, would fall into the "earth" category on the four-element model. Reflexology will help to stimulate the thyroid function and increase circulation to the extremities, making you feel warmer.

## The Thyroid as a Power Center

The thyroid is associated with the healing faculty of power, especially creative power. In ancient times, the thyroid gland was considered a third ovary! It was believed that a woman could create ovarian trouble by using negative words!

The thyroid is an energy center that controls all the vibrating energies of the body. Therefore, it is wise to watch what you say and understand how your words can have an effect on your health. All the vibrations of the words you speak come out past the thyroid gland and through this energy center in the throat.

The body forms to these vibrations, so speak, act, and think positively and your body will respond. Greet the world each day with positive words, and tell yourself how good, happy, successful, healthy, and strong you are today. Your body will listen!

### Foot Note

In glandular body typing, the thyroid body type is tall and thin with long fingers, arms, and neck. When overweight, these people hold the weight around their middle section (spare tire) and crave carbohydrate foods like cookies and pastries. Thyroid types tend to be emotional and like to express themselves. Cher and Daryl Hannah are both good examples of a thyroid body type.

# The Gonads: By Dr. Phil D. Glanz

The reproductive organs do more than just help us procreate, although they are not necessary for our own survival. The ovaries and testes are parts of the glandular system that take their commands from the pituitary gland in the brain. (See—sex really is mostly in the head!)

Hormonal messages from the gonads command our sexual response, control hair growth, regulate menstrual cycles, keep the skin luminous, and give us a sparkle in our eyes. Imbalances in the reproductive organs can show themselves in the following ways:

➤ Cramps

➤ PMS

➤ Menstrual irregularities

➤ Infertility

➤ Hot flashes

➤ Miscarriages

➤ Ectopic pregnancies

➤ Frigidity

The uterus and prostate gland are also part of our reproductive system. Sometimes women who experience imbalances, or even cancerous conditions, in the reproductive organs will have a radical surgery called a *hysterectomy*. A *full utero-ovarian hysterectomy* is when surgeons remove the uterus and ovaries of a woman. Of course this surgery makes it impossible to conceive children.

The removal of the ovaries may also plunge women into *menopause*. Menopause is when the female body has stopped producing eggs for procreation. The hysterectomy was originally so labeled because the reproductive organs create hormones that, when imbalanced, can make a woman feel "hysterical." "Ectomy" means removal of. So, surgeons believed that if you removed (ectomy) the source of the problem (hysteria), then the woman would be okay! Reflexology can help you through menopausal symptoms by stimulating the balance of the other endocrine glands to make up for the lost ovary functions. See Chapter 23, "Keeping Your Glands in Order," to see how reflexology has helped with these problems.

**The Sole Meaning**

A **hysterectomy** is the removal of a woman's uterus. Sometimes a **full utero-ovarian** or **total hysterectomy** will be performed, which also removes one or both of the ovaries. **Menopause** is when a woman's ovaries stop producing eggs. The ovaries discontinue their hormone production, which can lead to dry skin, emotional instability, hot flashes, and heart palpitations.

# Get over Being Teste with Me!

**Question:** Why do mice have such little balls?

**Answer:** Cuz' most of them don't know how to dance.

*Ovaries* are two almond-shaped glands about an inch long that are located on the right and left sides of the pelvic area in females. These little glands are responsible for helping shape the female body, regulating the menstrual cycle, producing eggs (ova) for making a baby, keeping the skin supple, and helping the calcium and other minerals in the body keep in balance.

The *testes* are two small, round glands each held in a sack-like pouch located on the outside of the man's body. They are responsible for the production of hormones and storage of sperm. The hormones produced by the testes help in the construction of the structural system and are also responsible for mental attitudes and aggressiveness.

**Tip Toe**

A good way to remember the location of the ovary reflex is to remember your Os. The **o**vary/ testicle reflex point is located on the **o**utside of each heel. The ovary and testes reflexes are interchangeable depending on the sex of the person you are working on. Remember "Get over Being Teste with Me!" to remind you the points are the same.

The reflex location for the ovaries and testes are the same on each foot. The ovary/ testes spot is a small, round spot found at just about the center of the flat part of the outside of the heel, just below the ankle bone. Using your thumb or pointer finger to find this spot, you will locate somewhat of an indentation. This spot should not be overworked and is usually tender on everyone. Press on this spot for three seconds, then release, then repeat two more times.

On each hand, the ovary/testes reflex is located on the inside of the wrists on the pinky finger side, just below the heel of the hand. The same goes for both hands.

One of the most widely studied uses of reflexology has been for its use in relieving PMS symptoms. The results have been positive. Reflexology seems to help lessen severe symptoms of PMS through relaxation and stimulation of endorphins. Reflexology can also help with the pain associated with cramping before and during menstruation.

Find out more about using reflexology for PMS in Chapters 2, "Why Do I Want My Feet Rubbed?" and 23. The figure in Chapter 23 also adds the specific points to work when experiencing PMS symptoms and shows the fallopian tube/spermatic cord reflex area, which is also a part of the reproductive system. A wonderful technique for relieving menstrual cramps with reflexology is shown in Chapter 15, "How to Touch."

### Foot Note

The gonadal body shape is a typical shape among women and, in rare cases, men. The gonadal, or reproductive, body type carries excess body weight in the hips, butt, and outer thighs, although their tummies are usually taut. This type is smaller on top than on bottom, similar to a pear shape, have long, slender necks, smaller feet, small ankles and wrists, but are tallish. These people are attracted to rich, creamy foods, tend to be creative, crave affection, and have "rich" tastes. If you are a gonadal you will need to stimulate your pituitary, pineal, and thyroid glands to stay balanced. Also, stay away from the fatty foods and eat more fruits and vegetables.

## Uterus on to Prostate Health

The *uterus*, also known as the womb, is a pear-shaped organ suspended in the pelvic cavity that is specialized to allow an embryo to become implanted in its inner wall and subsequently to nourish the growing fetus. Problems with the uterus include:

➤ Miscarriages

➤ Endometriosis

➤ Cramps

➤ Hemorrhages

➤ Adult acne

Red raspberry is an herb used historically to help strengthen the walls of the uterus for the prevention of miscarriage. If you are getting acne, see your OB-GYN to test your hormone levels.

The *prostate* gland is a male accessory sex gland located just below the bladder. Its purpose is to secrete an alkaline fluid as part of the semen. The prostate gland is shaped like a donut, wrapping itself around the proximal end of the urethra snug up against the urinary bladder's exit.

Problems with the prostate often involve enlargement of the gland, putting undue stress against the neck of the bladder and impairing urination. This usually occurs in older men, but is mostly preventable with a holistic lifestyle. Along with reflexology, the mineral zinc and the herb saw palmetto have been used with success to help the prostate gland.

As the ovary and testes share the same reflex spot, so do the uterus and prostate. These points can be found on the inside middle of each heel, just below the ankle bone. Press and hold this point for three seconds, release, and repeat two more times. This will usually be a tender spot on both males and females.

The prostate/uterus reflexes can also be found on the inside of the wrist, just below the bottom joint of each thumb.

This is a point to work if someone is dealing with prostate trouble and waking up in the middle of the night to urinate. For women, this spot can be held when experiencing menstrual cramps, or in labor to help relax the uterus. This spot should not be worked heavily if you are pregnant and have had trouble previously carrying to term.

**Tread Lightly**

Prostate trouble is one of the most common ailments among middle-age men. By age 50, 20 percent of American men have enlarged prostates, and by age 60 over 50 percent have it. (Statistics taken from Dr. Bernard Jensen's *Chemistry of Man* [Bernard Jensen, 1983].) Therefore men should get regular prostate checkups after about age 40.

## Doing Some Tubing

One other reflex area that deserves a special mention under the reproductive system includes the fallopian tubes/spermatic cord reflex. The fallopian tubes are found in the female body and are the tubes that lead an egg (ovum) from the ovaries to the uterus for fertilization. Women own a pair of these tubes, one from each ovary, that come together at the uterus. The spermatic cord in men is the cord that runs from the abdominal cavity to the testicles.

The reflexes for these areas are located on both feet, running over the top of the foot from ankle to ankle, kind of like a strap that connects the uterus/prostate point to the ovary/testes spot. You can work this area in many ways, including finger and thumb walking (see Chapter 14, "Let Your Fingers Do the Walking") or by stimulating the area with a special rotation move (shown in Chapter 15).

The hand reflexes for these areas are not shown on my charts here, since they are located around the front part of the wrist. But when you work around the base of your hands, all around the wrist areas, you will be stimulating your fallopian tubes/spermatic cord reflexes.

There are many uses for reflexology when it comes to the glands, including the relief of PMS and prostate enlargement, glandular balancing, stimulating late periods, and stimulating the thyroid into action, which boosts metabolism. Now that this chapter is "ova," we can dive into the next section, on the techniques of reflexology.

## The Least You Need to Know

➤ The reproductive system and glandular system, for our purposes here, include the ovaries or testes, uterus or prostate, thyroid and parathyroids, and fallopian tubes or spermatic cord.

➤ The thyroid regulates metabolism—a slow metabolism could mean an underactive thyroid and hyperactivity could be caused by an overactive thyroid.

➤ The thyroid is associated with our center of power; the words you speak have an affect on your health and life, so be positive!

➤ The ovary and testes area are tender on most people and should not be over-worked.

➤ The uterus and prostate reflexes are also tender spots, and moderate manipulation of this point may benefit menstrual cramps and/or prostate enlargement.

# Part 3
# Tools and Techniques for Feeling Good

*Now that you can locate all the parts and know how they function, you need to know the secret techniques of reflexology.*

*This next section will cover several hands-on techniques and introduce instruments that some reflexologists use. So read on to get more in touch with yourself!*

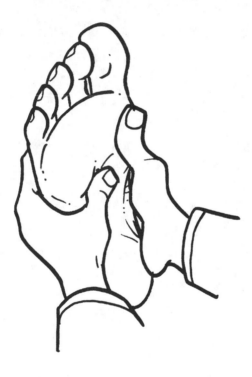

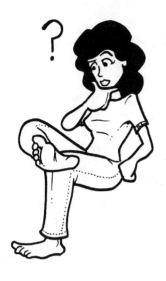

# Digging In:
# Where Do I Start?

Now that you've learned where most of the main reflexology points are and what the corresponding organs do for you, you want to prepare to get your hands on a partner, right? This chapter will take a macro look at how you get set to work on a mate, friend, or family member, and gives you a general idea of how a typical routine is performed. You need to know where and how to start, so let's take a look at the first steps.

## Taming Aunt Gretta

Whether it is speaking in public or practicing anything new in front of others, we all occasionally experience a certain amount of stage fright. The same kind of freeze-up might occur the first time you practice reflexology on someone else. You might be especially nervous if you work on someone like cynical, grouchy, old Aunt Gretta, who commonly refers to reflexology as "that witch doctor stuff."

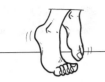

**Tip Toe**

When I am nervous, such as when I am speaking in front of a group or doing something new, to help my anxiety I try to imagine that everyone in the room owes me money. The old tip about imagining everyone in his or her underwear never seemed to work for me!

(Note how she was willing to promptly whip off her beige-colored knee-highs, hop up on your chair or table, and let you practice on her anyway.)

Don't let her grouchiness intimidate you! Once you are done, she will be more soft and kind, and if you're lucky, she will doze off and remember nothing, while you get to practice on a real live person! And at the worst, she will have something more to complain about to the rest of your family, which is free publicity if nothing else.

This chapter will give you a basic orientation in how to give a reflexology treatment so that you don't get caught staring open-mouthed and dumbfounded at a bare foot. The next two chapters will help you learn the method to use for touching a foot and show you the typical "moves" and techniques to make your treatments effective and pleasant.

By the way, having your mouth open and gazing dumbfounded into space is clear body language that you are hungry for more information. So read on!

# Hand Me That Foot

Before we begin, I assume that after reading this book you will not go out and hang a sign on your door declaring that you are a reflexologist! This book is meant to be a natural and safe self-help book. It is also meant to give you some general tips for practicing on your friends and family. It can also be used as a reference guide, or even a prerequisite when you decide to take a hands-on course on the subject.

**Tread Lightly**

Proper training to become a reflexologist is the only appropriate way to go. Check out Appendix A, "Reflexology Schools, Teachers, and Associations," if you are interested in becoming a reflexologist.

Even after reading this book and taking a bona fide course in reflexology, it is still important to have some volunteers to practice on before you practice on the public. So at the next holiday gathering, stretch those fingers and search out those volunteers! Reflexology treatments make great gifts and can even ease any potential family bickering that can spoil a good time. Your family and friends will be grateful, and you get some experience to boot.

There are lots of different things you will see when visiting the office of a professional reflexologist. You may see reflexology charts on the wall, framed certifications, or other credentials, a music player, essential oils and a diffuser, towels, maybe a massage table or a reflexology chair. All these make an office professional. Now, at home you won't have to go to all that trouble to work on yourself or your partner, but it will nicely add to the atmosphere of the professional.

At home, you can have your partner lie in their bed, on a couch, or prop them up comfortably in a La-Z-Boy or other comfy chair. The important thing is that you are both comfortable.

You should sit at your partner's feet, and for your best angle, their feet should be about central to your diaphragm.

Personally, I work on one foot at a time and keep my body centered around the foot I am working on. My normal treatments last about one hour, but you don't have to practice that long on someone to get results and make someone feel good. Even five minutes on each hand or each foot makes a nice session and is a loving way to connect with a family member. Remember that babies should not be overworked. A total of 10 minutes is adequate.

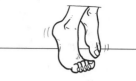

**Tip Toe**

If you are uncomfortable when giving reflexology to someone, you will interrupt or distract from the session by constantly having to shift and fidget in an attempt to make yourself more comfortable. Always situate yourself in a comfortable position before starting the session to avoid this problem.

## Time for a Quickie?

Here's a quick 10-minute routine that covers both hands and feet and can be used for people of any age. You can use this routine to get some quick relaxation and rejuvenation. With these moves you will not be working any specific reflex points purposely, but you will be giving some general relaxation to the whole body. These moves are like squeezing the whole body and giving it a stretch, kind of like you would before you begin an exercise class.

(In the next chapter we will actually get into describing the details of each technique, but to get you started, these few techniques are simple to understand. I have also referred to a few photos you can look up for further clarification.)

A quick 10-minute routine for amateurs to introduce reflexology to family members:

➤ After finding a place for your partner to lie back, make sure the back of their knees are supported with a pillow or cushion of some sort, so the back is not strained and the knees are not hyperextended (I will emphasize this point over and over in this book). You should find yourself a comfortable chair or stool that positions you slightly lower than your partner's feet.

➤ First, choose a foot and gently squeeze the foot with both hands, starting at the toes and working your way down to the heel (see Chapter 16, "Third Time's a Charm," to get an idea of how to grasp the foot). Make sure you don't pull or pinch the skin while you are giving it this gentle squeeze. Repeat this move three times.

➤ Rotate the foot on the ankle using one hand to support the ankle while you hold the ball of the foot in the other hand (see Chapter 15, "How to Touch"). Rotate three times one direction and then three times the opposite direction.

➤ Support the base of the toes by holding the ball of the foot and with the other hand grasp one toe at a time and gently rotate each toe three times in one direction and then three times the other direction (see the "Tootsie Rolls and Rotating Toes" section in Chapter 15 for a detailed description on how to perform this move). Be sure not to pinch the toes too tight; you don't want to squeeze the toenail and make it uncomfortable. Grasp each toe tip just snug enough to hold onto it while you rotate it in a circular motion.

➤ Repeat these three moves on the opposite foot. This whole process should take about a total of five minutes to do both feet (two and a half minutes each). The majority of the time is spent on rotating the toes.

➤ You can spend another five minutes on the hands. Take one hand and use your fingers and thumb to gently squeeze the webbing of the hand between the hand bones. The area between the base of the thumb and pointer finger feels especially good to most people (see Chapter 5, "In Your Defense: The Immune System," to locate the upper lymphatic reflexes). This area of the hand will stimulate some of the upper lymphatics, the thyroid, the parathyroid, and even some of the bowel. You can spend a little extra time here, since it feels good to most people.

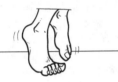

**Tip Toe**

If you or a person you are working on is experiencing a headache, firmly squeeze the webbing between the thumb and first finger for up to one minute. This has worked for my clients many times in less than 45 seconds. If the headache is still not alleviated, try drinking a full glass of water.

➤ Squeeze the webbing between the rest of the fingers one at a time. This works the upper lymphatics, chest/breast, and lungs.

➤ Finish off by squeezing each fingertip gently, which affects the brain and sinuses. You should have spent about two and a half minutes on each hand, to complete a total 10-minute mini-treatment! At this point, your family member will probably beg you to take a reflexology class so that they can be your practice volunteer!

## Timing Is Everything

Whether using this book to practice on yourself or family members, or practicing reflexology as a trade, the timing of your sessions is important. The time you would like to spend working on yourself or others should be determined up front. This is easy for the professional, since they usually have a predetermined fee and time. However, even when you are just experimenting with reflexology, you should determine the time you want to spend in advance and make sure that you balance your work on both sides of the body. But you don't want to spend your time watching the clock.

**Tread Lightly**

Using any type of alarm, such as a high-powered foghorn, to signal the end of a reflexology treatment is not suggested. This will most likely annoy your partner and break them out of the euphoric mood that you worked so hard to get them into.

There are different ways you can time yourself until you get comfortable with your own rhythm. You might want to consider using a kitchen timer to time yourself. However, some people might be annoyed by the ticking sound of a timer, so if you use one, just make sure that the noise really won't bother them. If it does, keep the timer outside of the room you are working in so all you hear is the "ding" when you are done.

You can check the duration of a CD or music tape that you choose to play during the treatment. Try to get CDs that match the amount of time you want your typical treatment to last. You can coordinate a treatment to the length of the CD, which is a nice way to "conduct" business. This is especially true if the music has a type of crescendo in it. During the crescendo you can do your most vigorous work and then drift back down into the relaxing techniques and finish up on the last note. It sounds really corny, but if you give it a try you might get into it!

The reason you want to stay on track with timing is so that you don't spend too much time on one foot. If you run out of time, you won't be able to do an effective job on the opposite foot. This can leave a person feeling unbalanced. Reflexology will relax the muscles in the body. You will feel a difference in the side of the body that has been worked on. Therefore, to stay in balance, both sides should always be worked equally, whether you are working on yourself or a friend.

I had one therapist tell me that she tried this experiment on her husband. They wanted to see how important it was to do both sides of the body in one treatment. Marilyn worked on her husband's left foot and lower leg and did not work on his right side at all. When they were done, her husband stood up, took one step, and fell over! This experience shows how important it is to keep balanced by working both sides equally!

If you are working with only one point for a specific result, you should also work the same point on the opposite foot or hand. (Remember that most reflex points and areas are located on *both* hands and feet.) You can divide your treatment between the feet and hands any way you like. A good way to break down an hour treatment is to practice 20 minutes on each foot and then finish up with 10 minutes on each hand.

Should you begin practicing professionally, you can also offer half-hour treatments to clients at a little more than half price. These less-expensive treatments offer clients with a smaller budget a chance to come more often. With a half-hour session, you can spend 15 minutes on each foot and forfeit working on the hands.

## Make Yourself Comfortable

Once you and your partner have agreed upon how long the treatment will be, you have to choose your location. Later we will cover all the fluffy, atmospheric-type things that enhance treatments, but for now we are just going to cover the basics of getting comfortable.

Whether your subject is sitting in a chair or lying on a couch, bed, or massage table, you will want them to sit back and be comfortable or lie on their back. Read more on chairs used for reflexology in Chapter 17, "Tools of the Trade." (I cover all the tips on getting positioned in that chapter, too.) If the person is lying flat on her back, support her knees by putting a pillow under them to make sure the knees are slightly bent. Keeping the knees fully extended puts strain on the kneecaps and the back, which can cause discomfort. You don't want people leaving more uncomfortable than when they came in!

### Foot Note

After a reflexology session, a physical difference in the recipient's body can be felt and observed, not only by the recipient but also by others! An experiment I use in classes to demonstrate this is to have my students work only on one foot as I explain the techniques. After about 15 minutes I have them all stand and try to guess (on a different person) which foot was worked on. The hint is to look at the shoulders. Ninety-nine percent of the time, the shoulder on the side of the body that corresponds to the reflexed foot is significantly "lower" (more relaxed) than the opposite shoulder!

If you don't have a massage table or a reflexology chair to use, you can improvise by utilizing a bed, a couch, or any type of chair that your partner can recline in. You will sit facing the soles of your partner's feet. (See the photo of me working on my husband in Chapter 22, "Reflexologists as Sole Practitioners," to see how it looks to be positioned correctly.) After you ensure that your subject is comfortable, you will need to get situated yourself. Sit at the base of their feet and low enough that the tips of their toes are about level with your solar plexus. This position will give you body leverage if you are working on someone who requires deep work. We will talk more later about specific finger techniques.

# Making Contact

One of the first things you want to do when working on someone is to establish contact with the foot. Gently lay your hand on one of their feet as you get yourself situated. Which foot you choose doesn't actually matter, but you probably want to touch the foot you intend to work on first.

You are making an initial contact to let the person know you are there. This first contact tends to put your client at ease, especially if your touch is gentle. (A stinging smack to the bare foot may not be the way you want to establish your first contact.)

## *Work Your Way Down*

Now that you've got that foot in your hand, what do you do with it? One helpful hint is to start at the top of the foot and work your way down. This way you won't miss anything.

**Tread Lightly**

Try to make sure your hands are warmer than the foot you are working on. Eventually both your hands and your partner's feet will warm up while you work, but you don't want them to jump at your first contact because of your icy cold fingers! Try rubbing your hands vigorously together to warm them up first.

By the top, I mean the top to you, which from your vantage point will be the toes, known as the *distal* part of the foot. You will want to work with each toe like it is its own separate little foot. The toes correspond to the sinus and head area. Many of us suffer with allergies. By working the toes first, you might just be able to give some sinus relief right away.

Move on to the ball of the foot, down the body of the foot, and end at the heel. Then you can get the sides of the foot and you won't forget anything! The last part of this chapter will outline a longer routine for you to use. After you learn more specific techniques, you can refer to this outline as a general guide for giving a more in-depth session. But just remember to start at one end and work your way down and you will cover the territory.

# *Come Down Off That Ceiling!*

Everyone has their own level of pain tolerance. The levels that different people can tolerate can be dramatic. One person may not even think you have started on them when you have been digging your deepest and exerting pressure into their reflex points, while another will practically jump off your table at the slightest amount of pressure!

Everyone is different, and you will need to learn how to use enough pressure to be effective, but not brutal, to some sensitive tootsies. Likewise, you will need to use your best judgment on how deep is too deep, even when your subject doesn't seem to be experiencing discomfort. Whether they tell you to go deeper or not, you should not go beyond what is reasonable pressure. If you have hands of steel, too much pressure could cause damage or bruising.

### Foot Note

Some people have high pain tolerance because they may have already experienced a lot of pain in their lives. They have developed a higher "pain threshold" in order to cope with the things they have been through. With that in mind, I wonder what it would have been like to work on Evel Knievel's feet!

# Reaching the Depths of Your Sole

Just like in a relationship, you don't want to scare someone off by getting too deep too fast! Get to know your subject and their foot before you dive right into the depths of their soles.

Some other factors can help you decide whether to go deep or not. You should always take a case history before a treatment when doing this professionally, but we will address that in later chapters. For now, the following information will help you get a "feel" for your subject:

➤ Find out if the person has had reflexology before.

➤ If they have had reflexology before, ask what they liked about it.

➤ Find out if there was anything that they especially did not like about their previous treatment.

➤ If they have never had reflexology before, ask them if they have had a massage.

➤ Question them on their preferences for deep or gentle massages.

The answers to these questions can help you determine how deep the treatment should be.

The condition of the foot will give you a clue as to how deep you can go. For instance, if the foot is light in color, soft, and very flexible, you might not want to jump in deep right away. This person might have a delicate constitution and may not need, or be able to tolerate, a hefty treatment.

On the other hand (no pun intended), a foot that looks like it has been barefoot most of its life and is heavily callused may need deeper work to be effective. This is not always the case, however. Going slowly is your best bet, and be sure to ask your subject to tell you if the pressure is uncomfortable or if you need to go deeper.

**Tip Toe**

Some people will not be comfortable taking their socks off, but this is okay. You can work on your own or another's feet through the socks. However, if the socks are dirty, offer them a clean pair of cotton socks to make the treatment more pleasant for you.

## Down to the Bone

Some areas of the foot are not appropriate to work deeply. You never want to work deeply directly on a bone or on the joints. When I talk about a deep pressure I generally am talking about working on the muscle layers of the foot. The ball of the foot and the heel are sometimes callused and harder. Therefore, to be effective you will probably apply more pressure to these areas. The midpart of the foot contains a majority of organ reflex points and the pressure will vary.

You don't want to go deep enough to give your subject a cramp! This may happen when you are working on the instep. If it does, help them to stretch out the cramp and then go back to the instep more gently. The deeper you work, the *slower* you will need to apply pressure. You don't want to make anyone feel like they just stepped on a rock. Applying the pressure slowly allows the body time to adjust.

**Tread Lightly**

As with anything, looks can be deceiving. I have worked on feet that appeared to be delicate and be sensitive that were just the opposite. On the other hand, a few very callused feet have been very sensitive to my touch! You never know, so make sure you customize your pressure for the client and not your own prejudices!

# *That Feels Yummy: A Relaxing Technique*

Remember that pain causes tension, so anytime we have done something that has caused discomfort, we want to re-relax the body. Yummies, a reflexology technique so named by my first reflexology teacher, Isabelle Hutton, is a good way to do this.

*"Yummies" is a technique of rubbing the ball of the foot back and forth between both hands.*

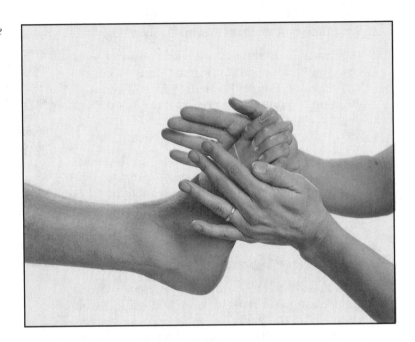

**Tread Lightly**

If you cause someone to yell when hitting a tender spot, don't allow your hands to jerk away from them, but follow this regime: *Stop* pushing, back off slightly, and hold the spot for a moment. The body will adjust to the pressure. Then give them a "yummy," which tends to make them forget they ever had any discomfort!

Yummies is a technique whereby you place both of your palms on either side of the ball of the foot, and gently but vigorously move your hands in opposite directions, rolling the foot loosely between your hands. In this technique, one hand goes forward, or away from you, while the other hand moves toward you. Repeat this motion for about five to 10 seconds, making sure your hands do not slide on the skin to prevent "skin burn" (due to friction). This technique will relax the body, especially the ankle and calf muscles.

# When Your Feet Bruise but Your Ego Doesn't

If your subject has a tendency toward anemia or if they bruise easily, work more gently on them. You don't want them to go home with bruises, even if the treatment felt good. They will have to make up excuses to their neighbors that their reflexologist really does care deeply for them. They will have to justify why they continue to go back even though they end up with bruises every time.

I had a client tell me that her first reflexology experience, with another practitioner, was effective but brutal. After her first treatment she had bruises up and down her shins for two weeks. She could barely walk the following day! I asked her why she wanted to get another reflexology treatment after that experience and she said she felt that the treatment helped the rest of her body feel better anyway.

A full assessment on this woman showed her to have a low blood count, and she also bruised very easily. Therefore, I did not work on her vigorously, but I was effective enough to keep her coming back for more. We also worked with her nutritionally and she began taking an algae supplement, liquid chlorophyll, and yellow dock to feed her body herbal sources of protein and iron.

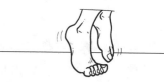

**Tip Toe**

Black cherries, barley grass powder, liquid chlorophyll, green algae, and yellow dock have all served well for many to build iron reserves in the body and bring back a higher red blood count. See your holistic nutritionist, herbalist, or other natural specialist to help you with a program suited to your needs.

The program changed her appearance and vastly improved her energy levels. The dark circles under her eyes went away and she enjoyed her newfound energy. Eventually I was able to work much deeper on her feet without the consequence of bruising.

## Another Embarrassing Story

Another good question to ask someone before you start working on them is if they have any old injuries of the feet or hands. Never work deeply on old injuries. I learned this lesson "firsthand" with someone who asked me to demonstrate reflexology on him at a luncheon. I acquiesced until his hand began to turn red and swell!

Embarrassed, I apologized and attempted a get-away. He then told me that he had injured the hand 20 years ago. The good news is that his inflammation subsided and he reported a renewed flexibility thereafter! Could it have been that my

**Tip Toe**

I find that my women clients are more sensitive just before their periods and not as sensitive during other times of the month. I have to adjust my pressure to fit the need at the time. You will become aware of this for yourself, too.

short use of reflexology was just what his hand needed to complete healing? No matter—please learn what I did from this experience:

➤ Always ask about old injuries before starting.

➤ Never begin work haphazardly on someone—be professional, even if you are not yet a reflexologist.

➤ Never work too deeply on an old injury.

## Smoothing the Way

Occasionally you will run into someone who, no matter how hard you push, no matter how deep you go, will always ask you to go deeper. Many times these people will have a lot of callus built up on their feet. This makes it harder for you to work on them and also makes them less sensitive to your treatments.

Suggest that they purchase a pumice stone and use it to rid themselves of their built-up calluses. The pumice treatments help make the feet more supple and sensitive to treatments.

My aunt Alice, a nationally certified reflexologist in Colorado, has another trick up her sleeve. She offers her clients a foot wax dip before their reflexology session. She says that these hot wax treatments for the feet not only make the foot feel fantastic, but also serve to exfoliate the skin and soften it up before reflexology.

**Tread Lightly**

If part of your foot has an injury, infection, bruise, or other foot type ailment, do not work directly on that spot. The same holds true for anyone you work on. You can, however, work around the injured spot, which will still move lymph and circulation and can enhance healing. You can also work on the corresponding hand instead of the foot if the foot is injured, or vice versa for the hands.

## The Tender Spots Need Work

As you begin to work with reflexology, you will notice that you will find areas on the feet and hands that are very tender. Besides indicating any local problems (such as corns or warts), these tender spots generally are the areas that need the most work. When there is tenderness in an area, this usually means that there is corresponding congestion in the organ associated with the reflex point.

Many times you will be able to tell where the tender spots are because you will be able to feel crunchies in those areas. Sometimes you will feel "electrical sparks" shooting out of a particular point. When you feel these crunchies or electrical spurts, you might want to ask your subject if they can feel any particular sensation.

Occasionally a person will tell you that you are digging into them with your fingernail. Of course, you will have trimmed your nails already (we will cover the importance of keeping short nails in Chapter 14, "Let Your

Fingers Do the Walking"), so it will not be your nail that they feel. They also might ask you what type of tool you are using when you hit one of these crunchies.

Actually, what they are probably feeling is the sensation of a uric acid crystal being broken up in their foot. It is not you at all, but a release of built-up toxins that have accumulated in the foot. You can work on these areas until the tenderness subsides. This sometimes can be done in one treatment, but may take as many as three in one week to get rid of the pain and stimulate the corresponding organs into action!

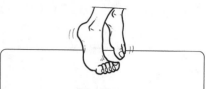

**Tip Toe**

Keeping fingernails trimmed is a good idea for reflexologists and all therapists who use their hands to perform bodywork.

In Part 4, "The Practice of Reflexology," where we go into more detail on tender spots and precautions, we will talk about when tender spots are not appropriate to work on. If you want details of some of the contraindications (when you shouldn't use reflexology) see the table in Chapter 15, which lists all the warnings for reflexology. But for now, the tender spots are your clues that they need to be worked!

# A Typical Routine

Now that you're starting to get comfortable, let's walk through a typical reflexology treatment. This is the first routine I learned early in my career, with some of my own refinements added to it. You can use this to practice on friends and family who volunteer to let you work on them. Once you learn all the techniques, you can come back to this treatment and use it as a guide.

You can use a typical routine like this for as long as you like, but since we are all creative beings and each person you work on will have different needs and requests, you will probably change this routine over time. I like to perform a generalized routine on each new client. When and if I find especially tender areas, I work on those areas until the tenderness subsides. Put your own creativity into your work and soon you won't be worried about what to do next!

➤ Begin establishing rapport with your subject and make a gentle contact with the foot. Question them about any injuries to the feet or hands that you need to be aware of. Make a general survey of the foot, ankle, and lower leg. Note any complaints that the person has.

➤ After grasping the foot with one hand, begin working on the big toe. The big toe corresponds to the head area and some people will even feel goosebumps on their scalp as you work on the toe. Proceed to the small toes, which cover the brain, sinuses, eyes, and ears. Work your way to the ball of the foot, which corresponds to the lung and heart area.

### Foot Note

Research scientists have found actual energy "spots" or areas that are different than normal energy (kind of like concentrations of energy) located under the skin at certain acupressure and acupuncture spots along the body! Some of these may be found on the soles of the feet. The researchers are using the acupuncture areas versus reflexology areas to try to validate this energy's existence; however, some acupuncture and reflex areas overlap, so keep your ears open to hear more on this exciting subject. Isn't it fun when science catches up with ancient "beliefs" and validates them for the skeptics?

➤ Work on the thyroid area, which is found all around the base of the big toe. Next work your way down the spine reflex and along the instep of the foot. The hip area is next; work your way from one side of the foot to the other. Cover each of the gonad points on either side of the ankle, and work across the top of the ankle to connect both points.

➤ Then, go back to the middle of the foot, working all the digestive and intestinal organs. Finish up the feet by "milking" the legs from the knees down and shake out the extra energy (see this technique in the next chapter under "Shake a Leg"). Proceed to the hands for a complete treatment.

➤ Leave the client to rest and go wash your hands. Come back with a glass of pure drinking water for your client and ask them how they feel.

The next chapters will give you the actual finger and hand techniques that you will use in this routine. Soon you will get really good at this and before long, good old Aunt Gretta will actually be bragging about you!

## The Least You Need to Know

➤ Before you get started, decide what kind of treatment you are going to perform (hands, feet, or both), how long it will take, and what position will be most comfortable.

➤ When you first start practicing reflexology, start at the top of the toes and work your way down. This will ensure that you cover everything.

➤ Everyone has a different level of pain tolerance. It will be up to you to use your common sense to determine how much pressure is enough.

➤ Always ask your subject if they have had injuries to the feet or hands before you begin working on them.

➤ Come back to the typical routine in this chapter when you have learned the actual finger techniques laid out in the next chapters, and use these techniques until you develop your own style.

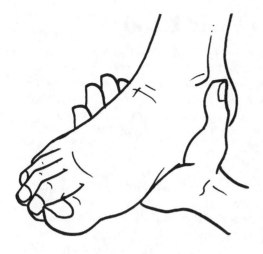

# Chapter 14

# Let Your Fingers Do the Walking

## In This Chapter

➤ Learn some of the basic techniques of reflexology

➤ Find out how to grip and support the foot

➤ Learn the joys of finger walking and thumb nibbling

➤ Understand facial clues from your partner that show when pain is not gain in reflexology

➤ Learn some lower-leg moves to complement a treatment

Did you know that the nursery rhyme "Rub a dub dub, three men in a tub" has nothing to do with reflexology? Rubbing is not really how reflexology is performed!

However, if you become a great reflexologist, you just might get to "rub shoulders" with some muckity-muck people (as some of my friends like to call them) who enjoy reflexology. I know at least one movie star couple who has a reflexologist make weekly house calls!

This chapter will show you that your positive attitude should be the only thing that rubs off on your client. Now let your fingers do the walkin' through this chapter.

### Tread Lightly

If you have a hand or finger injury, you shouldn't perform reflexology on yourself or others until you heal. You cannot be effective with an injury, and you may injure yourself further by applying pressure to an injured hand. You may want to use some tools on yourself, such as a foot roller (see Chapter 17, "Tools of the Trade"), until your hands/fingers recover fully.

# You're in Good Hands

First of all, always use both hands in reflexology. Remember that your goal is to help the person relax completely. They cannot do this if you are not supporting their feet or hands to stop them from moving away from your pressure. Gently support the foot from one side while you work with your finger and thumb techniques on the other.

For instance, if you are going to use a thumb-walking technique (we'll get to that in a minute) for the urinary system, which covers mostly the inside middle of the foot, you would want to thumb walk with one hand while you support the opposite side of the foot with the other hand. Check the following figure to see what I mean.

*Grasp the opposite side of the foot while working the urinary system reflexes.*

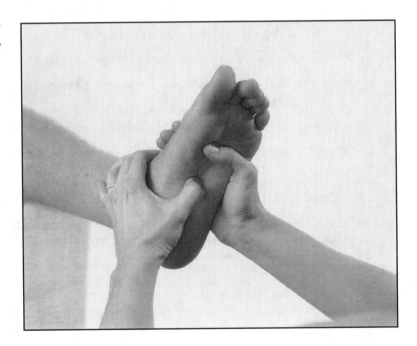

You want to use your supporting hand to secure the foot as close as possible to the area you are working on. For example, if you are working on the lung area (on the ball of the foot) with a thumb technique, you would use your other hand to support the top half of the foot, as shown in the following photo.

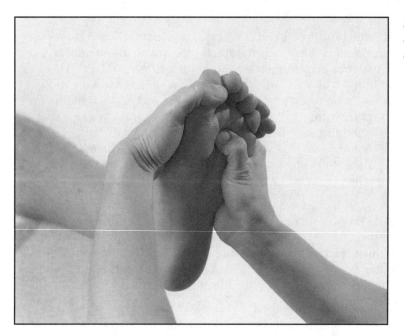

*Support the opposite side of the foot while working on the lung reflex area.*

By the way, you might have already guessed that a "rule of thumb" with finger techniques is that you keep your nails cut short! Sorry ladies, but the long fingernails just don't work well with reflexology. Keep them trimmed, and make sure the edges are well rounded so that you don't cause yourself or your subjects any discomfort.

Don't worry about not having big, strong hands or fingers for reflexology work. As you perform reflexology techniques, your hands will strengthen naturally. I will give you some tips in Chapter 21, "Healthy, Wealthy, and Wise: What You Need to Know," for things that will keep your fingers nimble. But for now, get your fingers into it and they will strengthen.

**Tip Toe**

Fingernails and thumbnails should be kept very short so that you can use your fingertips to stimulate reflex points and not your fingernails! Using your nails can cause discomfort.

# Finger Walking

Now let's take a look at some of the basic reflexology techniques. Reflexology is honest and straightforward, and so is its terminology. I like the simplicity of the reflexology terms, because they describe the technique and say exactly what they mean. The first one we'll look at is called *finger walking*, which is just what it sounds like.

The finger-walking technique is utilized in areas where it would be awkward to use the thumbs. Most of the techniques will feel very natural to you as you use them. For finger walking, you will use your fingers, mostly your pointer finger. To "get in position" put your hand out in front of you (left or right hand, whichever you are most comfortable with). Now take your middle finger and place the pad of the fingertip on top of the nail pad of the pointer finger. You will have effectively made a shape that resembles a capital "D." To use finger walking you will apply the tip of your pointer finger on the area of the foot or hand that you wish to work, and use the middle finger to "push down" on the pointer finger to apply pressure. The walking begins as you "inch" your way across a reflex.

If you imagine that your hand is dead weight—meaning that it is detached from your wrist and the rest of your arm (like "Thing" from the *Addams Family*), you can exaggerate the finger-walking technique by pulling or inching your hand along a flat surface by just using these two fingers. However, when you perform this technique on yourself or others, you will not drag your wrist across the foot, as in this example, but keep the wrist more level with the rest of your hand. With this technique the primary pressure will be under your pointer fingertip.

**Tip Toe**

Extra calcium and magnesium supplements have been helpful for many of my clients experiencing menstrual cramping. The essential oil of licorice root applied directly to the ovary and uterus reflex points has also helped me relieve menstrual pain almost immediately.

One of the primary uses for this technique is to walk around the top part of the foot from ankle to ankle. This area represents the fallopian tubes in women or the spermatic cord in men (see Chapter 12, "Sexy Stuff: The Glandular System") and also the pelvic area. If you were a massage therapist, it would be like massaging the lower back from one hip to the other. But this way you get a similar effect through the feet.

This area is good to work when a person has a sore lower back, sore hips, menstrual cramps, or any type of reproductive problems. Start from the middle of one side of the heel (around where the ovary/testes or uterus/prostate points are) and "walk" the fingers forward over the top of the foot to the other side of the heel.

Another way of using finger walking to work this same area is to hold the foot with both hands and place each pointer finger in the finger-walking position on either side of each ankle (inner and outer ankle where ovary/testes and uterus/prostate points are). In this position your thumbs will be under and below the heel of the foot. You can simultaneously finger walk up both sides and around the fallopian tube/spermatic cord reflex, with your fingers working their way toward each other. You will end when your fingertips come close to meeting in the middle (at about the top of the ankle). Just be sure not to pinch the skin when your fingers meet at the top!

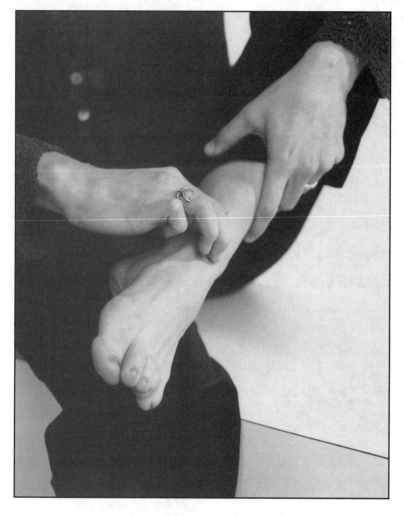

*Finger walking around the fallopian tube/pelvic region using a one-handed technique.*

Three main areas for using finger techniques are:

➤ For the fallopian tube/lower pelvic region

➤ For toe/finger squeezing

➤ For squeezing or walking along the lymphatic reflexes

There are no strict rules about when to use the fingers versus the thumbs, and you can use both all over the feet, ankles, hands, wrists, and wherever is comfortable. The next two photos will show you how to use your fingers for the toes and lymphatic system.

*Finger techniques for working the toes. This technique can also be used for the fingers in hand reflexology.*

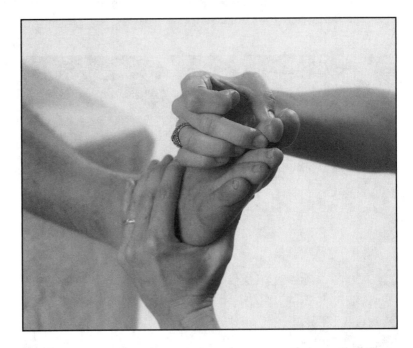

*Finger walking along the lymphatic system on the hand.*

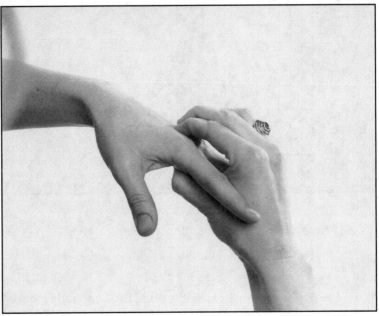

# Thumb Nibbling

*Thumb nibbling* is a term I use for the thumb technique that corresponds to finger walking (the correct term is *thumb walking*). Reflexologists use the term to describe a common technique that utilizes the thumb to stimulate reflex points.

The thumb is the most often utilized finger when giving treatments. The thumb is short and stout, which seems to give it more strength, and thus it can be used to stimulate those points that need deeper stimulation. If you roll the rest of your fingers into a loose fist and keep your thumb close to your fist, it will give your thumb more strength and leverage for some of the stimulation points we will use.

### Tip Toe

In reflexology your hands are your tools. Take good care of them and never do anything that is painful to you when performing reflexology. If you have arthritis in your hands and cannot perform reflexology on yourself at home, consider utilizing reflexology rollers, machines, or other tools between getting sessions from a professional.

Thumb nibbling sounds just like it works. The face of the nail will always point forward when thumb nibbling. You can pretend that the top of your thumbnail is like a "PacMan" (or Ms. PacMan if you prefer) eating his or her way across the crunchies of the foot!

Using the corner of your thumb to pinpoint deeper areas is good as long as your thumbnails are rounded. When you use the thumb or finger techniques, you will always "walk" with your fingernail in a forward motion (away from you). You'll find that this feels pretty natural.

A few of the many places you utilize thumb walking are:

➤ The central nervous system reflexes

➤ The digestive system reflexes

➤ The intestinal system reflexes

➤ The urinary system reflexes

➤ The respiratory areas

Check out the following photo to see an example of this technique used on the spine reflex. You can rest the fingers you aren't using on the opposite side of the foot when you are working in this location.

*Thumb walking along the spine reflex.*

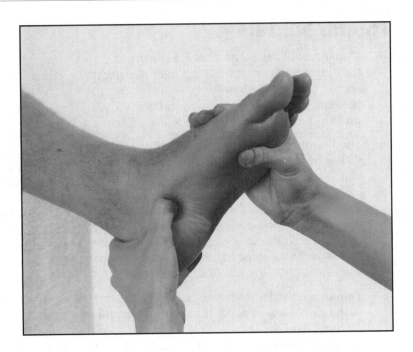

## Tip Toe

A tennis ball-size rubber ball makes a great hand exerciser and stress reliever. Squeeze the ball for a few minutes in each hand daily to build hand strength and keep your joints flexible. Here's a tip for stress relief: Buy a pale-colored rubber ball (or any other color besides red or orange, which can subtly inflame tension) and draw a big goofy face on it. Then name it. (Mine's name is Pulaski.) I take out Pulaski and squeeze him, he makes me laugh when I see him, and it eases my stress away!

# Pain Is Not Gain—Usually

Really, pain is not gain in anything we do—but a little discomfort sometimes helps us grow! The tender spots on the reflex areas, unless there is a local problem like a corn or a wart, are the areas that need to be worked. In Chapter 13, "Digging In: Where Do I Start?" we talked about the fact that everyone has their own pain tolerance levels, and you do need to be sensitive to them, but to be effective, you need to stir up a little discomfort every once in a while!

The pressure you exert when giving someone a treatment should be firm but not painful. Tender, like the almost-pleasant pain of a muscle ache or minor bruise, is okay. Pressure should be administered as deeply as the person can tolerate to be most effective. Look back at Chapter 13 for some more pointers.

Some people react to discomfort by saying "Wow, that's tender!" but if they say "*Ouch*! That *hurts*!!" you are going in too deep. Or, if you are a greenhorn, you may have inadvertently pinched the skin. You can also read the faces of the folks you are working on for a clue. This is especially true if you are using a chair and can see their faces when you work on them.

Use the following figures to help you read your client's facial expressions to see how you are doing. Figure A shows what someone experiencing bearable discomfort looks like. Figure B demonstrates that you have been successful at creating a euphoric feeling for your client. This will usually appear during the middle or end of the treatment.

If you are causing someone to look at you as shown in figure C, it more than likely indicates that you need to back off on how deeply you are working. Too much discomfort can bring out the worst in anyone!

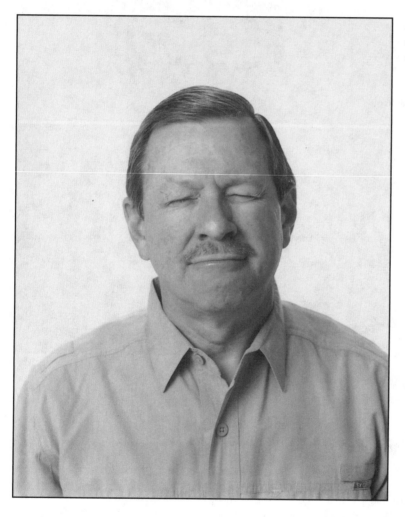

*Figure A: If your client looks like this, you are probably doing an effective job.*

*Figure B: Your client should look like this when you are finished.*

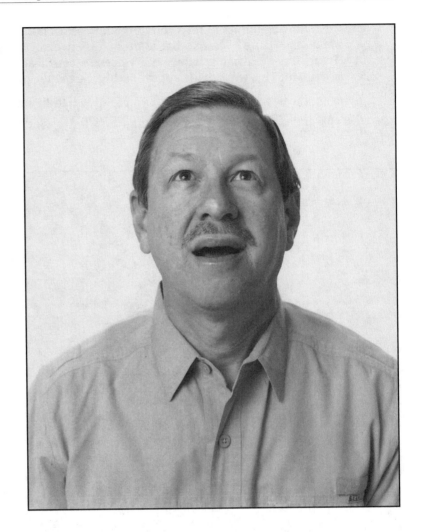

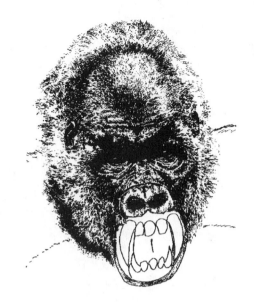

*Figure C: If you client looks like this, you are probably working too deeply. You might want to ease up on your treatment—or maybe run like hell.*

# Hooked on Reflexology

The preceding section should have given you a pretty good sense of how deep you can go and how to tell when to ease up. Now we are going to look at a technique that requires you to go pretty deep, and usually gets a distinct response.

*Hook and back up* is a technique mostly performed on those tough-to-get reflexes, such as the pituitary and pineal gland points (see Chapter 8, "What Nerve: The Nervous System"). They are glands in the brain, and their reflex points are located in the middle of each large toe, in the head area. These glands regulate myriad functions, so, needless to say, they are a popular spot to work on. Being endocrine glands, these glands also have a great influence on our hormones.

To access these points, you will need to "hook" your thumb into the location and then kind of pull upward and inward to stimulate the point, as shown in the following photo. This can be difficult to do, especially if you have fairly flat thumbs like I do. This is why some reflexologists will use a tool to find these points. (We'll discuss the pros and cons of tools in Chapter 17, "Tools of the Trade.")

**Tip Toe**

The pineal and pituitary glands are endocrine glands that regulate a host of functions in the body and may be helpful in regulating weight and controlling water retention, insomnia, and hormonal imbalances associated with PMS: acne, bloating, moodiness, and cravings. They are also used for dream enhancement.

**195**

To learn to do this technique with your thumb, you'll just have to keep practicing until you get it. You will know when you have found the pituitary and pineal spots because of the "electric shock" you will feel if you are working on yourself, or that your subject will no doubt tell you about, if you are working on someone else.

*Hook and back up technique: Use this technique to stimulate the pituitary and pineal reflexes. Be sure to support the toe firmly (not shown).*

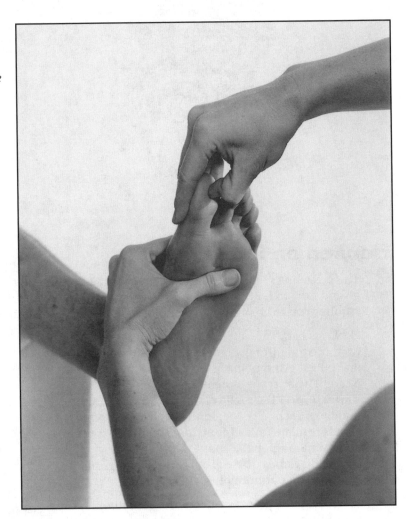

## Milk It for All It's Worth

A technique that you can end any reflexology session with is called "milking the leg" and can only be done if you are working on someone else. In other words, this one isn't a self-help technique, but it is nice for the person you are doing it to. Milking the leg is done just after you are done giving a complete reflexology session on the feet. Starting just below the knee, take both hands and wrap them around the calf. Gently squeeze both of your hands at the same time, loosen a bit, slide your hands down the leg toward the foot a few inches (without removing your hands), and squeeze again. Continue this process all the way down to the ankles, foot, and toes. This will take you about five to seven "squeezes," depending on how long the calf is.

You can work your way down, squeezing the foot in the same manner, and then "pull off" the energy at the tips of the toes with a grabbing motion. The best way to describe how to do this is to imagine that the person's leg is a rolled up, sopping wet towel. Your job is to squeeze the towel gently from the top all the way down, pushing all the water toward the end of the towel (the foot) and then pull off all the excess water at the bottom.

This technique is meant to cleanse a person's energy field, besides being relaxing to the body. Use this method to help pull out all the negativity and stress from a person.

### Foot Note

Milking the leg was a technique designed by one of my reflexology teachers as an extra treat for clients to cleanse negative energy and to revitalize the entire leg. The technique may not be covered in a reflexology class you take. Just as each reflexology chart you see will differ slightly, every teacher will have their own unique ways of teaching. So don't expect all classes to be completely identical, although most of the basics will be uniform, especially as the reflexology community begins to adapt specific standards. However, if you are lucky, you will get to learn some specialty moves from your instructors after you learn the basics.

## You're Pulling My Leg

To help stretch the lower back and help the person feel more relaxed after a reflexology treatment, you can gently pull on each leg. To do this, be sure to use both hands. When the person is lying flat on their back, simply grasp the underside of the knee with one of your hands and hold the bottom of the heel with the other.

Gently use your own body to tug softly at your subject's leg. You can do this by leaning your body back slowly in your chair. This technique will make the person feel that you have lengthened their leg a bit. Make sure that you do the same to the opposite leg. Balance is important! You can also shake the leg at this point, which is described in the following section.

## Shake a Leg

"Put your left foot in, take your left foot out, put your left foot in, and then you shake it all about! Do the hokey pokey and we turn ourselves about ... that's what it's all about!"

Not that I would consider reflexology hokey pokey (although some might), but shaking the leg at the end of a session sure seems to relax the entire body, and is a nice way to end a treatment. This technique is done very gently, and you will need to support the knee while you do it so you don't put extra *torque* on the knee. By torque, I mean any strain on the knee that makes it bend in a way it isn't designed to bend! This includes side to side and backward.

### The Sole Meaning

**Torque** is a turning or twisting force. In reflexology, you need to be careful not to torque the knee, since the knee is only designed to bend one way.

Support the back side of the knee with one hand, and rest the person's calf along the underside of your forearm. With your other hand, hold the bottom of the heel. With both hands, begin to gently shake the leg top to bottom and then side to side.

When you shake a leg side to side, you will be using the movement of your upper body more so than just your arms and hands. This helps the movement to be gentle and keeps the range of movement smaller. See the following photo to get a grip on how to shake a leg!

This is sure to be a hit with your subject. It helps to relax the whole body and can even ease tension in the lower back and hips.

Now you've learned how to support and grip the foot, how to finger and thumb walk, learned a few moves, and saw some general relaxation techniques. Now when you work on Aunt Gretta she'll think you've become a pro! Good job! Let's now build on all this knowledge in the next chapter where we really polish your skills and show you plenty more moves. Let's go!

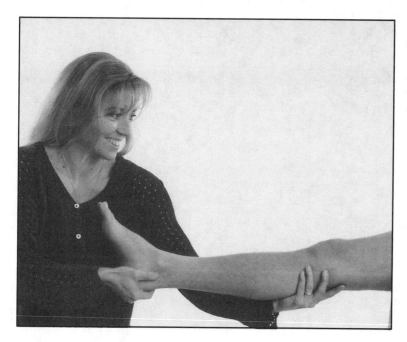

*The shake-a-leg technique. Be sure to support the knee when leg pulling or leg shaking. This technique is a great way to end a session.*

## The Least You Need to Know

➤ The terminology of reflexology matches the techniques and is quite straight-forward and easy to remember.

➤ Always use two hands when performing reflexology. One hand must always be supporting the foot or hand you're working on.

➤ Curl the rest of your fingers in when using your thumb techniques—this will lend the thumb more strength and support.

➤ Take clues from the person you are working on to determine how much pressure you should exert. Pressure should be as deep as can be tolerated.

➤ You can finish your treatment by gently pulling, shaking, and milking the legs from the knees down to enhance flexibility and relaxation and help clear negative energies.

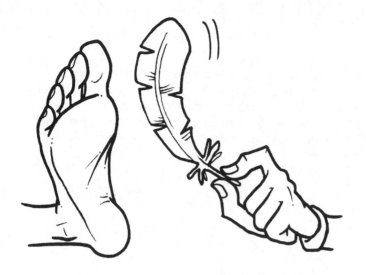

# Chapter 15

# How to Touch

## In This Chapter

➤ Gain insight into the subtleties of touch

➤ Discover the importance of maintaining contact

➤ Learn some circular and rotating techniques

➤ Find out what to do when working with an injured or ailing foot

➤ Learn the major contraindications for reflexology

Are you one of those people, like me, who love to have your feet rubbed? When I go to get a massage instead of reflexology, I ask the massage therapist to concentrate on my neck and then my feet. Even though she may not be a reflexologist, having my feet touched feels fantastic and relaxes me more than anything. However, once you have experienced a reflexology session from a trained reflexologist you will understand the powerful difference between reflexology and massage. You will also understand the differences between a professionally trained reflexologist and your partner who occasionally rubs your feet as a loving gesture. (Not that you should pass up that opportunity either!)

Massage works on the muscles and tendons and is a wonderful therapy, but reflexology works on energy, zones, and reflexes of only the feet, hands, or ears, and is a different experience. Let's take a closer look now at some of the similarities of touch that massage therapists and reflexologists *do* share, and then we will go into detail about when reflexology is *not* appropriate.

# A Healing Touch

Whether it's a personal touch, a touch of class, or a healing touch, touch is a very important aspect of our lives, central to reflexology in the same way it is important to touch the ones we love. Although you can use reflexology on yourself and gain beneficial results, having an experienced reflexologist work on you is an unsurpassed experience. When you work on someone or have someone work on you, there is an energy exchange that takes place between the touching of the feet and hands.

**Foot Note**

Our teacher encouraged us, after we had had much experience as reflexologists, to use our intuition when giving reflexology, keep our ego out of the way, and work the areas we "sensed" needed the most work. I find myself doing this with my clients at times. Something just "tells" me I need to work a particular spot. When I go to the spot, my client will usually look up at me and ask, "What's that?!" in response to the change in the feel of the area I work. I assume (although I cannot verify) that these intuitive areas that reflexologists learn to detect with experience are energy concentrations that need to be balanced through reflexology.

Touch is very important. In fact, it was discovered long ago that premature babies who were handled and stroked by their caretakers while in intensive care had a much greater survival rate than those who were not touched, or not touched as often. We are all connected, and we need to feel connected with each other. Touch is a way to establish and maintain this connection.

There is a difference between how I feel when I use my foot roller for reflexology and when my husband (my personal home-schooled reflexologist!) works on my feet. Subconsciously, you can convey messages through your touch. This is why I have dedicated a chapter of this book to the importance of touch.

It is not only important to touch correctly for health, but there are ways to touch professionally, and you will need to be aware of how to touch someone without making them uncomfortable. So onward through the techniques of touching!

# Keep Your Eyes on the Foot and Your Hands on the "Heel"

Giving reflexology sessions can be a thoroughly relaxing experience, and it can be easy to drift off. Keeping your eyes on the feet will help you stay focused and diminish the temptation to daydream while working on a person. This is especially true if you are working in a setting with a beautiful view out the window. If you gaze outside too long, you might find that you have worked your client's descending colon for 15 minutes (not necessarily a good place to find yourself)!

Even if you know the areas to work on by feel, it still helps to keep your attention on the foot and the areas that you are working on. You don't always have to stare directly at the foot or hand as you work, but keeping your gaze in that general direction is always a good idea. This will give confidence to the person that you are paying attention to them, and it will help you stay on track and appear professional.

Keeping both eyes and both hands always on the foot you are working on is a simple rule that will, more than likely, come naturally to you. As we discussed in the last chapter, one hand will need to be supporting the foot at all times, unless you are practicing techniques that use both hands at the same time. The next section will cover a couple of the two-handed techniques.

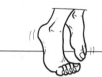

**Tip Toe**

If someone were working on your feet, would you rather have them intently watching what they are doing to you, or reading their mail as they work? Avoid being distracted while you work—remember that your goal is to help the person you are working on heal. They need your full attention to make this happen.

# Keep in Touch

When you first work on someone, you are basically introducing yourself (your hands) to their feet (or hands or ears as the case may be). Think about that for a moment. When we meet another person, we generally shake their hand. This is usually more true of men than of women, and it is more common in the American tradition, but nevertheless it happens worldwide.

When we touch another person information is exchanged through the touch. It is a subconscious process (although some of us make it a very conscious process) to judge someone by the feel of their handshake and the feel of their hand. Cold, sweaty, soft, or firm—all have different feels and mean different things to us.

**Tip Toe**

Kirlian photography reveals an electromagnetic field around all living creatures. Kirlian photography has been taken on the fingertips of a healer before, during, and after a healing session on another person. The energy of both the healer and subject was increased during and after the session!

**203**

# Don't Leave Me

When we make contact with another person in the physical form, we make more than just a contact. We exchange energy. Our cells communicate with one another. It is important that you try to keep that physical contact with the person's body throughout the reflexology session. When you are sending loving, healing thoughts to a person you are working on, their body will respond to you, and you don't want to break the flow.

However, there may be times when it is appropriate to break the flow. Your first concern should always be the person's comfort. Here are some cases when you may need to break contact:

➤ The need to use the restroom. This urge is often stimulated by the reflexology work you are doing.

➤ The need for a tissue. Sometimes your partner will release emotional tears during a session, or need to blow his or her nose, which also can be brought on by your reflexology work.

➤ The need for (another) blanket. Sometimes when a person lies still as you work on them they may get chilly. Stop and provide them a blanket so that they can fully enjoy the experience.

**Foot Note**

Many of my clients fall asleep while I work on them! Some say they try to fight it so that they don't miss any of the goodies, but they can't help themselves. One even took caffeine before he saw me because he loves the work I do so much he wanted to stay awake! He fell asleep anyway. I take it as a compliment that I have helped them to relax thoroughly, that they have enough security with me to be able to let themselves fall asleep, and that I have substantially gained their trust.

After making contact with the foot, if you break the contact completely, the body will respond to that change. It will keep your subject guessing at the subconscious level and will keep them from relaxing fully. If you do have to break off, start up again gently. Keeping at least one hand on the foot at all times is a way of not breaking contact. If you use music and you need to replay a CD, for example, try to use a remote control. This will allow you to keep contact with the person.

If you are using lotion or oil and need to apply some to your hands, then at least keep an elbow or a knee touching your client's foot while you get more lotion. It's like when you are driving and have to blow your nose—you use your knee for a moment to steer. Not that I would ever do a thing like that, officer, but the concept is the same!

Keeping contact during reflexology is like using the foot pedals on a piano. The foot pedals are used to keep the chords flowing. Without them, the chords do not blend together. Each time you lift your fingers off the keys and before you strike some new chords, you hear a break in the flow. This is the effect that you get if you are "pounding on the piano" or when you are playing allegro pieces like ragtime music. The touch you want to achieve with reflexology is like a flowing, smooth sonata. Keeping contact will allow you to create a relaxing, healing experience in which each touch builds upon the one before.

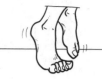

**Tip Toe**

Even if the person does not recognize it consciously, when you connect with them, they get a sense of security that you are there. That can be a very comforting feeling. This continuous contact will help the person relax and maintain a peaceful state.

## Good for the Sole

By the way, this contact-ual agreement you make with the foot is not necessarily just benefiting the person you are working on! You also get the benefits of reflexology as you work on another because your fingers are being stimulated. When you use your thumb and fingertip techniques, your brain and sinus area reflexes are being stimulated simultaneously.

The reflexologist always seems to benefit from doing this work. For instance, my body always responds positively after I work a day on clients. I feel energized, I feel clear and more alert, although I also feel very relaxed. I sleep better and my appetite is suppressed (meaning that I don't feel the need to overindulge in foods that are not best for me). Many times people comment afterward that I have a glow or my eyes look clear and bright after a day of giving reflexology. Reflexology not only gives the practitioner some physical benefits, but it may also be good for the soul. So, what I really am saying is "What's good for your sole is good for my soul." (I think that saying deserves a T-shirt!)

# Happiness Runs in a Circular Motion

So now we've learned about the energy exchange when you touch someone. Maybe that is why it feels nicer to have another work on you versus doing all your own reflexology work on yourself. Maybe somehow our bodies exchange energy and balance each other out in the process when we touch. In any case, now let's take a look

**Tip Toe**

The circle has always represented infinity, as it is a never-ending flow. When presented with a square or circle, those who think holistic or who tend to "go with the flow" many times choose a circle as their favorite shape, while those who may be more structured and organized will choose a square. Man needs straight lines in order to function in a more structured life. Nature is circular, and there are no straight lines in nature.

at some more wonderful techniques that you can use on your partner to induce relaxation. The following moves are all rotations and circular movements and will be like warm-up exercises for your body.

Circular motions are used in a roundabout way in reflexology. One of the first things you can do to loosen up the foot and to begin relaxation is called an *ankle rotation*. There are a few ways you can rotate the foot on its ankle. I have included some photos to show you how to hold the foot to perform these rotations. Remember that the foot does not revolve around you—you revolve around the foot!

## Ankle Rotation

The first and easiest way to perform an ankle rotation is the following:

➤ With one hand, cup the whole ankle like you are holding a large, hardboiled egg in your hand (support it, but don't squeeze too hard).

➤ With the other hand, grasp the ball (padding) of the foot. Do this by laying your four fingers across the top part of the foot just below the toes with your thumb across the ball of the foot, just below the toes.

➤ With the hand that is grasping the top of the foot, you will gently rotate the foot in a counterclockwise direction.

➤ Go s-l-o-w-l-y and stretch the foot as far as is comfortable for your partner.

➤ Rotate the foot three times counterclockwise, then three times clockwise.

Usually this will feel so good to the person that if you are not stretching it far enough they will "help" you by rotating the foot by themselves. Encourage them to relax if that happens and give them a wider stretch (circle). See the following photo for a look at this technique in action.

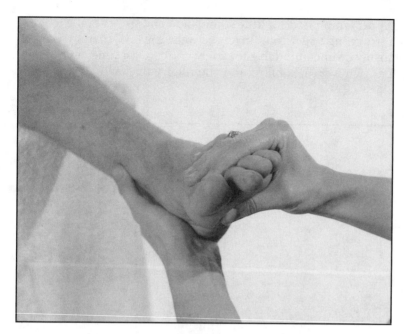

*Rotate the foot three times in a counterclockwise direction, then three times in a clockwise direction. Stretch the foot as far as comfortable.*

## Toe-Spreading Rotation

If the person you are working on has toes that have sufficient space between them, you can use another method for ankle rotation. The basic movements are the same, but the way you grasp the foot is different. Place your four fingers between the four spaces of the toes and then rotate, as shown in the next picture.

### Foot Note

An ex-ballerina client of mine loves reflexology, although she put her feet through torture during her dancing days. She tells me that her instructor would have the dancers place brillo pads in the tips of their ballerina shoes for motivation to keep their toes "up" inside the shoes! (And I thought high heels were bad!)

This method gives the upper lymph nodes a little stimulation and stretches the toes a bit. If you find yourself struggling to get your fingers between the toes, then bypass this method. It will probably be uncomfortable for your subject. Over time, reflexology sessions will help the toes gain more flexibility, and you can try this method in subsequent sessions.

*Use this method of ankle rotation if toe space permits!*

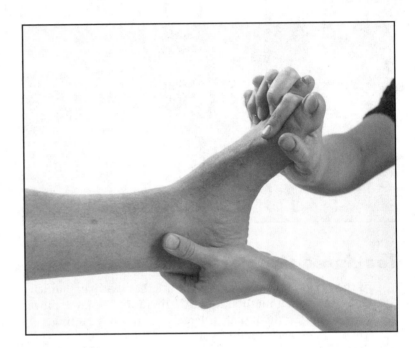

## Menstrual Relief Rotation

There is another form of foot/ankle rotation that you can use for relaxation and to stimulate the fallopian tube/spermatic cord/pelvic region (see Chapter 12, "Sexy Stuff: The Glandular System"). This is great for a stiff lower back or hips and for menstrual trouble or pain.

➤ Grasp the top side of the ankle from the front, with the webbing between your thumb and index finger pressing against the fallopian tube/spermatic cord region, as shown in the following photo. In this position, if your fingers are long enough, they will fall just about where the ovary/testes and uterus/prostate points are located on either side of the heel, which will stimulate these areas at the same time.

➤ With your other hand, grasp the top of the foot with the palm of your hand against the tops of the toes and your fingers overlapping the bottoms of the toes, kind of like you would grasp this book as you are pulling it off your shelf to read again! Use this hand to rotate the foot.

➤ When you get to the top of the foot in your rotation, rotate the foot into the webbing of the grasped hand to apply pressure to the fallopian tube/spermatic cord reflex.

You will also rotate the ankle three times in each direction using this method.

**Tread Lightly**

Reflexology should not be used in place of moving your body daily. Although reflexology is wonderful and stimulates the whole body, the feet were made for walking. Walking is one of the best exercises you can perform for the overall health of your body and your feet!

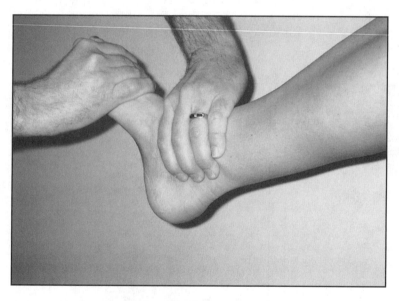

*This method is good if the person is having menstrual or prostate difficulties or a sore lower back or hips.*

## Finger and Thumb Rolls

Other circular motions involve using the finger and thumb techniques you learned in Chapter 14, "Let Your Fingers Do the Walking," and rolling them on the reflex points. For instance, the sex organ reflex points are excellent points to utilize finger and thumb rotations.

### The Sole Meaning

**Ovulation** occurs in females and is a term used to describe the time in a woman's menstrual cycle when the ovaries produce an egg and deliver the egg to the uterus to be (sometimes) fertilized. This process is controlled by the hormones secreted by the pituitary gland.

You can stimulate the ovary/testes point with the thumb or finger. This spot is on the outside of each foot about halfway between the ankle and heel (see Chapter 12, "Sexy Stuff: The Glandular System"). Find the area, apply a firm pressure, and rotate your thumb or finger on this spot without lifting it. Be sure that you are not just rotating your finger around the surface of the skin. You can try this technique on yourself easily by bringing up your foot, as shown in the following photo.

For the uterus/prostate point, which is in approximately the same location on the inside of the foot, you can perform the same technique using your fingers or thumb. Find the spot, press in, and rotate three times counterclockwise, then three times clockwise. You can also just press the point, hold it for three seconds, release, and repeat two more times. Both of these areas will more than likely be tender on most people. I find they are more tender on females the closer they are to their time of the month or near *ovulation* time. This spot is also great for someone who is experiencing menstrual cramps.

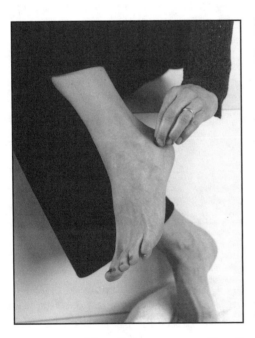 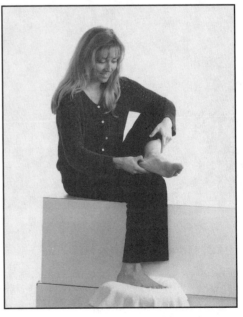

*You can use this technique on yourself easily or on others. Press in and rotate on each spot three times counterclockwise then three times clockwise.*

# *Tootsie Rolls and Rotating Toes*

Another rotating move that will get you rockin' and rollin' is what my teacher nicknamed "tootsie rolls." Tootsie rolls are another good warm-up technique to help the entire body relax and also can stimulate the sinuses to release congestion. Tootsie rolls and rotating toes can both be used to get a reflexology session started.

Tootsie rolls are just like miniature yummies (see Chapter 13, "Digging In: Where Do I Start?"). To make tootsie rolls, take each toe between the palm side of your fingers. Keeping your fingers straight, move each hand in an opposite direction and "roll" the toe between them. Do you remember

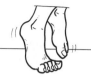

**Tip Toe**

Supplements that help curb sugar cravings include chromium (helps regulate blood sugar), licorice root (very sweet herb that can slightly raise blood sugar), and chickweed (mild appetite suppressant).

playing with Play-Doh when you were a child? Do you remember how to make snakes? You roll a blob of clay between your hands until it is a long snake-like piece. This is how tootsie rolls are performed!

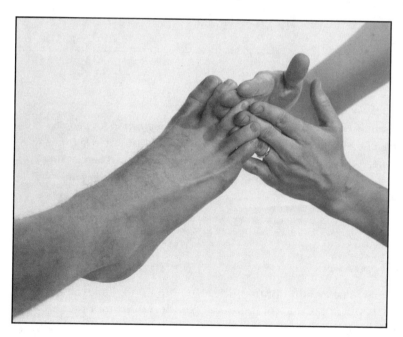

*Pretend you are making clay snakes while rolling each toe.*

A related technique involves rolling or rotating each toe and is fantastically relaxing. For this technique you will need to use one hand to give support to the ball of the foot at the base of the toes. Hold this part firmly. Grasp the baby toe at the tip and slowly rotate the toe three times counterclockwise and then three times clockwise. Since we are still imagining doing childhood things like making clay snakes, you can liken this toe rotating movement to mixing a Barbie-sized bowel of cake batter! If you remember, this technique is included in your 10-minute quickie routine in Chapter 13. Do this to each toe. Sometimes this will put someone to sleep right off the bat. Rotate the toes in a circle as wide as you can without discomfort to the client.

Remember the reflex for the head and neck is the large toe. Therefore, rotating the large toe is like doing neck rolls. If you feel crunchies as you rotate the large toe, this is a good indication of a stiff neck or that a neck vertebrae is out of alignment. Usually, after the rotations most, if not all, of the crunchies and crackling will disappear. The rotation will help loosen up the neck and may help it back into alignment. Sometimes pulsating, goosebumps, or a crawling sensation will be felt in the scalp or neck when rotating the toes—especially the large toe.

After rotating each toe, you can gently pull upward on the toes. Sometimes the toe will "pop" or crack. This might surprise the subject, but it should feel very good to them. This usually happens because the tootsie rolls and toe rotations loosened up the toes. If the toe was misaligned at all, a gentle pull will sometime cause the toe to go back into alignment. Do not do this forcefully. A gentle pull will most likely do the trick.

### Foot Note

In my experience, reflexology seems to be an effective pain-relieving session for people with arthritic feet. One of these particular clients gained great relief that would last for days after my sessions. At times, I accidentally would "pop" his toes, which caused him to jump. Afterward he would tell me how much better the "popped" toes felt, and he began requesting that I do it every time.

## No Pinching Allowed

When practicing reflexology be careful not to pinch or pull the skin. Reflexology involves techniques that apply pressure, rotations, and gentle, but firm movements. Pulling, rubbing, or pinching the skin is not what you want to do.

To avoid this, when you are moving up the foot or hand with finger or thumb walking, make sure you lift your fingers up just enough to let the skin fall back into place. Or use some talcum powder or a dab of oil to help your fingers slide over the skin. This is especially helpful when the person you are working on has very dry or scaly skin.

Touch is important, but how you touch is even more important. You will need to learn to be aware of every way your body is interacting with another. This is true for all types of bodywork. You need to be especially aware of what your other hand is doing when you are working on the body with one hand. For instance, when thumb walking across the lung reflexes, be sure that the fingernails of the supporting hand are not digging into the skin.

## Bedside Manner

I think a term that would fit what I am talking about here could be *bedside manner*, a term used to describe how doctors interact with their patients. You will need to have a good bedside manner to be an effective reflexologist. But a good bedside manner in reflexology is more than just acting and behaving professionally.

First of all, as you already know, keep your fingernails trimmed. Second, don't forget about warming your hands before you touch someone! Rub your hands vigorously together or keep a warmed towel nearby to heat up your hands before you start working on someone. This is part of good bedside manner, too.

**The Sole Meaning**

**Bedside manner** is a term used to describe how a doctor behaves in front of or toward a patient. Reflexologists also need to develop a good bedside manner to make the recipient feel comfortable, at ease, relaxed, and well cared for.

## Diamonds on the Soles of Her Shoes

Additionally, be aware of *both* hands and other things that might touch your client. For example, you probably want to take off any bulky jewelry that could interfere with a session. Your client won't like it if you get their leg or toe hairs stuck in your watchband! Ouch!

Because you are so focused on the techniques you are doing with one hand, don't become oblivious to the fact that a diamond from your wedding ring is sticking into your client's foot! Speaking of that, I wonder if that is where songwriter Paul Simon got the idea for his '80s hit "Diamonds on the Soles of Her Shoes"?

**Tip Toe**

Before working on a partner, always ask them to remove all their jewelry before you begin working on them. Not all folks are willing to take off their wedding ring, which is fine, so be sensitive to the issue. It is easier to work on a foot or hand with no jewelry, but you can always work around it if you must!

**213**

# Injured Areas: Don't Go There

The first rule in as a reflexologist—before you even get started with all these fun techniques—is to make a visual observation of the foot. You will need to look for injuries, cuts, and other ailments. As a reflexologist working professionally, you might make it a habit to chart all the conditions of the foot to keep records on the person you work on, and to chart changes in the tender spots you find. Like a dentist charts the teeth the first time he examines you, a reflexologist may create a similar record.

You do not want to work directly on any injured areas. It is also important not to work on someone else if you have any contagious conditions yourself, such as fungus growths (athlete's foot, for example, is a fungus that can grow on the hands, too). If you have a contagious ailment, it may spread through an open cut on your hand, so wait until you are over it before you work on others. Some reflexologists have worn sterile rubber gloves to work on folks for the protection of both the client and the reflexologist, although this is rare.

## Edema, Got the Dropsy's?

One contraindication for reflexology is working on a client with edema in the feet, more properly referred to as dropsy. Many of us hold excess water occasionally, especially women before menstruation. This type of edema is referred to as subcutaneous edema and is not very serious. Keeping the legs elevated usually corrects this condition.

But edema or dropsy is an excessive accumulation of fluid in the body tissues. This condition is serious because there may be collections of fluid in the chest cavity and in the air spaces of the lung (pulmonary edema) causing severe chest congestion. Edema may result from heart or kidney failure, cirrhosis of the liver, allergies, or drugs. If you have severe swelling of the legs, feet, and ankles from dropsy, do not work on these areas directly. Instead, work on the hands, and get to your medical physician immediately.

## Varicose Veins, Varying the Treatment

Most of us are familiar with varicose veins. Varicose veins are veins that are long and distended and can appear purple when you see them just under the surface of the skin. The superficial veins of the legs are most commonly affected. There may be an inherited tendency to varicose veins, but it is aggravated or can be caused by an obstruction of blood flow in the body.

The tiny broken blood vessels you sometimes see on your feet may indicate a problem with the circulatory system in general, and you should consider seeing a holistic health practitioner to help you strengthen your circulatory system nutritionally.

If you have knotty, irregular-shaped, or dilated varicose veins, reflexology would be contraindicated. You should not reflex these areas if you have them or if you are working on someone with them. You can work the corresponding part instead, but do not work directly on the area. For instance, when you find irregular varicose veins in the left foot, you can gently work the left hand instead.

Contraindications are warning signs. You will need to know them if you decide to become a certified reflexologist, nationally or internationally, and you should be aware of them even if you only plan to work on yourself or your friends. The major contraindications were touched on above and some more are listed in the following table. When you see these things, you should apply caution or choose to not to work on someone. Always refer your client or friends to their physician for any medical necessities! If you see an injured foot, you always have the option to work on the corresponding hand instead, and vice versa.

**The Sole Meaning**

A **contraindication** is a term meaning any factor that makes it unwise to pursue a certain line of treatment. For a light example, you would not give a massage to a person with a severe sunburn!

## Reflexology Contraindications

| Foot or Client Condition | Why You Shouldn't Go There | What to Do Instead |
| --- | --- | --- |
| Knotty, irregular-shaped, or dilated varicose veins | Reflexology may put too much pressure on these veins and break more blood vessels | Work around these areas or work the corresponding part instead (i.e., for varicose veins in left calf, work left forearm) |
| Severe swelling of the foot (edema) | Could mean insufficient blood flow and blockage of lymph system, could also mean heart disease | Refer this person to their doctor immediately and work the hands |
| Fractures, surgeries, or sprains | Could interfere with healing | Do not work directly on; work the same side corresponding part (i.e., wrist fracture on left wrist, work left ankle instead) |
| Contagious diseases or infections in either the client or practitioner | For the health protection of all involved | Wait until the infection has cleared |

*continues*

## Reflexology Contraindications  (continued)

| Foot or Client Condition | Why You Shouldn't Go There | What to Do Instead |
| --- | --- | --- |
| Open wounds | Health protection | Wait until the wound has healed (to facilitate healing, work the corresponding part far removed from open wound) |
| Ingrown toenails or corns | Can cause pain | Don't work directly on these areas; refer to podiatrist |
| Gout | Could raise blood pressure and cause discomfort | Work lightly and discuss the contraindication with the client; do not work on swollen area, instead work on kidneys, adrenals, and pancreas reflexes; refer to herbalist or holistic nutritionist for nutritional support |

Reflexology relies on the interconnectedness of the whole body and the energy zones (zone therapy) that run along our body channels (see Chapter 1, "What Is Reflexology?"). Knowing this, when dealing with a contraindication, we can still work on an area of the body that runs along the same energy lines, but on a different part of the body.

Say for instance you broke or sprained your right ankle. Your first goal will probably be to get someone to take you to the doctor for treatment. In the meantime, you can apply ice to the ankle (first aid), and then you can begin "reflexing" your right wrist to facilitate healing and possibly alleviate the pain in your ankle. During the healing process, working the corresponding wrist will help your ankle heal. Don't forget to work the other wrist too, however, since the body needs balance. But it is okay to work the corresponding wrist more, since that is the side of the body that will require more energy for healing.

To sum up, overall, be aware of both of your hands, pay attention to your client, keep in contact, and look for contraindications, and you will be on the road to becoming a very effective and appreciated reflexologist!

## The Least You Need to Know

➤ Keep your eyes on the areas you are working on to stay focused and to gain your subject's confidence.

➤ Keeping physical contact throughout a reflexology appointment will help your partner relax more thoroughly and will keep the energy exchange flowing.

➤ Be aware of both hands when performing reflexology. Be sure not to pinch the skin, and don't forget to remove your jewelry and have your partner remove theirs.

➤ Before performing any reflexology techniques you first need to observe the area you are going to work on. If you locate any injuries, cuts, ulcers, or other ailments, do not work there.

➤ Be aware of the contraindications to reflexology, and be sure to allow for them before you begin.

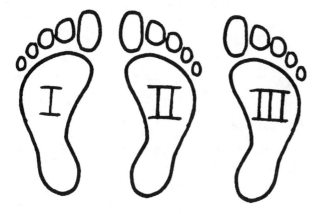

# Chapter 16

# Third Time's a Charm

---

**In This Chapter**

➤ Discover the mystery of the number three

➤ Learn why reflexologists do everything three times

➤ Understand how reflexology works on more than the physical level

➤ Find out how to use your knuckles, and how not to

➤ Learn some gripping, stretching, and twisting techniques

---

Well, now you know about all the rolling and rotating techniques and you find yourself relaxed and looking forward to more. Have you wondered why I keep instructing you to do each move and rotation three times? Well, even if you haven't wondered, I'm still going to give you some reasons in this chapter! After some philosophical talk on the mystery of threes, I'll introduce you to three new reflexology techniques you can use three times each to make you feel three times as good!

## Doing the Math

The meaning of numbers underlies everything in our lives. There are certain meanings attached to numbers that go deep into humanity's early beginnings, as taught in the Jewish Kaballa. Have you ever given any thought to how we use numbers in everything we do? Our modern world couldn't exist as we know it without this framework that numbers give us. Could our whole reality be a giant math problem? Imagine that!

For instance, you are now reading Chapter 16 and are on a certain page number and have been reading for a certain number of minutes or hours. You live at an address with numbers in it, and you need numbers to make a phone call. We all have some sort of identifying number, such as a Social Security number or a tax ID number. Names can even be broken down into numbers and then analyzed (as in numerology).

### Foot Note

Numerology is the study of numbers and their synchronicity in our lives. Here is a brief association that some have made to the base numbers:

| | |
|---|---|
| One—beginnings | Six—creativity |
| Two—union | Seven—luck |
| Three—balance | Eight—money |
| Four—structure | Nine—completion |
| Five—nurturing | |

Ten is considered one (1 + 0 = 1). In numerology, numbers are added together to get a one-digit number. For instance, if your address is 43 Pinecone Way, your number for your home would be 4 + 3 = 7. A place to live that will bring luck! This is just a generalization to introduce you to the concept. Consult *The Complete Idiot's Guide to Astrology* (Alpha Books, 1997) and *The Complete Idiot's Guide to Numerology* (Alpha Books, 1999) for more details on this fun subject.

Think about trying to buy this book without the use of numbers in the transaction! You'll never make it, will you? You will find this book in a bookstore with a certain address, in a certain numbered aisle, on a certain row number, with a certain price on it. Most places will charge you a certain percentage in tax, and you will need a certain amount of money to pay for it!

Reflexology is no exception. Most of our sessions will be timed to last a certain number of minutes, and we will charge a certain amount of money. Furthermore, we usually work with two feet and 10 toes. Reflexologists take this one step further, though, and use a particular number as a basis for their work: the number three.

## The Mystery of Threes

Why is it that the third time's a charm? And why were there three little pigs, three bears, three blind mice, and Three Stooges? Why do they say bad things happen in threes? Why do I only get three wishes and have to knock three times on the ceiling if I want you?

The mystery of threes has not yet been unlocked, although its roots can be linked to Christianity and the Trinity of Father, Son, and Holy Spirit. But most of us haven't really given much thought to the mystery of the number three. I like threes because they always give us a middle ground:

➤ Small, medium, large

➤ Past, present, future

➤ Short, average, tall

➤ Left, middle, right

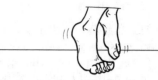

You can always choose the middle ground if you are unsure, but only if you have three choices to begin with. I like the middle choice for simple decisions because it can take the stress out of the decision-making process. The medium size is what the "average" person requires. People choose the middle ground for peaceful negotiations.

**Tip Toe**

If it's true that the third time is a charm, then using the rule of threes in reflexology will help you to have quite a charming practice!

Besides, the middle choice seems to be more balanced. Not that there is no validity in extremes, but the middle is usually where most of us function. Three may be a number that forces one to integrate. I see it as a peaceful number. There is black, and there is white. Both extremes are easy to understand because both are clear-cut. However, dealing with someone who is purely black or white in their thinking leaves no room for compromise. Many can live with some things in the gray areas.

**Foot Note**

In numerology, the three stands for the trinity, creativity, great strength, completion, and the integration of the physical, mental, and spiritual. It can be a complete number. You could think of the scales of justice. The scales need one scale on opposite sides and a middle piece that connects both.

In transcendental analysis there are three types of personalities, or aspects of ourselves: the adult, the parent, and the child. Each of these has distinct characteristics, but all coexist in each person. For example, you would not speak to a business associate the way you would to your young son! You would use the adult aspect of your personality with another adult.

For the purpose of reflexology, you will want to practice your techniques with the number three in mind. Each technique should be performed three times. For example, if you are doing rotations, rotate the foot three times each direction. When you are utilizing pressure points, press and hold three seconds, then release. Repeat for a total of three times.

The client should also be instructed to come see you three times in a row (such as three times weekly or once a week for three weeks, depending on the condition of the client) to get them off on the right foot. Then they should continue regular sessions for a minimum of three months for lasting effects.

# Body, Mind, and Sole

Physically, reflexology is beneficial to the recipient and the person who administers it. But it goes even further than just stimulating our mutual reflex points. It can also have an effect on all three parts of us: our body, our mind, and our spirit.

**Tip Toe**

An old wives tale says that whatever you do comes back to you three-fold. If you abide by this, then put out only what you wouldn't mind coming back to you three times as strong!

We talked earlier about the importance of touch and the energy that is exchanged. Touch can make a person's body feel good, and it also can positively affect the mind. When you are being touched in a healing way it can trigger a self-love response in your subconscious. The fact that you have allowed someone to care for you and help you heal means that you have taken time out to care for yourself. Self-love can have a positive effect on the immune system as well.

Why does reflexology work on the practitioner's spirit? Well, when you are taking care of someone with reflexology, it is usually because you have an inner urge to help people or a calling to heal. I believe that this inner urging or calling comes from the spirit or soul. Anything that you feel in your heart and soul that you need to do should be expressed.

The heart is the seat of the soul and cannot give you messages to do harm. Of course, the heart/soul's desire always need to be tempered with the intellect. But there should be no denying your deep calling to do what you are meant to do. Your heart will communicate with you.

**Foot Note**

English doctor and homeopath Edward Bach believed that reality begins in the ethers. When we are in tune with these messages, or when we follow our intuition, we are at one with our purpose in life. If we choose to ignore these messages, we go against our purpose in life and experience illness, accidents, and other problems. According to Bach, illness and "bad luck" are the divine's last attempt to wake us up and show us we are not living the life we were meant to live. On this theory, Bach created his famous flower essences, meant to help us attune to higher frequencies and ease us back into alignment with our purpose, which changes our health.

# Knead Me, Heel Me

Although it's a cute pun, reflexologists really don't knead anybody! (Although most *need* their clients, and hopefully their clients need them!) Kneading is really more a term for kneading dough, and massage therapists also use this term loosely as a play on words for their work, too.

Reflexologists use their hands as their tools to work on their clients. There are some reflexologists who employ tools in their practice, however, and we will cover that subject in depth in the next chapter. But for the most part, the reflexologist's hands are their biggest assets. Some reflexology organizations prohibit the use of knuckles during a reflexology session since they consider the use of knuckles a tool or because they believe knuckles can exert too much pressure on a client.

If you prefer deep work and wish to work on yourself at home, feel free to use your knuckles, foot rollers, or any other tools you want as long as you use your own common sense to determine what is helpful for you and what might hurt you. You know your pain tolerance better than anyone, and hopefully you live in a free country where your privacy is not infringed upon to help yourself at home in whatever legal manner you wish!

## Knuckling In

Some of the self-help techniques you can apply in reflexology can be done with your knuckles. The knuckles can exert much more pressure than your thumb or fingers alone and should be used carefully if you choose to use them on a family member.

223

**Tread Lightly**

Some reflexology organizations consider the use of knuckles outside the scope of reflexology. Therefore, if you use your knuckles, use them on yourself only or exert your own judgment and become a reflexologist and join the ranks of those who advocate occasional knuckle usage. The goal of the healer should be to unify and promote professionalism and care amongst practitioners, not to divide over specifics.

I especially like to use my knuckles to work my heel. The heel represents the lower pelvic region and hip area. To use this method, you can perform a kind of knuckle walk with the middle knuckle of your pointer finger of one hand while you support the ankle with the other, as shown in the following photo.

Use your knuckle and walk across from one side of the heel to the other. This technique really helps stimulate the circulation to the various areas. This is a great therapy if you have trouble with any of the following:

➤ Hip pain

➤ Lower-back pain

➤ Pelvic troubles

➤ Hemorrhoids

Just for fun, if you are a Three Stooges fan, you may want to say "Knuck, knuck, knuck" as you knuckle walk across your foot.

*Knuckle walking: A great method if you have hemorrhoids or hip, back, or pelvic troubles.*

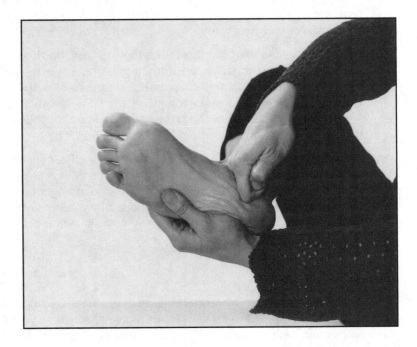

## I Can Breathe Clearly Now

Another method that utilizes the knuckles is great for the respiratory system, chest, lungs, bronchial tubes, diaphragm, back, and neck. To use this technique, follow these steps:

➤ Support the metatarsal bones (top of the foot) with one hand.

➤ Bend all four fingers in toward the palm of the other hand, but don't touch your fingertips to your palm as you would with a fist.

➤ Gently press your knuckles into the padding of the foot below the toes with one hand as you support the top of the foot with the other.

➤ Hold for three seconds, release, then repeat two more times.

Take a look at the following photo to see this technique in action.

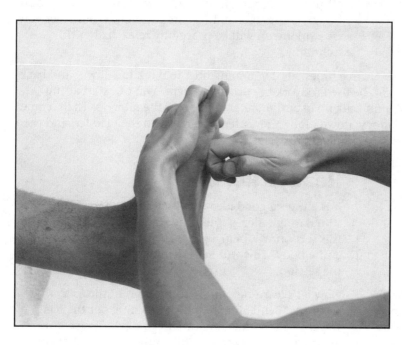

*This technique can aid the chest, lungs, bronchial tubes, diaphragm, back, and neck. Hold for three seconds, release, and repeat two more times.*

# Up, Down, and Back Again

Another great move that comes in threes is walking up the spine reflex. When we discussed the spine in earlier chapters, you learned that the spine gives us structure, but it also houses the main nervous system cables, putting it in both the structural system and nervous system categories. Working this reflex is wonderfully relaxing, and although this reflex can be worked indefinitely, you should remember to cover it at least three times.

Thumb walking is great for walking up the spine reflex. Start at the bottom of the heel with your thumb and walk all the way to the top of the large toe. When you get to the top, turn around and "walk back down" again. Up one more time and you are through. Whomever you are working on will be peacefully relaxed after this technique.

**Tip Toe**

In general, working a certain reflex area three times will help give balance to your reflexology sessions. You can always go back after you have reflexed everything three times and work more on the tender spots, since these are the areas that will usually require more work.

You can always get your "three times" in if you remember to work up, down, and back again. This technique can be used to work the urinary system. You can start at the bladder reflex area, thumb walk up over the ureter, and on to the kidneys. Then, come back down from the kidney, down along the ureter tube reflex to the bladder, and then one more time back up to complete the cycle.

# Ready? Relax!

It is always a good idea to loosen up the feet before stimulating reflex points. The stretching techniques in this section will help a person relax their legs, feet, and entire body. This will help them get more benefit out of the session.

**Tread Lightly**

Never push or shove the foot in any direction it does not want to go, nor farther than what is comfortable for your subject.

Now let's learn *three* more techniques in the following sections: "Bend and Stretch" (stretching out the feet to get them warmed up for reflexology), "Twist and Shout" (a spinal twist you'll be sure to shout about), and "Wringing Out the Stress" (another squeezing and wringing technique for relaxation).

## Bend and Stretch

The first one we are going to learn is a stretching technique that helps the person's whole leg relax, especially the back of the calves and hamstrings. This technique also gets the feet and ankles loosened up and helps increase circulation and prepare the person to respond better to reflexology. Here's how to do it:

**Tread Lightly**

Be careful not to pull or tug on the hair on the legs whenever you are practicing techniques where you are touching the lower part of the leg.

➤ First, cup the underside of the heel in the palm of your hand. This is the same grip we used to rotate the feet in the last chapter.

➤ Next, grasp the top part of the foot with your other hand. This is also the same grip you used with the rotation techniques. Be sure to not squeeze the foot on top and pinch the skin! The grip should come naturally. Your hand will grasp the outside of the foot around the ball with your thumb resting on the inside padding of the ball of the foot.

➤ Pull the top part of the foot toward you slowly as far as is comfortable for the person. Hold for a moment to allow the muscles to relax into the stretch. Instruct the person to exhale as you stretch the muscle.

➤ Do not grip the heel tightly. Let it move naturally with the stretch.

➤ Then push the top of the foot gently back toward the person as far as it will go. You can use the heel of your hand to push at the pad of the ball of the foot to get a good stretch. Hold this position momentarily. You do not want to hold this position for too long, as it could cause the foot to cramp.

➤ If the foot seems very stiff, try one of the rotating techniques from Chapter 15 first or a yummy, then try this stretch again. If the person has a lot of tension in their legs this stretch will help them to be more flexible.

And I bet you'll never guess how many times you should do this stretch. You're right—repeat this procedure three times back and forth on each foot. You can see this technique in action in the following two photos.

*Stretching technique step 1: Stretch the foot forward (toward you) and hold momentarily to let the muscles ease into the stretch.*

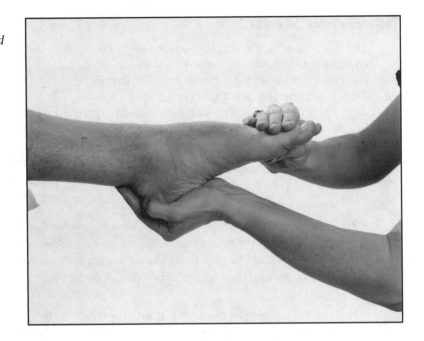

*Stretching technique step 2: Push the foot gently back (toward subject's knee) and hold only briefly to avoid causing a cramp.*

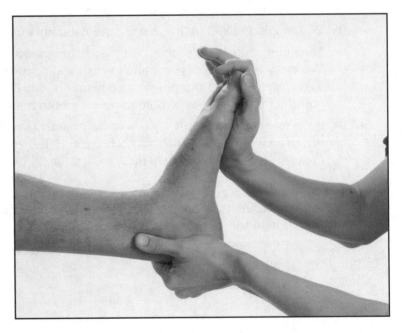

# Twist and Shout

Next is a twisting technique used by practitioners to relax the body. It can even have an effect on the alignment of the spinal column. In fact, we call it a "spinal twist"!

To perform this technique, take a look at the next two photos and follow these steps:

➤ Grasp the top (dorsal side) of the foot, just below the ankle. Both of your hands should grasp the foot firmly and your thumbs should be resting on the inside sole of the foot, just above the heel.

**Foot Note**

You can adapt the bend and stretch stretching technique to suit the four directions if you'd rather. Here's how: After stretching the foot to the front and then the back, stretch the foot to the inside (medially), while steadying the heel. Then move the foot laterally as far as the recipient will allow. Do each stretch the same number of times. You have done the four directions. Now rotate the foot in a circular motion counterclockwise, then clockwise.

➤ Begin moving the hand closest to the toes in short, firm motions, twisting the foot from side to side. Keep the other hand firmly holding the rest of the foot.

➤ After a few "twists" move both hands slightly up (toward the toes) and twist again. You can work this motion all the way up to the top part of the toes.

➤ Once you get to the toes, you can begin the same motion back down toward the heel again.

➤ And, you guessed it, you will go back up one more time for a total of three times on each foot.

This technique will help relax all the back muscles and is extremely rejuvenating to the entire body.

*Spinal twist starting point: Begin at the heel and work your way up, slightly, twisting the hand closest to the toes. This works the entire spinal region.*

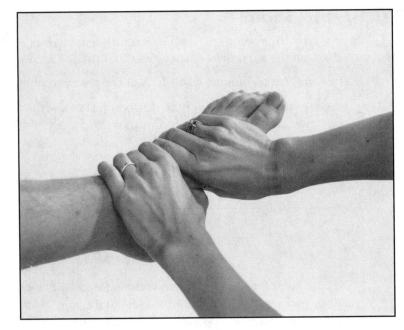

*Spinal twist ending point: When you get to the toes, work your way back down again to the heel, and then go back up one more time.*

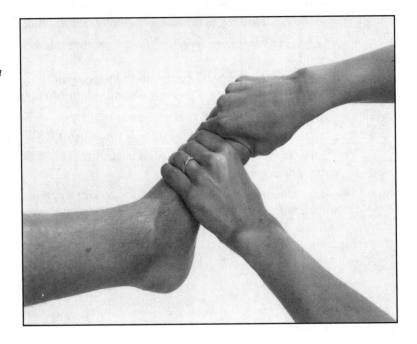

# Wringing Out the Stress

The third relaxation technique covered in this chapter involves wringing the foot. This will open up the lymphatic system and is good for any type of chest congestion. For this technique you can imagine the foot is a sopping wet towel or mop. Your job is to wring out the excess water. (Just remember that you don't need to squeeze it dry!) Does the wringing technique ring a bell with you? It should. It is similar to the spinal twist, but is slower and involves more squeezing.

To perform this technique:

➤ Lay your fingers across the top part of the foot.

➤ Place your hands one just above the other, reaching in from opposite sides of the foot. In this position your thumbs will be on the plantar (underside) surface of the foot.

➤ Gently squeeze both hands as you slightly turn each hand in an opposite direction.

➤ Move slowly upward and repeat two more times, moving from the ankle on up to the toes each time.

**Tip Toe**

When you are squeezing and stretching the foot in these and other techniques, keep in mind it is the same as squeezing the whole body, kind of like hugging! When you hug someone, squeezing too tight is uncomfortable, but if you squeeze too lightly you appear insincere—so go for the third choice, which is *just right!*

The following photo will help you get a grip on things. Be careful not to pull the skin on this one!

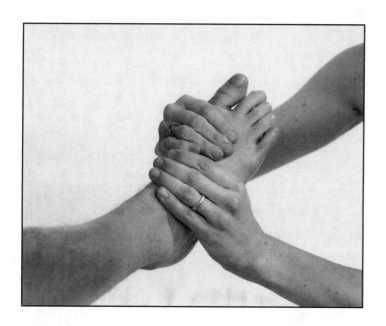

*Wringing the foot: Pretend the foot is a sopping wet towel and you are to wring out the excess water.*

I hope that these three new techniques, stretching, twisting, and wringing, will bring you and your partner a great deal of pleasure, and that pleasure will be experienced threefold by making you healthy, wealthy, and wise!

---

### The Least You Need to Know

➤ The number three symbolizes the integration of the physical, mental, and spiritual aspects of a person, which is a goal of reflexology. Reflexology not only works on the physical body, but can have far-reaching, positive effects on the mind and spirit.

➤ In reflexology you practice each technique three times on each foot or hand.

➤ You can use your knuckles if your thumbs are tired. The knuckles can be used to exert more pressure along tougher areas such as the heel. Be aware, though, that this is not considered a legitimate technique by some people, and be conscious of your subject's needs.

➤ Twisting, wringing, and stretching the feet are all great techniques for bringing more flexibility to the leg, foot, and ankle and can enhance a reflexology session by helping the person relax.

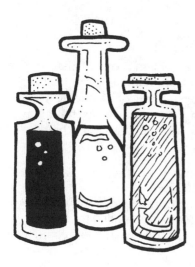

# Chapter 17

# Tools of the Trade

---

## In This Chapter

➤ Learn how essential oils can enhance reflexology treatments

➤ Consider some warnings about the use of tools in reflexology and hear about the pros and cons

➤ Find out about some of the tools that reflexologists use

➤ Learn about professional chairs and tables

---

A milestone in the evolution of man is when we discovered how to make and use tools. If this is true, then is a reflexologist who uses tools more evolved than one that doesn't?

Well, probably not, but there are some earnest differences on either side of this issue. From the use of lotions and oils on the foot to wooden probes, there are reflexologists that swear by them and swear at them!

Here we will take a look at some of the controversy regarding tools and give you a brief look at some of them. Some of the tools are designed for self-use, but if you want to get nationally certified in the United States, you better leave your tools at home!

Next, we'll take a look at aromatherapy (the use of aromatic essential oils). If you are not interested in becoming a reflexologist by now, then you won't hurt my feelings if you skip the section on the pros and cons of utilizing tools in your reflexology practice. But catch up with me again when we talk about some tools that can be used for home use when we get to the "Tools You Can Use" section.

# Oils, Potions, and Lotions, Oh My!

The use or application of essential oils during a reflexology session is considered beyond the scope of reflexology practice, probably because aromatherapy can be its own separate practice. Aromatherapists have a deep understanding of the medicinal uses and application of essential oils. Reflexologists are not aromatherapists, but many become both. And some reflexologists just utilize the oils on a casual basis in their work area. Let's take a look at why the use of essential oils is so popular with reflexologists.

Some of the largest pores of the skin are on the soles of the feet. As we saw earlier, our skin not only eliminates waste materials (sweat), but also absorbs what is applied to it. Since the pores are larger on the sole, they can absorb whatever is applied to them more efficiently than other areas. Makes you really want to watch what you step in, doesn't it?

But there are some very nice things you can absorb through your feet, like essential oils. The use of essential oils is a whole topic in itself, probably deserving of its own *Idiot's Guide*. I think one of the greatest uses of essential oils is as an application on the feet and hands. And what better time to apply them than before or after a reflexology treatment?

The use of essential oils involves the principles of *aromatherapy*, the therapeutic use of smells to gain a positive, desired effect on the body and the emotions. The oils can be used in a number of ways, including the following:

➤ Applied directly to the skin

➤ Diffused in the air

➤ Put on a cotton ball and inhaled

➤ Dabbed on the tongue (only *some* oils can be used in this way, such as peppermint or spearmint; many oils can be toxic if taken internally)

➤ Added to bath water

➤ Added to massage lotions, shampoos, and other beauty products for enhanced smell or medicinal purposes

**The Sole Meaning**

**Aromatherapy** is the therapeutic use of aroma to gain a positive, desired effect on the body and the emotions.

Essential oils, derived from plants and flowers, trees, bark, roots, and leaves, are the distilled essence of the plant. These oils can be used as medicines and should be chosen carefully. (See Chapter 3, "Reflecting on History," for a list of some favorites.)

Essential oils vary greatly in their quality, so if you want the pure stuff that gives you therapeutic benefits, you will have to investigate this yourself. See Appendix B, "Supplies and Where to Find Them," for some connections, or consult your local aromatherapist.

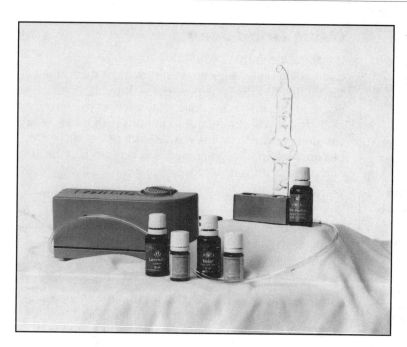

*Aromatherapy essential oils and diffuser: Essential oils can complement reflexology treatments.*

# Lovely Lavender Oil

Lavender oil is one of the most widely used oils in the world. It is effective for dozens, if not hundreds, of ailments from dissolving scars on the skin to relieving PMS. This oil has been used most commonly to induce relaxation, and some use it as a sleep aid.

Diffusing lavender in the room before you give a reflexology session to someone who is stressed can be a good way to assist their relaxation. A dab or two applied to each foot before or after treatment can also help someone relax into the benefits of reflexology.

Lavender can also be useful for headaches. Rubbing a tiny bit on the temples or base of the skull can help relieve tension in the face, jaw, and head. Other oils that are known for their relaxing benefits include:

➤ Chamomile

➤ Tangerine

➤ Angelica

➤ Jasmine

➤ Orange

**Tread Lightly**

You should always ask your partner to smell an oil before using it on them. The aromas have different effects for different folks and just because something smells good to you doesn't mean it smells good to someone else. Get permission before you share your oils!

### The Sole Meaning

A **hertz frequency** is a measurement of vibrational frequency and energy levels. Everything is composed of energy and therefore has a certain vibration. These frequencies are also measured in kilohertz (kHz). For example, a normal, healthy human ranges in frequency from 62 to 78 kHz. It is believed that we are receptive to colds at 58 kHz, to flu at 56 to 57 kHz, to cancer at 42 kHz, and at 25 kHz, death begins. Grade A essential oils start at 52 kHz and go clear up to 320 kHz, and may help us raise our own frequencies!

## Using Good Scents

If you decide to share your oils with someone you are going to do reflexology on, you should let them smell the oil first to make sure it agrees with them. If you don't do this first, you could get a reaction you weren't ready for! If you choose not to use oils with others, you should consider them for yourself as a practitioner. Pure oils are high in *hertz frequencies* and can facilitate health and protect us from airborne germs.

Usually people come to see me who are ailing in some way. In order to protect my own immune system, I wear one of my protective oils such as angelica or frankincense—or as my husband jokingly calls it, "Frankie scents." Also, diffusing the oils in your reflexology room can keep airborne germs at bay.

Another tip for using essential oils in reflexology is to put a few drops on a warm, wet washcloth and "wash" your client's feet before you begin. The hot cloth will warm the feet, which feels good. Tea-tree oil is antifungal and antibacterial so this helps protect you from any unseen bacteria on your client's feet! Or you can add a few drops of oil to a warm footbath prior to the reflexology session. After you wash the feet, make sure you wrap one of them in a warm towel while you are working on the other. This will ensure that the foot won't get chilly during the therapy.

### Foot Note

New equipment developed by Bruce Tanio of Tanio Technologies (also head of the Department of Agriculture, University of Washington) was used in a Johns Hopkins study to determine the frequency of humans, food, and the relationship of frequency to disease. Holding a cup of coffee dropped one man from 67 kHz to 56 kHz, down to 52 kHz when the coffee touched his lips, and down to 48 kHz when he drank the coffee! Another test dropped a man from 65 kHz to 48 kHz by holding a cigarette, and down to 42 kHz when he smoked it! Other tests proved negative thoughts drop frequency as much as 12 kHz. Positive or prayerful thoughts raise our frequency, so keep thinking positive!

# The Tool Debate

Lotions, essential oils, knuckles, wooden probes, and electronic tools utilized during a reflexology session are all prohibited or considered beyond the scope of practice for many reflexology association members. Although I do not personally use tools in my practice, I do stand firmly in the middle on the issue and will present the information without prejudice. However, I do use some of the tools shown in the photographs in this chapter on my own feet and hands, and I thought you might want to try them, too!

My interest in the controversy over the use of tools by reflexologists prompted me to include this material to let you consider whether there is a controversy at all and if so, why. I like to get to the bottom of all matters, especially ones that leave me with a question mark! I find that when everyone understands the whole picture, we can usually live together better or *at least* agree to disagree.

To present this information to you so that you can go into this field more informed, I interviewed two different people, who I hoped would lend insight to the tool issue and put a rest to the rumors! The first is well-known tool advocate Zachary B. Brinkerhoff, III, Director of the Modern Institute of Reflexology in Denver, Colorado, and the other is Barbara Mosier, Director of a national certification organization, the American Reflexologist Certification Board (ARCB) in Littleton, Colorado. You will hear from them both in this chapter.

### Tip Toe

Flying west anytime soon? Believe it or not, there are reflexologists at the Salt Lake City Airport and at Denver International Airport. What a great way to fill up your layover time and unwind from a hectic day of travel! I have heard that the one in Utah uses essential oils in his work—so give both a try and tell them where you heard about their practice!

## Using Whatever Works

Tool advocates say that tools can make reflexology more efficient. The tool advocates believe in a "whatever works" philosophy. Advocates also say that not all people can perform reflexology effectively or deeply without the use of tools to stimulate the deeper pressure points. They say that the proper utilization of tools can open up the practice of reflexology to those who may not be able to apply pressure to specific points effectively and can make a nice enhancement for the tool users' clients.

Advocates of wooden probes and even electronic devices designed to be used during reflexology treatments say that these tools offer the reflexologist

### Tread Lightly

Some say that using tools overworks and damages the reflexes and their corresponding organs, throwing the body into a very heavy cleansing process.

a way to get the job done more effectively in a shorter amount of time and will save the reflexologist's finger joints in the long run.

Dr. Zachary B. Brinkerhoff, III, Director of the Modern Institute of Reflexology, personally utilizes and instructs reflexologists in how to properly use tools in their practice. He says, "It's the '90s, and we are into modern practice. If a reflexologist can do a better job by utilizing tools, then I believe that he or she should retain that freedom of choice."

## All Thumbs

Reasons for opposing tool or other applications to the foot vary. Lotions and oils are restricted by some of the major reflexology organizations because they believe that lubrication may cause a reflexologist to slip off of a reflex point.

There are many schools, teachers, and certification programs available that will privately certify you, and there are also some organizations that are not related to a specific school that will certify reflexologists who can prove a high level of hands-on competency, a large volume of documented hands-on work, and a high score on a written reflexology exam. These boards will help unify the practice of reflexology by setting national standards for the practice.

To qualify for certification you must prove that you have actually taken a training course in reflexology. These boards are nonbiased and therefore do not discriminate or favor one school/teacher or type of training over another, as long as you prove that you understand the concept, theory, and practice of reflexology and anatomy and pass their testing procedures.

Since the ARCB is one of these boards, and is working toward setting national and international standards for reflexology, I wanted to understand how the issue of tool use was viewed. Barbara Mosier, the director of the ARCB, was kind enough to grant me an interview. When I questioned her about the controversy over the use of tools for reflexologists she stated,

> "There is no controversy over the use of tools. ARCB tests on the American standard thumb- and finger-walking techniques only. Testing on the use of tools is outside our scope of practice, as ARCB does not have the knowledge or expertise to test the skill level of applied technique and client-patient reaction with the use of tools."

### Foot Note

I met a Chinese couple while traveling and the wife claimed she gave her husband a foot reflexology treatment by pounding on his soles with her fists! I heard no complaints from the husband and both were smiling. In Taiwan I have seen sharp wooden probes in reflexologist's hands that I would run from! But I think the bottom line comes down to touch. Let's not loose the wonderful energy exchange we get from touching one another.

Maybe there is no issue on tools after all, but for now I stand in the middle, advocating freedom of choice, personal responsibility, and high standards of professionalism. I have seen all sorts of slants on reflexology and have not heard of any being harmful. I hope that reflexologists can and will unite on this subject so we can continue to promote the practice as a whole, and not in fragmented pieces. If tools are just an issue that the national certification boards choose not to recognize, then you should use your discretion, and, for that matter, you should use your discretion for anything and everything! If your goal is certification in the U.S., however, you might want to understand the position of the board you are testing with first.

So to sum up, I've put together a table for you on the pros and cons I have heard from both sides of the fence. I hope this helps in keeping your view balanced, too.

| Tool/Application | Pro | Con |
|---|---|---|
| Lotions | Makes some finger- and thumb-walking techniques smoother; better feel for client | Practitioner may slip off point |
| Essential oils | Can serve therapeutic effect and enhance reflexology session; can serve as antibacterial protection for client and practitioner | Practitioner may slip off point |

*continues*

*continued*

| Tool/Application | Pro | Con |
|---|---|---|
| Wooden probes and nonpowered tools | Saves practitioner's joints; enhances some techniques for practitioner when used for stimulating certain "tough to get" reflex points; requires less strength from practitioner | No feedback for practitioner through touch; may go too deep |
| Electronic machines | Time effective; can stimulate faster healing by performing deeper percussion/ stimulation | Harmful to the delicate balance of nature; loss of human touch; loss of need for practitioner; too harsh; creates rapid and unwanted cleansing reactions in recipient |

My advice is for you to carefully use all the tools you like on yourself. But most important, learn how to use your hands and fingers as tools, and remember the importance of healing that comes with touch. Then if you choose, take some training from a competent school or teacher who teaches the proper uses of tools before you utilize them.

**Tip Toe**

Some reflexologists utilize lights with various color gels for the application of color therapy before, during, or after a reflexology session. Color is energy and works by affecting the energy around you.

## Tools You Can Use

Now that we've looked at the pros and cons of using tools, let's take a look at a few of the tools themselves. Many things can be used as tools, from everyday items to those designed especially for reflexology, and you can find tools that are designed for a wide variety of uses.

Some reflexology tools, such as wooden foot rollers, are used as self-massagers. Foot rollers are usually wooden and resemble rolling pins with grooves carved into them. They are meant for rolling beneath your foot while you work or sit and are great for using under your desk while you are busy working at your computer!

# Havin' a Ball

There are rubber balls with pointed rubber tips that folks use to work on themselves. I find that the rubber points are especially useful for stimulating the pineal and pituitary reflexes on your own thumbs. Remember these spots? They are located about in the middle of your thumb pads and your large toe pads. You will know when you find the spot because you will feel a "zing" when you hit it. You can also rub the ball between your hands for an allover stimulating effect.

You might notice a metal tool in one of the photographs in this chapter. This instrument is called an acupressure device and is commonly used to work specific acupressure or reflex points on the ears. The tiny ball on the end prevents puncturing the skin. Study up on the acupressure points on the ears to see what it might affect before deciding to try it.

### Foot Note

Just the other day at a restaurant we noticed a waiter had his ear pierced in the strangest place, not on the earlobe itself, but through the little projecting area in the middle of the ear closest to the face. I don't know what the technical term for that part of the ear is, but I remembered from my chart at home that it corresponded to the stomach. We questioned the waiter about his earring, and he said that he had it pierced recently. I then inquired how his stomach was, and he said that actually it hadn't felt so good since his piercing! What do you think? Coincidence or synchronicity?

Here's a list of some nonpowered tools that some use to stimulate reflexology areas on the feet and hands. (If you can't wait to get your hands [or feet] on some of these, check out Appendix B, "Supplies and Where to Get Them.")

➤ **Wooden probes:** All shapes and sizes from pointed to dull-ended to three-pronged, such as the Happy Massager

➤ **Wooden foot rollers:** Used to roll under your feet while sitting or standing

➤ **"Buzz" balls:** Rubber balls with pointed rubber tips to roll in between your hands or under your foot

➤ **Wooden rollers:** Wheel-like devices similar to pizza cutters, used for rolling over reflex areas

Actually, I consider the corner edge of my coffee table my personal self-reflexology tool. I have also been known to use a rubber pencil eraser on myself to stimulate some tender spots.

*Some tools of the trade used by reflexologists.*

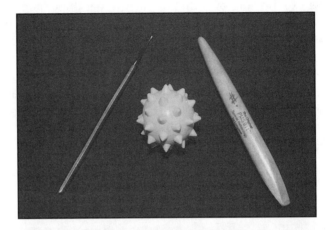

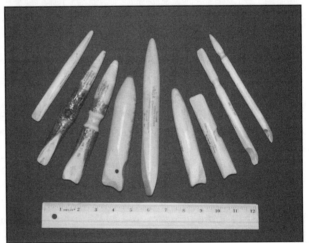

## Probing the Subject

There are several types of wooden probes that can be used to stimulate reflex points, but when using a probe you should be careful not to push too hard. You will need to get a feel for the probe you work with and pretend that it is just an extension of your own finger or thumb.

The disadvantage of using a piece of wood while working on another person is that you may not get the same feedback you would using your own thumb or finger, although those experienced in using probes say that they can in fact detect "crunchies" and other feelings using probes.

Pencil erasers are another tool that some reflexologists use, although they are obviously not designed for reflexology. The hard, small rubber eraser on the end of an unsharpened pencil seems to be a perfect probe for reaching spots that need a more pointed pressure technique.

Students of the late Eunice Ingham claim that Eunice would use a pencil eraser at times on her students to demonstrate stimulating pressure points. For someone with relatively flat thumbs like me, it is difficult to stimulate my pituitary and pineal points without the aid of a rubber-ended tool.

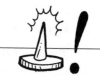

**Tread Lightly**

If you decide to work with a wooden probe to stimulate reflex points, be careful not to push too hard. Get a feel for the probe you work with and pretend that it is just an extension of your own finger or thumb.

# Plug-In Tools for Toe Jammin'

Now, it's time to go beyond your average, nonpowered, wooden, handcrafted reflexology tools and examine the Tim Taylor version—HIGH POWERED plug-in tools.

This could definitely be considered a manly man thing, but the machines do not discriminate. Now let's get plugging and turn up the juice. Oh, and by the way, these plug-in tools are never to be used while you are in a moving automobile or immersed in water.

## Reflex Pro Machine, Percuss-O-Ramma!

The Percuss-O-Matic is a pneumatic-powered "jackhammer" that is used to deliver between 600 and 10,000 impacts per minute to the plantar aspect of the feet or palms of the hands.

The Percuss-O-Matic is similar to the Reflex Pro, which is a solenoid-powered linear percussion device that can complement finger techniques by working all the reflexes in the toes, ankles, and the dorsum of the foot. This machine has six speeds from 60 to 3,600 impacts per second!

These machines are both handheld percussive massagers that produce a lineal, piston-like action for focused pulsation. A suction cup–like end works the foot. The Percuss-O-Matic is especially intended for use on the heel, but can be used over the entire foot.

Zachary B. Brinkerhoff, III, of the Modern Institute of Reflexology says, "Percussion massage energy is not only designed to increase blood circulation through reflex stimulation, but to stimulate the negative DC electrical circuitry of the body, which incites repair and regeneration at the cellular level."

## Electric Foot Rollers

Electric-powered foot rollers are used by some to prepare the subject for a clinical reflexology session by releasing adhesions in the joints, ligaments, tendons, and muscles of the feet or hands. These machines are excellent for home treatment between visits to the reflexologist. Some foot rollers are floor-mounted machines designed for use while lying on your back. You rest your feet or the back of your ankles (Achilles tendon) on the roller when lying down or sitting with your legs stretched out in front of you.

Similar to the foot rollers is the Chi Machine, designed also as a floor device that you rest the back of your heels in as you lie on the floor. This machine "shakes" your legs and claims to have positive effects on the spinal column, stimulate aerobic activity, oxygenate the body, and increase lymphatic flow, which aids the immune system. This is a noninvasive gentle rocking of the whole body which massages internal organs and aids digestion and elimination, energizes, and relaxes.

## This Machine Sucks

The VacuFlex is a machine used by South African reflexologist and author Inge Dougans. This machine is a piece of equipment that resembles astronaut boots! Both feet are put into the VacuFlex at the same time. This device uses cupping, acupressure, and vacuum suction to produce stimulation for feet that are in poor shape. Dougans claims it is especially helpful for epileptics or folks whose muscles tend to cramp or spasm during hands-on reflexology.

Low- and high-powered lasers are also being used to stimulate reflex points on the feet, the hands, and the

**The Sole Meaning**

The **Reflex Pro Massager** is an FDA-approved therapeutic percussion massage appliance. This machine is the evolution of the original Percuss-O-Matic invented in 1944 by Robert C. McShirley, Sr., then modified by Dr. Clemet T. Wittman, D.N., who founded the Modern Institute of Reflexology.

**Tip Toe**

The next time you are in a Jacuzzi, try concentrating the jets on the soles of your feet and the palms of your hands. You'll be amazed at how good this can make you feel!

ears. Laser light can facilitate a change in energy frequencies and help heal the body energetically. I see this could be one of the up-and-coming healing modalities since we all are becoming more and more aware of the light, color, and vibrational aspects of our universe.

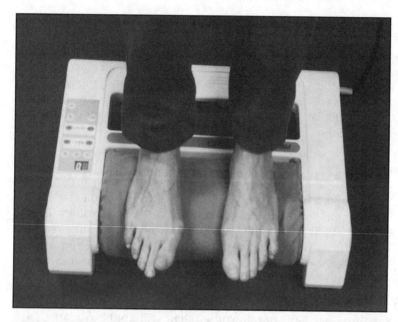

*Some high-powered tools used for reflexology: a foot roller (top) and the Percuss-O-Matic (bottom). (Photo compliments of Modern Institute of Reflexology)*

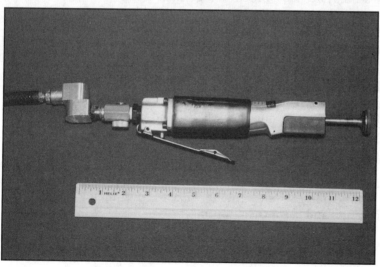

**Tread Lightly**

Beware of giving up your individual freedom to choose by trying to make personal opinions into governmental issues. Leave the government to rule over the big issues, not everyday choices. Keep reflexology in the hands of the good people who practice it by supporting those you agree with, and not fighting against those you disagree with.

As you can see, there are many devices that can be used to render reflexology-style treatments and achieve similar effects. It will be up to the practitioner to go with what they feel best doing. However, I suggest you start out learning and using the pure hand-to-foot techniques first.

It will also be up to each client of reflexology to find the practitioner that they are most comfortable and happy with. After all, this is what makes holistic health unique. Reflexology and natural health are all about empowering others to take care of themselves naturally. Empowerment is self-responsibility. If you aren't comfortable with a particular practitioner, try someone else until you find the one who works best for you.

# Pull Up a Chair

Back in Chapter 13, "Digging In: Where Do I Start?" we got you prepared and situated to give reflexology. Back then I assumed that you were at a family reunion and were working on Aunt Gretta on the couch or a bed. However, if you are going to become a reflexology pro, you will want to gather up some supplies for your work to help get you prepared for starting your own practice.

The first requirement is that your subject be comfortable. If you travel as much as I do to see clients, sometimes a massage table or reflexology chair will not be available. In these cases, both you and your subject will have to improvise. I have performed reflexology on folks lying on couches, in La-Z-Boy chairs, and on the floor. These can all make comfortable places for you and your subject if you are creative.

Remember that another requirement for positioning yourself is that your subject's feet are centered with your torso when you sit at their feet. This gives you the best position to administer pressure. Make sure that you are comfortable as well. If you have to reach too high or too low to work on a foot, your arms will tire and you won't be as effective.

## Tables and Chairs

If you use a massage table, have the person lie on their back. Then place something under their knees to keep them from overextending. I like to cover up my clients, which makes them feel secure and keeps them warm.

Sometimes a person will move about or fidget if they are uncomfortable or will lift their head up to talk to you. Try to make them comfortable. It is important to discourage the person from lifting their head, which will put strain on their neck and keep them from relaxing completely. If they must hold their neck up, prop them up with more pillows, or move them to a chair.

If you use a reflexology chair with a locking mechanism, have the subject lean all the way back and lock the chair in place. The advantage of working on someone in a chair is that you get to watch your subject's facial expressions. This will help give you clues as to how they are doing and, more important, how well you are doing.

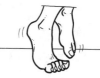

**Tip Toe**

When subjects fidget on your table or chair, try to make sure they are comfortable. If they continue to fidget, tell them "Even my honest clients lie still." See if they won't get your drift and try to relax into the treatment.

Utilizing a reflexology chair versus a massage table where the client lies on their back is up to the practitioner and the client. I find that the chair seems to encourage more of a casual session, since the chair keeps the person you are working on facing you. This position naturally prompts folks to chat with you. The massage table keeps them lying down, and clients may feel more comfortable drifting off or closing their eyes while you work on them.

Some people who have breathing difficulties such as emphysema or severe asthma may not be able to lie flat and will usually require a chair or a way to be propped up. Other than client requirements/preference, the use of a chair or table is really up to you.

## Some Favorites

Among my favorites are LaFuma chairs, designed so that when the person leans all the way back their feet come up to the perfect position for practicing reflexology. Hand-made in France, these chairs are not cheap, but are extremely comfortable.

They also fold up nicely like a beach lounge chair and make it easy for you to take to your family gatherings, health fairs, or to make house calls. Many massage tables these days are also portable. Go with what you are most comfortable with or what is most convenient for you.

*The LaFuma chair (left) and a reflexologist's knee chair (right).*

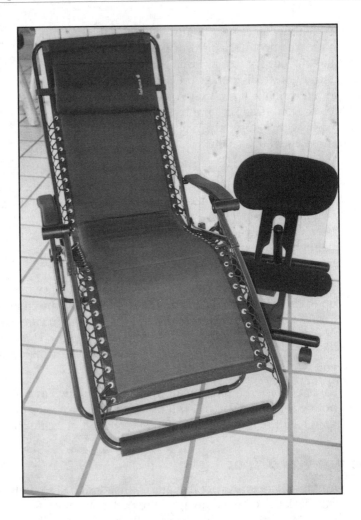

**Tip Toe**

Soaking an injured wrist or ankle in a tea made from comfrey has helped many heal quickly. Comfrey is an herb that may be purchased in bulk at your local health food store or herbal shop.

A great chair that I find works well for the reflexologist to sit in is a type of chair that has rollers and two pads, one for your knees and one for your bum. These chairs are designed for you to kneel in, keep you somewhat low to the ground, and give your knees some padding. The position keeps your back straight, which is better overall for your posture and spinal health.

Ultimately, the most important thing to remember is that whatever kinds of chairs, tables, or tools you choose to use, they should be comfortable for you and the people you work on. See Appendix B for places to find tools, chairs, and tables. And have fun putting your own personality into your work!

## The Least You Need to Know

➤ Aromatherapy and the use of essential oils on the feet are excellent additions to reflexology and can facilitate emotional as well as physical healing.

➤ Reflexologists should use their own fingers and thumbs as their only tools to learn how to practice reflexology. After that, the decision to use tools should be a personal one. As a client, choose a practitioner and techniques you feel most comfortable with.

➤ There is an abundance of tools, both powered and nonpowered, utilized by reflexologists worldwide. Use your own discretion about which tools, if any, you choose to work with.

➤ Reflexologists have a wide range of professional tables and chairs to choose from. They are designed to position the client's feet at about solar plexus level.

➤ When choosing tables, chairs, and tools, keep the comfort and safety of both the client and the practitioner in mind.

# Part 4
# The Practice of Reflexology

*We've talked a lot about how to practice reflexology on someone in a general sense. Now let's learn how to read a foot! In a way it's like palm reading, but instead of the palm you will read the sole.*

*When you start working on other people's feet, you will naturally be exposed to many different types of foot problems. Remember, you are not a foot doctor so we won't be getting into diagnosis, but it would be to your advantage, as well as your client's, to know how to recognize some of the foot ailments you are going to see.*

*Then we will end this section with some tips to start you off on the right foot if you'd like to have a career in reflexology. Here you can learn some of the extras that can make your sessions more holistic and keep your clients coming back for more!*

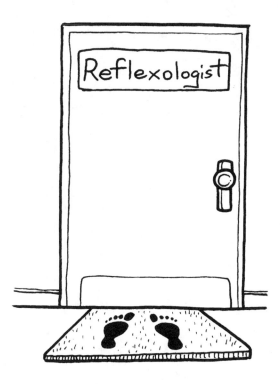

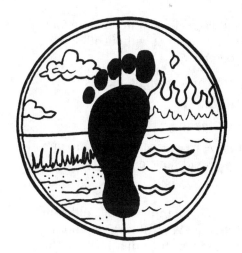

# Chapter 18

# Finding Balance: The Elemental Foot

> ## In This Chapter
>
> ➤ Discover how to relate the condition of the foot to the four elements
>
> ➤ Understand some imbalances and what might cause them
>
> ➤ Learn how to best handle imbalances in foot conditions
>
> ➤ See how feet reflect imbalance in the rest of the body

Becoming a reflexologist can be an interesting journey, since you will work with many different types of people one-on-one and see many different feet. You will begin to make associations with conditions of the feet and the condition of a person. You may also get to understand more about the four elements and the balance they serve in all aspects of our lives. Let's take a closer look at how observing the feet can help the thoughtful observer learn something about the foot owner.

## The Four Elements Revisited

In this chapter we will again take a look at the four-element model we discussed way back in Chapter 4, "The Foot at a Glance." You will be able to put all the foot ailments you encounter into one of the four categories on the chart. This is intended to help you understand the "nature" of the problem you are dealing with.

When you understand how the elements interact with each other, you are better able to discover an appropriate solution. Fighting fire with fire doesn't put out the fire. But throw on some earth and you will see much better results.

### The Sole Meaning

Air, fire, water, and earth make up all four basic elements on our planet. Nothing can exist without all four present. The **four-element model** is used as a tool to teach a philosophical way of seeing the elements in everything we do.

You need a balance of each element in your life for health. The world could not exist without all of the elements working together:

➤ The sun (fire) to provide light and heat

➤ The air to breathe

➤ The water to drink

➤ The earth to give us a place to stand and provide structure and provide an element to grow food from

You will learn how to look at things from a different perspective in this chapter. We will look at various conditions of the feet and see how they relate to the four-element model and learn how the model can help us deal with an imbalance of the elements in the body.

*This chart shows some foot conditions associated with each element. The condition is caused by an overabundance of the element.*

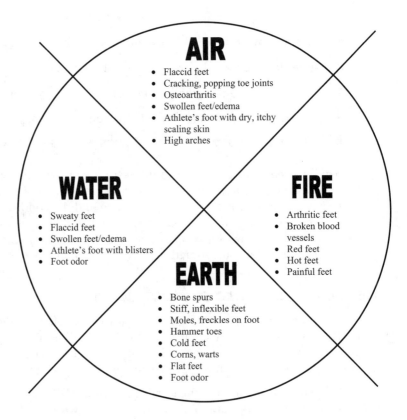

**AIR**
- Flaccid feet
- Cracking, popping toe joints
- Osteoarthritis
- Swollen feet/edema
- Athlete's foot with dry, itchy scaling skin
- High arches

**WATER**
- Sweaty feet
- Flaccid feet
- Swollen feet/edema
- Athlete's foot with blisters
- Foot odor

**FIRE**
- Arthritic feet
- Broken blood vessels
- Red feet
- Hot feet
- Painful feet

**EARTH**
- Bone spurs
- Stiff, inflexible feet
- Moles, freckles on foot
- Hammer toes
- Cold feet
- Corns, warts
- Flat feet
- Foot odor

# Air: Snap, Crackle, and Pop

Snap, crackle, and pop isn't just for breakfast anymore. These noises can also be heard during a reflexology treatment. They usually can be heard or even felt when working with the joints. They are the same noises that you hear during an adjustment at the chiropractor.

The noises you hear are usually just little air bubbles in the synovial fluid between your joints. When the toes or ankles are rotated or maneuvered just so, these little bubbles can be squashed and will pop—hence the sound. If you are working on someone who has arthritis or a degeneration of the bones, the crunching, snapping, and popping noises could actually be the joints rubbing together. If this is the case, then the person will usually hear these sounds each time they walk barefoot, and usually the feet will be very sore or tender to the touch. Be very careful when working with degenerative bone conditions. Always use a lighter touch with these people.

**Tread Lightly**

When working with someone with a degenerative bone condition, work lightly to avoid unintentionally breaking a weakened bone. People with osteoarthritis or osteoporosis have porous bones that are vulnerable to breaking.

## *Tiny Bubbles*

Other times, you may hear crunchies that are actually the breaking up of uric acid crystals that have accumulated on the nerve endings at the bottom of the foot. When you squash these crystals with your thumbs, fingers, or knuckles, you may be able to hear them crackle if they are large enough. Feet and hands that crack, snap, and pop can be thought of as having too much of the air element, indicated by the little air bubbles in the joints.

If you have lots of popping and cracking in all of your joints, including your feet, hands, back, neck, and jaw, it could mean that you have a trace mineral imbalance. All the minerals in the body work together to keep the body in balance. When there is a deficiency of mineral intake in the diet (a common occurrence now with our mineral-depleted soils) it will cause a mineral imbalance in the body. The body will take what it needs from our reserves of minerals in the body, such as calcium from the bones or magnesium from muscles, to get what it needs to balance.

**Tip Toe**

Here's an example of using the four-element chart to find a balance: Too much fire causes hot, dry conditions. What is better to cool off a hot, dry condition than a little cool water? Note that the fire and water elements are opposite to each other on the chart. Keep these principles in mind as you use your four-element philosophy.

## *Striving Toward Balance*

Remember that the body is always striving toward balance. On the four-element chart you can go to the opposite element for a clue as to how to handle any condition. For instance, too much air will leave a person lacking structure, an earth quality. This might manifest as porous bones (air spaces in the bones) such as osteoporosis.

Look at the element chart. Earth is opposite air. What could be more helpful to those with porous bones than a little more strength in their structure? Structure is a characteristic of earth. What could be earthier than minerals from our earth like calcium and magnesium? Minerals are known to support our structural system. See how it works?

### Foot Note

A person with osteoporosis or other bone degeneration should consider seeing an herbalist or nutritionist who might help them get the right type of herbs rich in minerals, like alfalfa or colloidal minerals. Juicing organic fruits and vegetables also supplies an abundant amount of useable minerals.

# Water: Puff, the Magic Ankles

When you first look at the foot and see that it is swollen in certain areas—or just plain swollen all over—ask the person if they twisted or sprained their ankle recently, which could be a cause of the swelling. Make sure that before working on someone with swollen ankles that it doesn't fall under one of the contraindication categories (see Chapter 15, "How to Touch").

If neither of these conditions are true, then your partner more than likely has an overabundance of the water element. This is especially true if the person also has a puffy face and fingers. You may suspect that the person is holding excess water in their entire body. If this is so, it could mean sluggishness in the urinary system or the lymphatic system. This can happen when a person has been sitting or inactive all day.

# Work Those Lymphs

When the ankles are swollen, be sure to work on all the lymphatic areas between the metatarsals and the lower lymph areas all across and around the ankles. The next area you should work on is the urinary system. The kidneys could be ineffective and potassium levels could be low. Stimulate the kidney and bladder areas, and note any tenderness there.

Instead of having too much water, the body could be holding onto water because it is in a state of dehydration! When the body consistently is not getting enough water, it can have a tendency to hold onto fluids. This will go away after drinking enough water daily for the body to let go of its stash.

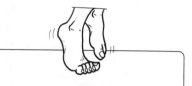

**Tip Toe**

Water retention can mean either that the person has too much water or, ironically, that the person is on the verge of dehydration and the body is holding onto water to protect itself. Either way, the urinary and lymphatic systems need to be stimulated to help this condition.

# Go with the Flow

In my experience, someone who has swollen areas on the feet when they come in for reflexology will not have swollen feet when they leave. Reflexology will help stimulate the lymphatic system and get things moving again. The following can also help relieve water retention:

➤ B-complex vitamins

➤ Juniper berries

➤ Parsley

➤ Dandelion root

➤ Cornsilk

➤ Buchu root

And, surprisingly, the person suffering from excess water should be encouraged to drink plenty of water before and after their session. This helps keep things flowing smoothly.

### Foot Note

In a group of reflexology studies compiled by the American Reflexology Certification Board, a Danish study revealed that reflexology treatments have a pain-relieving effect on acute kidney stone complaints. The study shows that 9 out of 10 patients in the therapy group experienced no pain following the treatment.

# Earth: Stiff Toes, Stiff Neck

Many times you will observe a pair of feet that have toes that are curled in and feel very tight or stiff. If you ask the person to spread their toes out you will usually still not be able to see any space in between the toes.

When you try to perform tootsie rolls on these types of toes, it will feel more like rolling a pencil between your fingers! On the element model, this could be considered too much earth: too much structure, stiffness, and rigidity. Earth is the hardest of all elements and the most solid.

### Tread Lightly

Be *very*, very gentle with stiff, crackley toes, as these stiff toes could break while you are performing reflexology! Be sure to support the toes well with the other hand as you are using your fingers to very gently rotate the toes one at a time.

## Curls My Toes

Fear can also make the toes curl. Many times, when we are afraid or unsure, we will curl our toes under our feet. We will look at the personality features of the foot in the next chapter, so more on that later. Physically, stiff toes will correlate to a stiff neck, and even compression on the brain.

Often, toes like these are women's toes. Because of the pointed toe boxes so popular in women's shoes, many of us female folks have shoved our tootsies into these spaces for years. The results are overwhelmingly stiff toes and stiff necks!

## Earthy Moves

The best therapies for these stiff, tight toes are full toe rotations, tootsie rolls, and the knuckle technique (where you push your knuckles into the padding of the ball of the foot). This will open up the toes and the spaces in between and get some circulation and flexibility back to these areas. See Chapter 16, "Third Time's a Charm," for a refresher and photo on using the knuckle press technique.

Another good way to help these toes spread out is to put your fingers between as many toes as you can while doing an ankle rotation. In a way, you are trying to get air (space) in between this dense, earthy condition to break it up and spread it out (opposite elements on the chart).

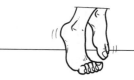

**Tip Toe**

With dry, cracking type feet, there is also a deficiency of the water element. Some popular mucilaginous herbs (high in the water element) include aloe vera, marshmallow, and slippery elm.

# More Water: Those Slimy, Sweaty Feet

Sometimes you will see a pair of feet that are sweating profusely. Kind of like a wet fish, these feet are difficult to hold onto. Sweaty feet are an obvious overabundance of the water element in the body. Since the pores on the feet are the largest, this is a convenient place for the body to eliminate moisture.

The problem with excessive sweating is that the body can only eliminate water for so long. Eventually there is the danger of the well running dry, so to speak. Balancing the water element is definitely a necessity.

## Working Up a Sweat

Conditions that cause excessive sweating in the feet can be linked with nervousness or a great amount of stress. When we are nervous or stressed, the body is more likely to sweat. Work on this person's nervous system and adrenal glands. Of course, the urinary system is part of the water element, so work on the bladder and kidney reflexes also.

The best way to perform reflexology on someone who has an overly wet condition of the feet is to work with a clean, absorbent cotton sock on the foot and work through it or use a terry-cloth towel over the area so that you do not slip off the reflex pressure points. If this is something you are not comfortable with, you can also try applying some cornstarch or talcum powder to the feet to help dry them before working on the reflexes.

## Drying Out

When there is too much water in the body, it will require a little bit of warmth (fire) to evaporate and balance the water. Make sure you use a lukewarm washcloth to bathe this type of feet before you start. The cloth can be somewhat dry and adding a little golden seal powder to the cloth will help dry up and may slightly disinfect the feet before you work on them.

# Fire: Feet That Flame On

A bright red foot is a good indication that there is an overabundance of fire in the feet. Red is a color that is associated with fire. There is a lot of blood going to an area that is red.

Excessive heat is also another clue that a person has too much fire. For instance, the clients that I see who have arthritic feet with much pain also have very red, hot feet. There is no need to warm up my hands before working on these people. Inflammation is an overabundance of the fire element. Think of the word "inflame"—it actually describes fire!

## Back in Circulation

There may be a problem with the circulatory system when you observe hot, red feet. Fire, manifested as inflammation, could be caused by the circulation stagnating in the inflamed area. The blood is failing to circulate well enough to move the inflammation away from the swollen areas. Reflexology will benefit these conditions since it aids the circulatory system.

Since the circulatory system falls within the fire category, you should take a look at the health of the entire circulatory system. Is it inefficient? Why is the blood going to the feet and then staying there? Is there a blockage somewhere in the veins or arteries that is inhibiting the free flow of blood or could it be another condition such as arteriosclerosis? Does the person have hemorrhoids? Hemorrhoids are just swollen veins in an inconvenient place.

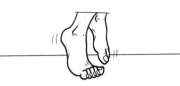

**Tip Toe**

Astringent type herbs are herbs that tighten tissues and usually have a drying effect on the body membranes as well. Some popular drying (air type) herbs include sage, white oak bark, and witch hazel.

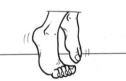

**Tip Toe**

To reflex the area for hemorrhoids, you should first work the entire colon, since hemorrhoids are usually caused by constipation. Then work on the reflex corresponding to the rectum, which is the area on the left foot and left palm where the colon ends—this is just below and slightly overlaps the bladder reflex.

Use reflexology with the goal of improving circulation. The techniques that stretch and maneuver the feet gently but vigorously, such as yummies and rotations of the toes and ankles, will aid a person with an imbalance of fire. It will help get the fire moving to other areas. Also work the heart area on the padding of the ball of the left foot.

## Cooling Off

A nutritionist, or someone competent in helping with nutrients or herbs, can be sought out for advice on how to help strengthen blood capillaries and balance circulatory problems. I have seen people make great progress in helping their circulatory systems with the use of the following:

➤ Lecithin, a food supplement that keeps cholesterol in balance in the body

➤ Psyllium hulls help keep dietary fat from being absorbed and cleanse the colon

➤ Liquid chlorophyll provides natural minerals

➤ Omega-3 oils

➤ Vitamin C

➤ B-complex with extra niacin and B6

➤ Hawthorne berries, an herb used historically for the heart

➤ Coenzyme Q10, a nutrient to support the oxygenating abilities of the circulatory system

**The Sole Meaning**

**Lecithin** is a substance produced by the liver if the diet is adequate. It is needed by every cell in the body and largely makes up cell membranes; without it they would harden. Lecithin protects cells from oxidation, protects the brain, and is a fat emulsifier. Supplements are usually derived from soybeans, which contain a fair amount of lecithin.

Since you don't want to add fuel to the fire, you should not attempt to keep the foot snugly wrapped up in a heating pad as you might with someone with cold feet! This can only aggravate the fire condition. A cool approach is much better.

Cooling aromatherapy would be a good choice for someone with too much fire. A cool aromatic such as peppermint or birch oil would be appropriate. You might also want to wash their feet with a cool, wet cloth with a little birch oil on it before their treatment to sooth the inflammation and cool the fire condition.

Can you see how you can use your understanding of the elements in your reflexology treatments? Next we will take a look at the personality side of the feet. You can keep the four elements in mind for this one, as each element definitely has its own "personality."

## The Least You Need to Know

➤ You can use the four-element model to understand which element the body is lacking or overabundant in as you observe the condition of the feet.

➤ Usually an overabundance of one of the elements is corrected by adding more of its opposite element on the chart.

➤ Popping or cracking joints can indicate too much air. This is balanced by earth. Too much earth, however, can cause stiffness.

➤ Sweaty or swollen feet indicate too much of the water element. Work the lymphatic system and use a warming and drying element for balance.

➤ Fire or hot conditions in the feet can indicate a problem with the circulatory system and can be helped by cooling elements.

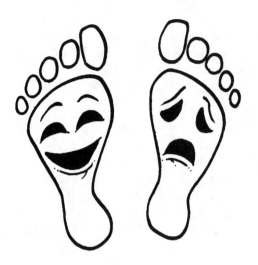

# Chapter 19

# The Personality in the Feet

---

### In This Chapter

➤ See how your feet can show the path you've walked in life

➤ Learn to recognize more elemental conditions of the feet

➤ Discover what the lines on your feet say about you

➤ Find some indicators of wealth on the hands and feet

➤ See what your moles and freckles may be telling you

---

Our feet carry us through life, and by observing their physical shape and condition we can gain insight to how we walk through life. Do we skip merrily or just shuffle along? Have we traveled a "hard road" or have we floated or even been carried through life?

Here we will take a peek at what the condition, shape, and signs on the feet and hands might reveal about the way we walk the earth, the way we think, and maybe even the lessons we need to learn. What type of footprints do you wish to leave behind?

## High Arched and Up in the Clouds

Do you walk on your toes? Do you like to tiptoe through the tulips? Do you have high arches? In foot personality analysis, a person with high arches is the dreamer, inventor, the thinker, and one who has his head in the clouds! High arches would fall into the air category on the four-element chart (see Chapters 4, "The Foot at a Glance," and 18, "Finding Balance: The Elemental Foot").

The high arches keep a person up in the air. People with high arches usually like to travel, especially by air. People with their head in the clouds can think up things that some of us cannot fathom. They are visionaries who make great consultants to companies who want to see the "big picture." These people can help us get prepared for the future through their ability to see beyond today. Sometimes they are ahead of their time.

# High Achievers

People with high arches many times have high ideals and high expectations of themselves and others. They are forward thinkers and actively take part in life. Living in the clouds makes it easier for high-arched people to change directions quickly and easily, and our high-arched friends can confuse us at times when they quickly switch directions.

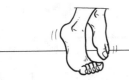

**Tip Toe**

High-arched people may require more earthy foods to keep them grounded! Earthy foods include root vegetables, beans, nuts, and supplements like calcium, magnesium, and iron.

High-arched folks spend much of their time up in the air, where there are no landmarks. The high-arched person feels free and unencumbered because of this, but it can drive the more grounded, earthy people a little crazy! Many people with high arches work in the computer industry, an intellectually dominated, forward-thinking, technology-driven market (although there must have been some fallen arches that did not foresee our Y2K problems!).

# Walking on Air

High-arched people enjoy flight and many become pilots, hang gliders, and skydivers. They can't get enough of taking their feet off the ground! Usually, these folks walk with a bounce in their step and are not as concerned about the mundane matters of life. They are more focused on ideals and creativity.

They can be natural experts in engineering design, since they can see how everything fits together in the "big picture." But they probably won't want to work physically building the pieces.

**Tip Toe**

If a high-arched partner comes bouncing into your life, get ready for some stimulating intellectual conversations while you're packing your bags for the trip you will be going on together—the high-arched of the world love travel!

Reflexology is a great therapy for folks with high arches because it tends to "bring them back down to earth" and can be very grounding and comforting to those who are intellectually driven. Reflexology can help these people get more in touch with their bodies.

# Flat-Footed and Down to Earth

The opposite of high arches is flat feet, which are feet with no arches at all! In contrast to the high-arched folks, flat-footed folks are more grounded. People with flat feet feel a real connection to the earth. They enjoy being in the forest, out in nature, and like the feeling of their feet on the ground. People with flat feet can enjoy reflexology because they are in tune with the physical pleasures of the body—more so than the high-arched folks.

Sometimes flat-footed people have a feeling of being unsupported. These people sometimes feel that they are carrying more responsibility on their life path. Flat-footed people may feel a drive to achieve and may be overburdened with this responsibility.

## Earth Mothers

Having such a strong connection to the earth, many times flat-footed people work with organizations that are earth-oriented, like protecting the rights of indigenous peoples or working to protect the environment.

Flat-footed people need to be careful not to become martyrs and to let themselves break free of their self-induced burdens sometimes. A good reflexology treatment utilizing uplifting aromatherapy oils, such as a mixture of bergamot and pink grapefruit on the temples, would be an excellent therapy for the flat-footed person.

### Foot Note

Although flat-footed folks will enjoy music that is more earthy, such as Indian flute music, they should be encouraged once in a while to listen to harp or piano music. Music by Bach or Mozart falls more in the air element and will help disconnect a flat-footed person from his worries over the plight of the earth and its inhabitants.

# What Makes Your Toes Curl?

In the last chapter we talked about the stiff-toes-stiff-neck scenario in the feet. But other than too much of the earth element or tight toe boxes squashing the toes together, why do people hold their toes curled under? In a word: fear.

Since the toes represent the head area, curling the toes under is a subconscious protective position. It can be like hiding your head in the sand or covering your face. Pay attention the next time you are watching a spooky movie: Do your toes curl?

On a day-to-day level, when you are unsure about something or are fearful or not ready yet to face the music, so to speak, you might be curling up your toes to "lessen the impact" of what you are hearing or seeing. Curled toes can also be a metaphor for gripping or hanging onto persons, things, or events too tightly. The need to trust and let go is key for those with curled toes.

## The Sole Meaning

A **callus** is a thickened portion of the epidermal layer of the skin. Repeated friction or constant pressure to the foot or hands causes calluses.

# The Callused Personality

A callused sole doesn't necessarily mean a callused soul, but could indicate a callused personality! *Calluses* are common on the foot. They occur naturally the more a person walks barefoot or wears ill-fitting shoes.

A real callus is thick skin on the foot caused by constant friction or pressure on the area. In life, when we are exposed to constant struggles, abusive situations, and irritations, we can become callused or hardened to those situations or emotions.

Calluses on the skin or in our personality are meant to protect us from the outside influences that hurt us. Someone who had a hard life but has become stronger in spite of it may have callused feet. Calluses are not just the body's way of toughening up, but metaphorically are the personality's way of toughening up those areas of our lives that have been abused.

## Foot Note

More than likely, when you meet a person with extremely callused feet they will be crunchy on the outside but soft in the middle. People who have been through great pain in their lives are usually the people with the greatest character and strength and also the deepest compassion for others. When you get past the callused layer in the personality, you will find that these people have hearts of gold.

To deal with calluses on the feet, administer foot-baths with Epsom salts added to the water to help loosen the dead skin layers. Then a pumice stone or some other abrasive material can be used to remove the calluses. If you are giving reflexology to a very callused foot, you might want to have your subject soak their feet in a footbath first, or consider a wax dip, which softens the feet before a session.

See where your calluses are and think about them in terms of the areas of the body they reflect. Do you have a callus on your large toe, representing the head area? Did you experience a great amount of verbal or mental abuse in your past? Does your heart area have a callus? How does this relate to your affairs of the heart? The heel represents your lower body or reproductive areas. Could issues over children, or not having children, contribute to a callus on the heel? Think about these things, deal with the issues, then pumice those suckers away!

**Tread Lightly**

When a callus is on the side of the large toe, it can push the toe sideways and create headaches or stiffness in the neck. This can also lead to the formation of a bunion, which we will talk about in the next chapter.

# Filled with Emotion: Swollen Feet

Physically, a very swollen foot and ankle can indicate edema or lymphatic congestion. But what if the feet and ankles have always been, and still are, puffy? This usually indicates that a person holds water easily. Proper minerals, exercise, ample water intake, and reflexology should correct this problem, but swollen feet can also have an emotional connection.

In our four-element chart, water relates to emotion (see Chapter 4). Holding onto water could indicate that a person has a hard time expressing emotions and is, therefore, holding onto them. These emotional camels could be very sensitive due to the fact that they are "filled with emotion" much of the time.

**Tip Toe**

The water-retentive person should try to come up for air sometimes, take things a little more lightheartedly, and work to prevent water retention to help with their emotions. Sometimes, retaining water can put pressure on the brain and make us feel more vulnerable, sensitive, and emotional, as with PMS. Again, minerals, water, B-complex vitamins, and reflexology can all help release excess water.

Often, loved ones of this type of person will plead with them to "let it go," which is really what the lesson is. This person needs to learn to release repressed emotions, to let things flow and roll off their back, and not take everything personally or so deeply. This is easier said than done, but is a good growing experience for the person with water-retentive feet.

The person who retains water/emotion will have a tendency to brood or be hurt deeply by things people say or do to them, even when the intention of others was not to hurt them. They can cry easily or hold onto hurt or depression for long periods of time.

# Hot or Cold, Wet or Dry?

Hot feet indicate an excess of the fire element. People who have warm hands and feet are usually warm all over. They can be considered hot-tempered, hot-headed, or thought to have a very warm heart. Hot feet, of course, can indicate painful conditions of the feet, but here we are addressing the fiery type of condition in the personality.

Usually, hot feet can mean a person is very passionate. He or she may love romance. These people can get fiercely angry, but usually the anger will be gone as soon as they are done expressing themselves. Hot feet usually belong to willful people. Heat comes from the blood. The blood is near the surface in those with hot extremities.

The fire energy in these people usually runs on the surface. They may wear their hearts on their sleeve, so to speak, and be influenced very easily by a "pretty face" that appeals to their sexual or romantic inclinations. Stamina may be short-lived, however. They are fast to ignite a creative idea or plans and also like the idea of making a fast buck. Hot feet can mean impatience.

Remember that if a hot-footed hot-head ever gets angry with you, they will forget about it shortly after they express it! Don't hold onto this scolding—especially if you are a water-retentive person! Let it go, because more than likely, the hot-foot already forgot about it!

**Tread Lightly**

Cold feet can mean slow circulation or metabolism. Consider anemia or low thyroid activity. Be sure to keep the feet warm and offer a blanket. Feet exposed to cold can lower the body temperature and make someone feel cold all over.

## Cold Feet Run Deep

Cold feet and hands can indicate a person who keeps their emotions on the inside. They are not as expressive with their feelings as a hot-footed person. They can have more poise and remain calm and controlled even in emergency situations.

The cold-footed person has deep-running emotions. This can make them more insightful and self-reflective than those who immediately express their thoughts. Introspective is a good word for chronically cold-handed and -footed folks. On the physical level, check for an underfunctioning thyroid or anemia if the body, hands, and feet are chronically cold and fatigued.

# Never Let Them See You Sweat

Remember in the last chapter when we talked about wet feet meaning an imbalance in the water element? Water relates to our emotions, and releasing too much water, in a metaphorical sense, may mean that a person is not sensitive to life issues. They let their emotions "run out at the bottom," and, therefore, life is not too meaningful. They may be out of touch with the deeper meanings of life.

They can also be people who have had trouble in the past having their emotions validated and therefore are nervous about what they feel is proper. Sweaty feet can belong to nervous folks who have a need to share their emotions but feel they cannot. This leaves them at odds with what they really want to express and what they fear they may lose by this expression. Chronically sweaty feet could be a person's discreet way of letting out their emotions without having to express or intellectualize these feelings.

# Dry to the Bone

If you have a very dry or scaly foot, you should check for dehydration or any problems with the urinary system. Dry-footed people could have a dry sense of humor and tend toward dry conditions such as itchy, dry, flaky skin, dandruff, psoriasis, sneezing, and nervous system conditions. Good things to feed the nervous system and protect the brain and immune system include the following:

➤ Fish

➤ Lecithin

➤ Vitamin E

➤ B-complex

➤ Egg yolks

➤ Essential fatty acids

➤ Zinc

Dry feet are related to air, and the air element relates to the head and nervous system. Too much air can indicate mental illness or disorders and can mean a vulnerable immune system.

**Foot Note**

Metaphorically speaking, calluses on our sole can indicate calluses on our soul. These invisible soul calluses can shut us off from our full potential of experiences and child-like exuberance. Calluses can indicate a need to break free from self-limiting ideas and fears that deaden our expression.

# Footloose

Loose feet that are overly flexible and lacking in tone can indicate very open, flexible people who go with the flow of life. Sometimes they are blamed for being unorganized because they lack any form of rigidity and structure. Some amount of structure is required for organization.

These people may not show up on time for appointments, which doesn't really bother them. Type B personalities are usually the owners of very flexible feet. They are easy to get along with because they usually take things in stride, but don't expect them to meet you on time!

## Fancy Free

A loose-footed person may have a hard time taking a strong stand on issues. These people can get along with others very well. Flaccid feet fall into the water and air categories on the four-element chart.

Water and air take on the shape of their containers. These people need to be aware of ill-intentioned people who may manipulate them. Loose feet can be a sign of being too lax about life and affairs and can show the need for more discipline in thoughts and ideas and discernment in judgment of people who have an influence in your life.

## What a Stiff

On the opposite side of the coin, a foot that is stiff and rigid and has a hard time loosening up may have a personality to match! Rigid feet can mean rigidity or very structured thinking. These people can have a hard time "letting loose," and can probably really use a good reflexology session, along with a good laugh.

They tend to be very pragmatic, stable, and solid, which makes them just the kind of folks you would want to handle your accounting and do your taxes. These people will usually have strict schedules and regimes and will always be on time, if not early. These are people who are very reliable, but also not ones to take many things lightly.

On the negative side, these people lack the ability to let things fall though the cracks and can become too set in their ways and therefore miss out on experiences that would expand their minds or enhance their enjoyment of life. Everyone needs to have some fun and loosen up once in a while—work on getting to these people's sense of humor and help them relax—but be sure to keep your appointments with these folks and be on time!

# Connecting the Dots: The Future in Your Feet and Hands

Chinese doctors, palm readers, personologists, and others have interpreted lines or crevices in the skin for years for clues to health and personality. There are some who can read the lines on your feet to assess your health. This book does not go in-depth into this subject, but I have included some of these interpretations here just for fun.

These ideas are based on the premise that the lines in the feet and hands are usually caused by mental or nervous tension in the body. When we are nervous, many times we will wring our hands; when we are angry, we clench our fists. We are usually much less conscious of what our feet are doing, but they, too, react in response to our emotions.

In my reflexology work, the most significant lines on the feet that I look for are any lines along the spinal column reflex, which is along the arch of the foot. When there are many lines running across this, it could indicate central nervous system tension, stress, and mental strain.

Usually, a person with many of these fine, short vertical lines has a personality that changes easily. One moment they can be high spirited, and at another moment they are feeling blue. Usually, these people are very dynamic, and when they are feeling well they push themselves to the limits and run themselves down very quickly. The goal of a person with many lines up and down their spinal reflexes is *balance*.

**Tip Toe**

A plantar wart is caused by a virus in the body. Some reflexologists link the location of a plantar wart on the foot to a virus in the part of the body the wart corresponds to! An interesting concept that might be worth checking out!

**The Sole Meaning**

In Chinese assessment, a line running down the earlobe means that a person could have a genetic tendency toward heart disease. Don't panic if you have one; just make sure you take extra good care of your heart and circulatory system!

# A Fortune at Your Fingertips

Looking for money? Here are some fun things to look for:

➤ Lines that wrap completely around the wrists can be called "bracelets of wealth." They are found more on women than men. Maybe women really do control all the money! The more bracelets, the more wealth!

➤ The second toe is considered to be the wealth toe. If a second toe is longer than the large toe, this can indicate there is wealth in the person's future. Some believe this is the toe of intelligence. Many times, intelligence and money go hand in hand.

➤ Look for a large "M" on the palm of your hand. This can mean good luck in money or in marriage—or both!

➤ Curl your hand up into a fist with your fingertips facing toward you. Look for the pointy fold sticking out the side of your hand just below the pinky joint. This is called your pocketbook. If the skin is thick and full, this could indicate that your money purse will be filled up and bulging with money!

I've seen a lot of lines in my days as a reflexologist, and you'd be surprised at how often these prove to be true.

# Say It with Freckles: Larry, Curly, and Mole

Moles and freckles are just a concentration of pigment on the skin. Energetically, a concentration of pigment is a concentration of energy in the body. Therefore, some believe that anywhere a mole or freckle is found on the feet or hands indicates a concentration of energy in the corresponding body part, which is density (excess earth) in that area.

**Tip Toe**

I had a client who had a large freckle on her left ovary reflex on the heel. Just to test the validity of the idea that moles or freckles can indicate a genetically inherited condition, I asked her if her mother had any type of female problems. She said her mom died of ovarian cancer!

If you find moles or freckles on your feet or hands, consider the reflex point you find them on. This can be a sign of a genetically inherited congestion in the corresponding area. You may want to consider an internal cleansing program designed to cleanse the particular organ. The moles or freckles won't usually disappear, but you might want to do something that will decongest the particular part just for preventative medicine's sake.

For example, if you find a freckle on the ball of your foot and also one on the top of your foot, you might think about your lung and chest area. There may be a concentration of energy there. You can work preventatively on yourself by avoiding living in a heavily polluted environment and staying away from smoking! Since the freckle is also on the chest reflex, make sure you go in for your mammograms if you are a woman.

Get plenty of exercise that stimulates your upper lymphatic system. Take up a form of aerobic exercise that increases lung capacity and consider taking a supplement such as mullein, slippery elm, or lobelia if you get hoarse or are prone to laryngitis or other upper respiratory congestion. Most important, use reflexology to rub out those tender areas in the lung and upper chest reflexes!

### Foot Note

One of my massage therapists told me that a freckle on the bottom of my foot meant that I was condemned as a witch in a past life and burned at the stake! I wonder if my freckle was the last ash that was left. (Don't ash me, I'm just the reflexologist.)

My husband has a freckle on the bottom of his foot in exactly the same place as I do. We take this coincidence to mean that we are of the same soul and were meant to be together. Either that or he was a warlock who charred along with me! How's that for a smokin' relationship?

### The Least You Need to Know

➤ High arches can mean a person is intellectually driven. Reflexology treatments can help this person come down to earth.

➤ Flat feet can mean a person feels heavy with responsibility and unsupported. Help this person melt their burdens away with reflexology.

➤ Calluses on the feet can mean that a person has had much adversity in life and has built up resistance, but they are usually soft at heart.

➤ Rigid feet can mean a rigid personality. Help the person loosen up with reflexology.

➤ Freckles or moles can indicate a concentration of energy in the corresponding body part.

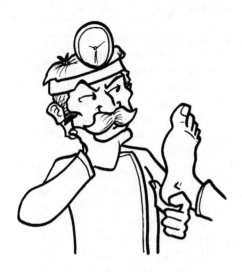

# Chapter 20

# Podiatry Matters

## In This Chapter

➤ Discover how to identify some common foot problems

➤ Find out how to deal with athlete's foot

➤ Learn about bone spurs, hammer toes, bunions, and more

➤ Discover the importance of wearing proper shoes

➤ Learn some natural remedies for some common foot conditions

"Time wounds all heels."

—A sign seen in a podiatrist's window

By now you may have worked on everyone's feet in your family, and hopefully have been experimenting on yourself, too! But, besides all those metaphorical and philosophical ways to look at feet, how do you identify an obvious physical problem? This chapter will help you identify what some of these problems are and how you can avoid getting yourself into any of these conditions in the first place. Now take off your shoes and follow in my footsteps…

## The Doctor Is In

Remember that a reflexologist is not a *podiatrist* (foot doctor) and should never give medical advice or diagnose conditions. However, as a reflexologist you will gain familiarity with many conditions of the feet.

This chapter will give you a holistic view of some common foot ailments. It will also describe these ailments and their probable causes. I will offer you some tips to help you and your clients help themselves with natural remedies. Otherwise, you can refer them to a foot specialist. It doesn't hurt to find and build a relationship with a good podiatrist in your area if you plan to set up a reflexology practice.

Dr. Robert Timm, a podiatrist from Colorado and teacher of foot joint realignment and reflexology, says, "Reflexologists need to understand that not all sensitive areas are reflex points that need stimulation. It could be a local problem such as Morton's neuroma, plantar fascitis, a tumor, a plantar wart, osteochrondritus, a malpositioned joint, a cyst, arthritis, a corn, or a callus caused by a joint that is misaligned, however slightly."

**The Sole Meaning**

**Podiatry** is the health profession that cares for the human foot. The doctor of podiatric medicine is called a **podiatrist** and examines, diagnosis, and treats diseases, injuries, and defects of the foot.

It will be important for a student of reflexology to understand and be able to recognize some of these local problems and know how to work with or around these ailments. We are going to discuss some common problems you may see, and touch on a few things that you shouldn't touch on!

# An Athletic Fungus

*Tinea Pedis* is the medical term for a condition we all have heard of called *athlete's foot*. Athlete's foot is a contagious fungal condition otherwise known as *ringworm*. The term "athlete's foot" came about because it has been a common condition among athletes who share locker rooms (barefoot) and showers. This ailment is also common in those whose feet sweat a lot or who are obese.

**The Sole Meaning**

**Athlete's foot** is a fungal condition that is actually **ringworm**. The medical name for this contagious infection is **Tinea Pedis**. The term "athlete's foot" was coined because it has been a common condition among athletes who share locker rooms and showers.

The fungus thrives in warm, moist areas such as showers and locker rooms. The fungus can be spread by contact with any surface, especially warm, moist surfaces such as showers that have been contaminated by an infected person. Wearing the same shoes or socks, walking in the same areas, or even touching the feet of another person who is infected can spread the fungus.

## Don't Sweat It

Symptoms of athlete's foot include itching, scaling, and even cracking of the skin. Sometimes small blisters appear. Treatment for athlete's foot varies from soaking the feet in potassium permanganate solution to applying commercial antifungal ointments or powders. Natural remedies include the use of tea-tree oil to rid the skin of the fungus.

The best preventative medicine against athlete's foot is wearing flip-flops into locker rooms and locker-room showers. Try to keep your feet dry, and don't keep sweaty socks on your feet for any length of time.

Since contagious infections of the feet and hands fall under the contraindications chart for reflexology, you will need to know how to identify them and will need to politely decline to work on a person with this infection. Don't assume that the person will tell you they have this condition when they set an appointment with you. Many times people are unaware that it is a problem and do not even know it's contagious!

## Bye-Bye Fungi

Your best bet is to send an infected person to a foot specialist or their family doctor, who can prescribe a treatment for them. You may want to suggest that they try tea-tree oil. Since tea-tree oil is antifungal and antibacterial, it has been used with success for many with this kind of ailment. A quality tea-tree oil applied to an infected area two times a day for 5 to 10 days or until the condition disappears has cured many of my clients of this condition. Tea-tree oil is also very drying and should help dry up blisters caused by the infection.

When you first observe the feet before administering reflexology, be sure to check the toenails. When someone is prone to fungal infections they can have fungus growing on the nails and not even be aware of it. Fungus on the toenails will appear as a flaky growth on the top and frequently under the nails. Sometimes it is yellowish in color.

**Tip Toe**

Historically, the inner bark of the taheebo tree has been used as an herb commonly called Pau D'Arco (Spanish term for "for everything"). It has been used to kill fungal infections internally and externally. Some make a tea of the bark and soak an infected foot or hand in the solution. Others take capsules internally. Some do both.

If you observe this on a client's toenails, use your discretion when deciding whether to work with them or not. As a preventative measure, you can choose to apply the tea-tree oil to your own hands before working on them and avoid making contact with the toenails. You can also choose to work on them through their socks. Otherwise, set an appointment with them after their infection is cleared up.

# Bone Spurs and Other Missteps

Bone spurs are a sharp projection of bone. These are usually caused because calcium is out of solution in the body. This is nutritionally caused by a trace mineral deficiency.

A person is usually very aware of a bone spur when they have one. Bone spurs are easy to identify by observing the foot. They can be seen as little, hard bumps protruding from the foot or hand and can be as large as a marble. They usually occur around the wrists or the heel of the foot.

When you see a bone spur, don't get spurred on to work on it! Some people have been known to smash their own bone spurs against a hard surface, breaking them up to be eliminated or reabsorbed by the body naturally

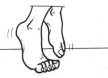

**Tip Toe**

Hydrangea is an herb used historically to dissolve calculus buildup and stones in the body such as kidney stones, bladder stones, and bone spurs. Hydrangea may be swallowed and usually comes in capsules. Some have applied the essential oil of birch to these areas and have claimed the spurs have disappeared with regular use in a matter of weeks.

afterward. I wouldn't suggest you do this to anyone (unless of course you'd like the nickname Dr. Crusher). When a bone spur is present, do not work directly on the bone spur. Work around the area.

## *Tool Time for Hammer Toes*

*Hammer toe* is an actual deformity of a toe or toes. Most often this occurs in the second toe (the wealth toe!) and is caused by fixed flexion of the first joint. In other words, the joint of the toe gets permanently fixed in a bent position and cannot be straightened.

**The Sole Meaning**

Hammer toe is an actual deformity of a toe caused by fixed flexion of the first joint. In other words, the joint of the toe gets permanently fixed in a bent position!

This condition can be very painful and usually (since most of us have to wear shoes every day) the pressure from a shoe on top of a hammer toe or toes causes friction and can create a callus or corn on top of the toe. This makes it even more hardened and painful. Consult your local farmer for less painful ways to grow corn!

When working on someone with a hammer toe or toes, flexibility will be an issue. Try to get the person to loosen up and work especially with techniques that stretch and rotate the feet. Do not work directly on top of the hammer toe or corn that might have developed there.

Don't try to force these toes to straighten out! This could be very painful for the subject. Now, over time, if the person wears correct-fitting shoes and comes for reflexology regularly, this condition may just work itself out! The problem is the tightness in the muscles keeping the toe in a bent position. Therefore, work on loosening the muscles around the metatarsals. But use extreme caution to avoid forcing the toes or hurting an individual with this condition. Toe rotations are also good to use on those with hammer toes.

## Not-So-Golden Arches

Some folks will have what is called *fallen arches*. No, these people are not fallen angels, but the arches in their feet have actually fallen, which can be a very painful condition.

Many times, there is a lack of muscle tone in the entire body when you see this condition. Those who gain a large amount of weight in a short period of time will often suffer with fallen arches.

When the arches fall, there could be torn ligaments or strained muscles in the bottom of the foot. So be gentle on folks with this problem. If you have fallen arches, try the following:

➤ Get some exercise.

➤ Walk barefoot in the sand.

➤ Use a foot roller daily.

➤ Use the toes to pick up small objects such as marbles or small rubber balls.

**The Sole Meaning**

**Fallen arches** can happen with prolonged standing or excessive weight, tearing or weakening the muscles of the arch of the feet and causing flat feet.

Sometimes orthotics prescribed by a podiatrist or even a chiropractor will help the person regain support.

# When Good Women Love Bad Shoes

"Shoes are required to eat in the cafeteria. Socks can eat any place they want."

—Sign seen in a Florida cafeteria

If the shoe fits, wear it. Literally, this should be a rule for all of us. Most of us wear ill-fitting shoes that cause corns, calluses, and deformation of the bones of the feet. Remember how much weight our feet bear. We need to wear good shoes to allow our feet to walk correctly and support us as we walk through life!

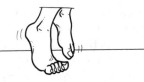

**Tip Toe**

Mom: "Cliff, you've got your boots on the wrong feet."

Cliff: "But Mom, these are the only feet I have!"

You've probably guessed that the females of the species are the ones most guilty of choosing shoes for looks and style over pure comfort. I am personally guilty of jamming my feet into all sorts of shoes as a young girl to hide my size 8½ flippers!

Make sure you pick shoes that have a wide enough toe box for the width of your feet. If not, the weight of the foot, especially when there is a lift or incline on the shoe, pushes the weight up to the ball of the foot. Then the toes are jammed together tightly into the toe box. This will cause deformities such as hammer toes or bunions.

Many times, these conditions require surgery, so work first preventatively. What would you do if you had to walk a mile in your own shoes? Think about that before you purchase your next pair.

## A Nation of Pronation

*Pronate* or *pronation* means the act of turning the foot so that the sole faces backward, causing the foot to come down on the inner margin. (Wouldn't it be easier to look in a mirror?) And then of course there is *supination*, which is the opposite of pronation, meaning the foot comes down on the outer margin.

**The Sole Meaning**

**Pronate** or **pronation** means the act of turning the foot so that the sole faces backward. **Supination** is the act of turning the foot inward so that the **medial** margin is elevated.

Here are some twisty-turny conditions our feet can be in that are the causes for much back pain:

➤ **Pronation-abduction:** The foot moving away from center midline of the body

➤ **Eversion:** Sole turning outward, away from midline of body

➤ **Dorsiflexion:** Foot turning toward top of foot and body

Any way you turn them, there is a nation full of feet that are walking incorrectly! A good sign that you are pronated is if you see more wear on one side of the soles of your shoes than on the other. Most of us do not walk perfectly and have some degree of pronation. This is why we have prescription shoes, orthotics, canting of boots, and sole inserts of all kinds.

## If the Shoe Fits

We choose shoes not necessarily for comfort, but for style and sometimes because our occupation requires specialty shoes that aren't necessarily anatomically correct. Your best bet to avoid these conditions is to work preventively by wearing shoes that fit correctly. Nowhere should your toes be squashed or your heel be slipping out of a shoe.

Birkenstock is known for designing their sandals anatomically correct, and other companies are springing up all over with the same idea. We have to help our feet walk correctly in order to make our life path easier.

You might want to consider working with a podiatrist who does foot alignment. A muscle imbalance in the legs and feet can cause pronation. A physical therapist or a fitness instructor may be able to help you locate and correct these imbalances. And of course, reflexology is exercise and stimulation of the feet, too, which may help you ease back into the correct position. Sometimes wearing orthotics is uncomfortable at first because of the adjustment the muscles in your the feet will make. Reflexology can help pull out tension in the feet and will help you adjust to the change.

### Foot Note

I once worked at a Colorado ski resort where we not only sold equipment, but custom-designed boots, putting an incline on the edges to give the owners a skiing advantage. This process is called *canting* a boot. We were instructed that if a customer asked us if we custom fit ski boots, we were to reply, "Yes, we cant!"

## This Little Piggy Had Corn

Little piggies may like corn, but your feet's little piggies think they are a painful nuisance. The medical term for a corn is a *keratosis*. A keratosis is any horny growth of the skin. The keratosis is caused by constant pressure or repeated friction on a toe. Corns are raised, circular lumps that are usually yellow and resemble a kernel of corn. The base of the corn is at the surface, and the tip lies in the deeper tissue of the skin. Sometimes the corn is attached to bone!

### The Sole Meaning

**Keratosis** is any horny growth of the skin. The most common ones are warts and corns.

281

Many times, corns need to be surgically removed. The cause, again, is ill-fitting shoes! So, don't be corny, wear proper shoes. When you are working on someone with corns, do not work directly on the corn itself, as it may cause pain to the bone it is attached to.

# Do You Cry When You Peel a Bunion?

*Bunions* are another bone deformation of the foot. A bunion occurs when the big toe overlaps another toe. This condition sometimes results from a heredity trait called *hallux valgus*, although an improper-fitting shoe can also cause the problem.

**The Sole Meaning**

**Hallux valgus** is a deviation of the big toe at its **metatarsophalangeal** joint. This deviation causes what is known as a **bunion**. *Hallux* is Latin for "great toe," and *valgus* means "an overt positional deformity, turning away from the midline of the body."

Hallux valgus is a deviation of the big toe at its *metatarsophalangeal* joint. As a result, the bursa is enlarged and because it is an area often affected by constant rubbing, a callus develops over the area, which forms the bunion.

Bunions are more likely to occur in women than men. Tight shoes with high heels and pointed toes are likely to cause this condition. Commercially available felt pads can help relieve the pressure. If the bunion is extremely painful, a surgical procedure to realign the phalanges and remove excess bone tissue may be performed.

Do not push directly on a bunion. Bunions most commonly occur around the thyroid reflex area. Work the inside of the thyroid area and be gentler on the outside where the bunion is. Never try to force a toe back to its proper position. Be aware of the bunion and work around it, especially if it is inflamed.

# Grows (in) on You

Ill-fitting shoes can also cause ingrown toenails. An ingrown toenail is a condition in which the sharp end of a toenail grows into the flesh of a toe. It is most common on the big toe. The tissue around the toenail may become infected, causing discomfort.

**Tread Lightly**

Never work directly on any bone disorders of the feet such as bunions or hammer toes. Also do not push directly on bone spurs, corns, or plantar warts.

Trimming the toenails improperly can also cause ingrown toenails. Toenails should be cut straight across when trimming.

Since there is already pressure causing pain to the toe with an ingrown nail, do not apply any pressure to this toe when performing reflexology!

# Some Natural Remedies

Obviously, proper care of your feet is very important; after all, our feet carry us where we want to go. Wearing proper-fitting shoes and simple precautions can prevent most of the problems highlighted in this chapter!

When your feet hurt, you hurt all over, and it lowers your stamina and your spirits. Try reflexology as a natural healing therapy and consider some other natural remedies listed in the following table.

## Natural Remedies for Common Foot Ailments

| Condition | Natural Remedies | Reflexology Tips |
|---|---|---|
| Athlete's foot | Tea-tree oil applied one to two times a day directly to infected area (entire) foot or hand), morning and night. When condition dries up and clears, golden seal added to a bit of honey and beeswax makes a nice foot balm or salve to heal dryness. Prevent future infection by wearing flip-flops in community showers/locker rooms and keep feet dry when possible. | Reflex all lymphatic system reflexes and immune system components |
| Stinky feet | Zinc—up to 45 mg per day for the average adult. Remember, if you stink, take zinc. Pumpkin seeds or encapsulated herbs commonly labeled as herbal pumpkin also contain a good amount of a natural form of zinc, which may prove helpful. Liquid chlorophyll added to water daily will help to deodorize the entire body also. An activated charcoal supplement should be useful as well. | Work on the reflexes to the kidneys. Imbalances in the kidneys cause odorous feet. Work the reflexes to the whole urinary system, reproductive system, lymphatics, and all endocrine glands. |

*continues*

## Natural Remedies for Common Foot Ailments  (continued)

| Condition | Natural Remedies | Reflexology Tips |
|---|---|---|
| Plantar warts | Footbaths. Place both feet in very hot water, then very cold water. Alternate until hot water cools. DO NOT TRY THIS IF YOU HAVE A WEAKENED HEART OR HIGH BLOOD PRESSURE—the increase in circulation could cause problems. A teaspoon of colloidal (liquid) silver taken internally for 10 days may help kill viruses. Silver is a trace mineral that can be found at most health food stores or through herbal or other natural supplement distributors. It should be used only temporarily. Tea-tree oil applied topically to the wart after each footbath should prove helpful. The wart should be gone in a week or so. | Work lymphatics, immune, and liver reflexes. |
| Bone spurs | Usually occur because calcium is out of solution in the body, caused by a mineral imbalance. Supplement with a good herbal calcium and a multi-mineral supplement such as colloidal minerals or alfalfa. Hydrangea has been used historically to break up calcium deposits. Take until spur disappears, then continue supplementing with alfalfa or other natural mineral supplement. | Work parathyroid reflexes, heart, and small intestines. |
| Fallen arches | Foot exercises such as picking up small items with the toes, orthotics, and a weight-loss program. | Work the heart, small intestine, and kidney reflexes. |

Hopefully using these natural remedies can save you an unnecessary trip to the doctor, and you will have learned a way to help your feet and help yourself!

## The Least You Need to Know

➤ Athlete's foot is a contagious ringworm infestation of the foot that should not be touched. When you see this condition, reschedule a client after their infection clears.

➤ Never work directly on a bone spur, corn, or ingrown toenail, as this will cause pain to your client.

➤ One of the most important things you can do to avoid foot dysfunction is to wear proper-fitting shoes.

➤ Tea-tree oil has been used to clear up fungal conditions of the skin.

➤ If your feet stink, take zinc.

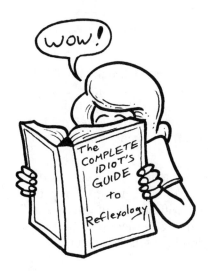

The COMPLETE IDIOT'S GUIDE to Reflexology

# Chapter 21

# Healthy, Wealthy, and Wise: What You Need to Know

## In This Chapter

➤ Learn what you need to know for a successful, professional practice

➤ Discover how to separate your feelings from your client's and keep a professional distance

➤ Find out how to eliminate negative energy and keep yourself centered

➤ Learn some exercises to keep your hands flexible

➤ Take a look at the possible future of reflexology

"The doctor of the future will give no medicine, but will interest his patient in the care of the human frame, in diet and in the cause and prevention of disease."
—Thomas A. Edison, D.Sc.

The late, great inventor Thomas Edison certainly could have been speaking of the holistic reflexologist when he spoke of the doctor of the future. This chapter will focus on how to be a professional reflexologist, although you can apply these tips no matter what type of natural therapy you choose to practice, whether you are a physical therapist, colonic therapist, aromatherapist, or herbalist.

Then, we will take a peek ahead at the possible future of reflexology and what the larger reflexology associations are advocating for the emerging practice of reflexology.

# Empathy, Not Sympathy

In reflexology, as in other fields, there is more than just physical technique involved in being a professional. It is a hard lesson to learn, but trying to keep your feelings separate from the people you work on is important for the health of a reflexologist or any health practitioner. Many of my colleagues in the natural health field tell me that they feel like a mental trauma therapist. They say they wind up listening to all sorts of troubles their clients are experiencing.

**Tread Lightly**

Reflexologists are not psychologists, medical doctors, or lawyers, although they often find themselves in a position to give advice to their clients. Don't do it. It can cause you legal trouble, and your advice may not be correct for the situation anyway!

There is a danger in this. The danger is that you, as the therapist, can take on the burdens and worries of your clients, since naturally, you will care about their well-being. You may even begin to give them your thoughts, opinions, and advice. If this happens, you can get yourself into big trouble!

As reflexology practitioners, we are not licensed psychologists or counselors. We may want to listen, but giving advice can be considered practicing medicine without a license or posing as a psychologist. Not only can this get you in trouble with the law, but you can unintentionally lead your client down the wrong path.

No matter how good you think your advice may be, you should keep it to yourself when dealing with your clients. Leave all legal or medical advice to those legally allowed to administer it. And if it is a moral issue, tell them to tune into Dr. Laura Schlessinger!

## *Would You Like a Shrink with That?*

Some reflexologists team up with psychologists and other counselors to complement the effects of their treatments. Psychologists, psychiatrists, and counselors who recognize that emotional blocks can be stored physically may want to incorporate a competent reflexologist into their practice.

Reflexology can foster the release of stored emotions and send a new vitality through the body. The counselor may find this therapy to be a catalyst to the progress of the patient's mental health.

If one of your clients is in emotional pain or needs to talk or cry, by all means let them. You should never make a person uncomfortable for displaying their emotions. Remember, you are doing bodywork on the person, and this can trigger the release of repressed emotions.

You may want to be prepared for this type of release to happen so that if and when it does, it won't take you by surprise. Keep a box of facial tissues in your room at all times. This is a simple thing to do to help you be prepared to support your client.

When a person who has released repressed emotions leaves you, make sure to take some time and clear yourself mentally. Take a deep breath, bless the person, and get ready to focus on the next person who deserves your full attention.

Some other tips for clearing yourself after giving a reflexology session:

➤ Drink a full glass of water.

➤ Wash your forearms and hands and visualize releasing the energy between you and the client.

➤ Smudge yourself with a bit of smoke from some burning purifying incense.

➤ Dab a bit of your favorite uplifting essential oil on each shoulder and the top of your head.

➤ Throw a pinch of salt behind your back (just kidding!).

➤ Say a silent prayer for the person who just left you, and know that there is always a reason for everything in the big picture.

## *An Epiphany of Sympathy*

Some of us will need to make a conscious effort not to obsess over the problems that our clients are going through. Since you will more than likely see hundreds, if not thousands, of people over the span of your career, you cannot afford to take on the emotional burdens of any of them.

Remember that you are a facilitator of healing. Keep your feelings separate from your work. This is the key difference between *empathy* and *sympathy*.

➤ **Empathy** is feeling compassion for a person's situation.

➤ **Sympathy** is actually taking on those feelings and becoming saddened or burdened by another's plight.

**The Sole Meaning**

**Empathy** is feeling compassion for a person's situation. Empathy is the emotion you should have for your clients as a professional reflexologist. **Sympathy** is actually taking on those feelings and becoming saddened or burdened by another's plight, which can get you in trouble.

Empathy is a must for a healer, but sympathy can get you into trouble.

# Keeping a Professional Distance

It is important that as a reflexologist you hold yourself in high regard by keeping moral standards and ethics in your work and even your personal life. (Again, see Dr. Laura for inspiration—or a tongue lashing, as the case may be!)

**Tread Lightly**

In all healing therapies, it is a bad idea to become involved with a client on a sexual basis. If this is a problem, end the professional relationship.

As with all healing therapies, it is suggested that the reflexologist not become involved with his or her clients on a sexual basis. In some states, professional massage therapists have to sign a form when going into practice that declares that they are not going to practice prostitution! How humiliating for the professional!

When a client begins to engage you in very personal conversations or begins to reveal their personal lives to you, it is a good idea to immediately guide the conversation back to reflexology. Encourage them to talk about nutrition or something else that you do professionally or something that the client is there to see you about—such as stress reduction, for example.

This is the best way to help keep your relationship with your client on a professional level. Politely guiding the conversation will help you avoid being embarrassed by listening to details about your client's private life.

## Avoiding Amateur Hour

Once you make reflexology your career, you will need to take it seriously as your source of income. Therefore, you probably won't want to start working on folks at parties just for fun. If you set this precedent, then you might find yourself expected to do it at parties for free after doing it all day as your business! It could also compromise the professional status that you are working to build through your practice.

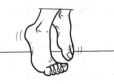

**Tip Toe**

Here's a tip for those of you who might have a future as a reflexologist. Even when you are first learning reflexology don't start out by mixing social situations with reflexology treatments unless you plan to work for free forever!

While I believe reflexology should always be a family perk, meaning that your family members should be able to be treated free when you are available, it is best to not offer your services free to friends and acquaintances, even if you really need the practice. I think it is okay to practice on your immediate family, but otherwise, practice in school or with paying clients. After your reflexology class, trade with your fellow class members for more practice.

As you learn reflexology, you might want to start off by offering your services in exchange for a donation until you feel qualified and comfortable with your skills, at which time you will set your professional fees.

# Reflexologists Charge by the Foot

I set my prices in line with the average cost of a massage therapist working in my area. I also increase my fees occasionally, for several reasons. Increasing your fees should be done as you gain skill and confidence in your work. You should also increase your fees as a reflection of the time and money that you invest over the years in school, seminars, and in other activities that add value to your services.

Don't worry about scaring off folks with your fees. You will attract the people who need you. Also, people like to know that they are paying for something of value. If you are confident enough to charge a decent price for your services, you will naturally be more valued as a practitioner and sought out by people who seek competent, valuable services.

**Tread Lightly**

Although you should not act as a counselor to your reflexology subjects, sometimes the person needs to unload as the session can stir up emotions for them. To stop or ignore the person would impede their healing release. Allow yourself to be a sounding board at these times, and treat what is said with confidentiality. At the end of the session, let it go yourself.

Adding extra services to your sessions can be an option you offer to your clients at an additional fee. Such services can include:

➤ A foot roller machine treatment

➤ Aromatherapy

➤ A foot wax dip

➤ Ear coning (before or after reflexology session)

➤ Biofeedback while they are receiving reflexology

➤ Use of the Chi Machine or other devices

➤ Jin Shin Jyutsu

➤ Color therapy

➤ Detoxification steam room session (after reflexology)

➤ A pedicure (if also a manicurist)

Always let a person know up front that there is an extra fee and what the fee is for these services. Taking a liberty with an extra service and then tacking on the surprise fee to a bill at the end of the treatment is not good business. Give your clients options and explain them sufficiently.

# Dumping the Bad Energy

A good rule for reflexologists, which also holds true for any type of health practitioner, is that you should only work on others when you are feeling well yourself.

As a reflexologist, you are helping to uplift a person. Our bodies have an energy field that works in a magnetic way. When we are well and exuberant, we give off energy. When we are ill or very down, our energy runs low. When our energy is running under par, our energy fields can actually take energy from others to balance us out!

This is why you say that someone "drained your energy" when dealing with someone who is severely depressed or cut off from their spiritual side. As reflexologists we need to have an overflow of energy so that it can be passed on to those we work with who are low in energy.

## *Making a Connection*

Getting this energy is a matter of being in touch with God, the Universe, or your Higher Self, whichever belief you hold. Energy is available to all of us, and it is a matter of keeping our hearts open and keeping our "connection" to our personal source of energy that can protect us from getting drained.

As a reflexologist you want to be a clear channel, channeling God's energy, or universal energy, through your own body and energy field so that when you work with others who need a little extra, they can draw it from you without you feeling the drain.

### Foot Note

When you are feeling low and come in contact with others who either have low energy or are not aware of how to tap into their source of energy, you can easily drain these people. This will cause them to feel worse than when they came to see you. If this happens, you might loose a potential customer. It is for your own and your client's protection that you choose only to work on people when you are feeling good.

You will have to come up with your own techniques that help you tap into your unending energy and keep you protected. Here are a few that people find useful:

➤ Some reflexologists meditate and surround themselves with white light before they work.

➤ Others ask their angels and guides to be with them.

➤ Some ask God, Jesus, Jehovah, or Buddha directly to guide, protect, and work with them.

➤ Some will use mental images or thoughts.

➤ Some use essential oils, which raise the body's frequencies.

Choose what works best for you. It doesn't hurt to perform your connection ritual every day—even when you are not seeing clients.

## Clearing Your Energy

Some reflexologists expand on their treatments and incorporate energy work such as Reiki or Jin Shin Jyutsu with their treatments. It is a good idea to let your clients know that you may perform energy work on them in case they have a personal or religious objection to any of these practices. Although these techniques are innocent enough, you don't want to scare off a potential client who could benefit from the physical effects of reflexology!

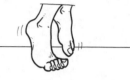

**Tip Toe**

Dried sagebrush has historically been burned and its smoke used by Native Americans and others to cleanse the aura (or energy around the body).

A technique my teacher taught me when I was studying reflexology works to clear the aura of the client when we are done with a treatment. This is not a reflexology technique, but it finishes off a treatment nicely. If you would like to try sweeping the aura, follow these steps:

➤ Pretend that you are using your hands to "push" or smooth out any tension or stuck energy surrounding your subject's body.

➤ Start at the feet, keeping your hands about three inches above the person's body.

➤ Sweep your hands up and over the top of their head and down toward the ground. Imagine that you are sweeping off excess energy that is not beneficial to the person, and it is going down into the earth to be purified.

➤ You can shake your hands as you would if you were shaking off excess water. Imagine that the person keeps all their positive energy as you do this.

➤ Repeat three times.

Be sure to explain what you are going to do before you start this, and get your client's permission. You don't want to leave them wondering what kind of odd modern dance performance you have suddenly decided to treat them to, after all. Most people will have their eyes closed but will be able to feel the subtlety of the energy moving around them.

# *Washing Up*

It is important that you wash your hands thoroughly after practicing reflexology on yourself or someone else and before you begin working on another client. This is common hygienic protocol for any type of work where you are touching another person.

To make sure that you don't energetically take on any of your client's toxic energy that you might have swept off, be sure to clean your hands and forearms up to the elbows and use cool water. This will ensure that you stay clean physically and psychically!

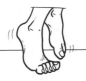

**Tip Toe**

Many manufacturers of massage tables and equipment will offer fitted sheets made specifically for massage tables. See Appendix B, "Supplies and Where to Find Them," to find out where you can look for these things.

**Tread Lightly**

Consult with an herbal specialist or holistic nutritionist to understand what supplements might be best-suited for your particular body. Many iridologists are also herbalists and can assess your genetic makeup by reading your eyes. Through their assessment they can help you find out what types of foods or herbs your particular body type might respond to best.

If you use a massage table, you will need to change sheets between clients. I use a pillow for my client's head, and I like to use a soft, clean towel over the pillowcase. Each new client deserves new towels and sheets. Be aware and be tidy and hygienic in your practice.

# Jack Be Nimble: Supplements and Exercises

You want to take good care of your entire structural system if you are a reflexologist. The structural system needs extra minerals for repair and regeneration. Some supplements that have been helpful for the connective tissues in the joints are chondroitin and glucosamine sulfate, which are supplements that help rebuild connective tissues.

Uña De Gato, also known as Cat's Claw, has been very helpful to me for my structural and immune system. My thumbs will swell occasionally when working on a lot of reflexology clients. The Uña De Gato I take eliminates the swelling and takes away the pain within 20 minutes. As long as I take my two capsules daily, I don't have this problem.

And don't forget your herbal sources of calcium. Alfalfa and liquid chlorophyll are rich in earth minerals. Alfalfa, the land plant richest in minerals, has roots that go deep into the ground. Liquid chlorophyll is made out of the "blood" of the alfalfa plant and is just as helpful for the structural system. All of these supplements feed the structural system, which includes your bones, muscles, and ligaments.

## Bend and Stretch

Reflexologists should also do exercises to stretch and strengthen their hands. Try the following exercises to stay nimble:

➤ Spread your fingers as wide as you can and hold them in this position. This opens up spaces between your fingers and lets blood and energy flow into your hands.

➤ Twirl your hands at the wrists as if you were twirling a baton to help keep them flexible and avoid carpal tunnel syndrome.

➤ Take a pen or pencil and twirl it between your fingers, passing it on to the next finger all the way across and back again.

These exercises will keep the fingers flexible and preserve them for a good, long career!

## Stand Up for Your Posture

In addition to hand exercises and proper nutrition, it is important to take care of the rest of your body. This includes practicing good posture. A good chair can help; see Chapter 17, "Tools of the Trade," for more on that subject.

When sitting at the foot of the massage table or reflexology chair, you should be sure that your back is straight. When you stand to work on the hands of your client, stand beside them and stand up straight. Make sure your table is at a convenient level for you. You should be able to stand comfortably next to the person who is lying on the table.

Keep your legs spread about shoulder width apart to give you a solid foundation. This will keep your back straight and help to keep you from leaning on one leg too long, which will tire you and over time can ruin your posture.

# Stepping into the Future with Reflexology

No one can predict the future (well, at least not with 100 percent accuracy!), but as far as reflexology goes, we can at least see what direction we are heading. The goal of many reflexology associations is that reflexology become a separate therapy apart from any other type of therapy, especially massage.

Currently, in 1999, reflexology really does not have its own status apart from massage. Many schools licensed as massage therapy schools also have reflexology programs. Some reflexology schools only teach reflexology, but are licensed by the state as massage therapy schools. In some states, you have to be a massage

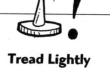

**Tread Lightly**

Massage therapy and reflexology are separate therapies. Try not to confuse the terms or practices in the same modality.

therapist to practice reflexology! Even in Canada, where reflexology is a widespread, popular, and common practice, it still seems to be blurred into massage therapy. Worldwide, reflexologists are working to make reflexology a separate therapy from all other modalities. See Appendix A, "Reflexology Schools, Teachers, and Associations," to find some reflexology organizations and schools that can get you started on your path to becoming a reflexologist.

# Massage Versus Reflexology

Many reflexologists are nurses or massage therapists who decided to specialize in reflexology. Some of us, like myself, are not massage therapists, nor do we have any interest in practicing massage therapy. (Not to say that I don't enjoy receiving it!)

Even though most of the training you will find in reflexology will be found at massage schools, reflexology is not massage therapy. The differences in the therapies are charted out in the following table, based on information produced by the American Reflexology Certification Board, which is a national certification board in the United States.

## Reflexology and Massage Contrasted

| Difference | Massage | Reflexology |
|---|---|---|
| History/originators | Per Henrik Ling (1776–1839) | Dr. William Fitzgerald (1872–1942) |
| Techniques and terminology | Tapotement, petrissage, effleurage, friction, vibration | Alternating pressure, thumb walking, finger walking, hook and backup, rotation on a reflex |
| Basic premise | Stroking restores metabolic balance within the soft tissue; works with superficial tissue | There are zones and reflex areas in the feet and hands corresponding to all body parts; works with reflexes |
| Application of techniques | To entire body; client undresses; oils, lotions, or creams used | Hands and feet and possibly ears; only shoes and socks removed; oils, lotions, or creams not used |

| Difference | Massage | Reflexology |
|---|---|---|
| Body of knowledge | Books on massage, massage schools, massage associations, and massage certifications | 40+ (now 41+) books solely on reflexology, reflexology schools, reflexology associations, and reflexology certification |

(Special note: Irish reflexologist Anthony Larkin claims to have the largest collection of reflexology books in the world—this one makes #100! See Appendix A for more.)

| Difference | Massage | Reflexology |
|---|---|---|
| Research | Unknown | Scientific research studies have been conducted in the U.S., Australia, and Denmark proving the effectiveness of reflexology |
| Definition | Massage is the systematic and scientific manipulation of the soft tissues of the body | Reflexology is the application of specific pressures to reflex points in the hands and feet |

*(Courtesy of the ARCB)*

## Reflect on This

Reflexologists should not be required to attend massage school if they have no intention to practice massage any more than a chiropractor should have to become an orthopedic surgeon. Orthopedic surgery is a different therapy with a different philosophy than chiropractic care, just as reflexology is different from massage therapy.

If reflexologists want their own mode of healing, they will need to separate it from massage and teach it in schools focusing completely on the holistic nature and theory of reflexology. In the future, we may see more schools specializing in reflexology as their sole curriculum and an increase in hours of practice and schooling required to become a professionally certified reflexologist.

## Foot Note

Currently, many schools require about 100 hours of documented reflexology sessions after you complete class to earn certification. The ARCB board also requires an additional 100 hours to qualify for national certification!

As this ancient, natural, safe therapy is introduced into modern days, unfortunately more and more folks will push for rules, guidelines, and laws to regulate it. But don't worry. If you are new to reflexology, you are on the cutting edge of the future of health care. You will always be able to take care of yourself and your family for the rest of your life, no matter where reflexology takes us in the future. Enjoy the ride and welcome to being self-empowered with reflexology!

As for taking reflexology into the future, keep your eyes open for the use of laser technology integrated with reflexology. The Modern Institute of Reflexology is working to stay on the pulse of this technology by incorporating the lower- and higher-level laser technology into their foot, hand, and ear reflexology curriculum!

And now it's into the future for the next chapter, which will guide your footsteps on the path to a successful reflexology career.

## The Least You Need to Know

➤ Learn to keep a professional distance from your clients so that you don't wind up in legal trouble or take on the burdens of the people you work on.

➤ Only work on a person when you feel good yourself to avoid transferring negative energy or illness.

➤ As a reflexologist you should take good care of your entire structural system by supplementing with minerals and doing your own hand exercises and stretches.

➤ Reflexology is different from massage. Keep your eyes open to see reflexology become a separate therapy in the future.

➤ No matter where reflexology goes as a profession, once you learn this ancient healing art, you are empowered to take care of your health naturally.

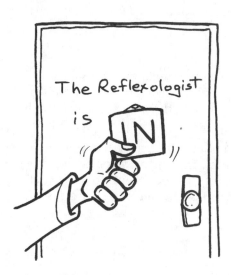

# Chapter 22

# Reflexologists as Sole Practitioners

> ### In This Chapter
>
> ➤ Learn how to start a reflexology practice
>
> ➤ Discover how to make reflexology treatments a holistic experience
>
> ➤ See how you can make your practice unique
>
> ➤ Find out how to cover your bases with a consent form
>
> ➤ Learn to keep a step ahead of the future reflexology laws

A reflexologist goes to the doctor. "Doc," he says pointing to his foot, "When I touch my colon reflex it hurts. When I touch my neck reflex it hurts. And when I touch my stomach reflex it hurts. Do I have some rare disease?"

"No," the doctor replies, "you have a broken finger."

This chapter is designed to help you get started in your reflexology career. It will also give you the bigger picture, to help you see reflexology treatments as a holistic experience, rather than a focused pressure on a single point. I will help set you up so that your practice in reflexology is unique, legal, organized, and successful, whether you have a home-based practice or work in an office.

Fortunately, it is rather inexpensive to start a reflexology practice, and you can become a sole proprietor in no time!

# Getting a Foot in the Door

To become successful in anything, the first step, of course, is to know your subject well. The rest is a matter of marketing, advertising, publicity, word of mouth, timing, and location. But the most important factor in determining the success of a practice is the sincerity of intent.

The bottom line, in my experience as a holistic health practitioner, is that word of mouth is the way you are going to build your business. The only way you get word-of-mouth business is if you take care of each and every one of your clients to the best of your abilities. Each person has unique needs and personalities, but everyone can see through you if you are not sincere.

## *Buy One, Get One Free*

As for the rest of it, cover your bases—be professional, on time, clean, and friendly. Let folks know you are out there with business cards, brochures, flyers, ads, or even articles in the local paper or magazines. Then make sure they can find you—get an answering machine or voice mail so you don't miss any potential business.

### Foot Note

You don't want to leave a poor impression when a potential client calls the number on your business card or in the Yellow Pages. If your three-year-old answers the phone or your customer gets no answer at all, you will probably lose business! Use a number where a client can leave a message or make sure you answer the phone yourself.

Initially, you might find that it can help to get folks in to see you if you offer specials or coupons. Ultimately, though, you want to build a practice on repeat business. To do this, you must connect with your clients. And to do that, you must have the following:

➤ Good intentions

➤ Sincerity

➤ A good knowledge of the therapy

➤ All your business bases covered

From there I encourage you to put your full personality, interest, and style into your practice.

## *Finding a Niche*

Some of you may want to specialize your practice. Maybe you love children and want to become a reflexologist who specializes in children. From there you might want to specialize even further by working with children with certain conditions like ADD, diabetes, handicaps, or asthma. You could even start teaching new parents how to work on their babies.

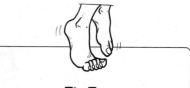

**Tip Toe**

When you have continued success with reflexology for a particular ailment or enjoy working with a certain type of person, you may have found a niche to specialize in!

Some of you might be into fitness and want to have an office in a health club and work on people with sports injuries. Maybe pregnant women hold your interest and you enjoy working on them. You might want to expand your skills to become a midwife and a reflexologist!

I know one reflexologist who specializes in working with the handicapped and especially those with no feeling in their lower body. The stimulation helps simulate walking in the nervous system and helps their entire body.

I enjoy the elderly and love to see the great responses I get from these people. Consequently, I volunteer my services at a local nursing home. I also make special house calls to do business with elderly people. But you can specialize in any group you would like without having to turn down other people that come your way.

Reflexology is universal. Just start working on people and let your heart guide you to your specialty. Usually it will be a certain condition or certain people that you have the most success with that will guide you to a specialty.

I like the combinations of reflexology, aromatherapy, and ear coning. I specialize in folks with allergies and ringing in the ears because I have had continued success with them. You will find your passion—the folks you were destined to share your healing abilities with will find you. Be open and let the world know you are here to serve!

# The Healing Atmosphere

Atmosphere can create a mood and enhance—or take away from—what should be a positive experience. Loud or irritating noises, offensive smells, uncomfortable temperatures, and bright, annoying lights can all take away from the effects you want to create with a reflexology session. Your office should be dimly lit to enhance relaxation. Burning candles add atmosphere. Try not to have vibrating or bright lights in your client's face as they lie back to be worked on.

The following photo shows me working on my husband on our back deck. It is nice to have a healing view, but it is not always feasible. We try to make our whole life holistic, so we have chosen a beautiful place to live. However, most sessions will be indoors, so try to give your clients a nice view to look at or lower the lights and give them atmosphere, depending on what you think is most appropriate.

*Now this is what I call a room with a view! Atmosphere is important when practicing reflexology.*

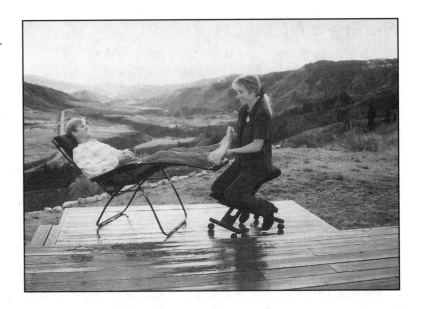

**Foot Note**

I once lived right on a huge lake, and my reflexology home office was a room looking out over the lake. My clients loved to watch the waves roll up and the swans and ducks paddle by as I worked on them. Nature is naturally relaxing. If you can't share a natural view with your clients, keep the room dimly lit, add candles and good smells, and you will induce relaxation in your client and yourself!

## Sounds and Smells

Begin collecting a nice array of soft, relaxing music to play while you are working on clients. Some good choices include Native American flute music, harp, and piano. Instrumentals are best. You can even have your client choose their favorite type.

The use of essential oils for aromatherapy is discussed in Chapter 17, "Tools of the Trade." It is best to purchase and use only the high-quality, grade A oils. Most over-the-counter oils are diluted with another less-expensive oil or synthetically produced and combined with a small amount of the real essential oil.

Many times, the synthetic materials in the oils will give people headaches or nausea. Beware of the quality of what you use. Many people are sensitive to smells, especially if they have lowered immune systems, poor liver function, or if they are pregnant.

## *Maintaining the Mood*

Once you've set the stage, begin working and be quiet! Remember that the client is paying you, and this is their time to be pampered. It is okay to talk with a client while you are working on them, but let the client initiate the talking.

Try to keep your answers brief. It is not an invitation to let them know your life story. If you engage your client in an intellectually stimulating conversation, it will keep them mentally focused, which will inhibit their relaxation.

# Working from Home

Fortunately, a reflexology practice is very easy to start from your home! All you need are the following:

➤ A massage table or reflexology chair

➤ A chair for you to sit on

➤ A private, quiet room

It is especially important to have a special room (other than your bedroom please!) that is dedicated to reflexology only. A separate room dedicated to your practice will give privacy and make the client feel comfortable. It will also alleviate the problem of unexpected guests such as delivery people interrupting you, kids or spouses coming in and disturbing you, and will keep any pets you might have from entering your work space.

**Tread Lightly**

Avoid applying synthetic or offensively strong smelling materials to the body because the skin absorbs what is applied to it. This can cause reactions and even leave a bad taste in your client's mouth, figuratively and literally!

**Tip Toe**

You can suggest a small donation for your reflexology services while still in school. This will help you attract business and get feedback on your techniques while you build confidence. It will give you a head start once you decide to establish yourself as a reflexologist.

If you can manage it, having a home-based practice with a separate entrance for your business is best. This is not possible for many, so if you can arrange it, make your office as close to the entrance as possible—just so you don't have folks wandering through your home to find their way in and out.

Once you pick your room and have it set up with all the essentials, it's time to decorate. Reflexology charts on the wall make great additions, as well as your reflexology certificate, business license, and any insurance policy you have to practice, if you like. And of course, all the "extras" that make reflexology a holistic experience should be included.

## No Pets Allowed

It is very important if you have pets to make sure that they have no contact with your clients! Many people are afraid of dogs—no matter how friendly! Keep dogs and cats in the backyard and away from approaching clients. A dog jumping up on a visitor's car can make you lose the client permanently.

Be meticulous about cleanliness in your house if you have an indoor pet. The pet should never be allowed in the room where you have your clients. Many folks have animal allergies, and you don't want them to leave your home/office in worse shape than when they came to see you! This is not good for repeat business!

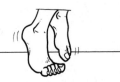

**Tip Toe**

Follow the same professional guidelines and behaviors for your home-based business as you would if you were leasing a professional office space. Making it easy and practical for your clients to visit you will keep your practice buzzing!

## Keep It Clean

Keep the pathway to the entrance of your home office clear. If there is snow, shovel it, and put down salt if there is ice. Keep toys, bikes, and all clutter away from the driveway and surrounding areas, especially during the times you are seeing clients. Try to have an obvious, designated spot for your clients to park if possible.

Additional insurance coverage on your home office for personal liability is something you will need. This will help to protect you from misfortunes, such as your clients slipping or hurting themselves coming to your home. You will have to contact your insurance company to get details on adding a policy to cover people coming to and from your house for therapy.

# Stopping Trouble Before It Starts

Legal issues surface in everything we do these days. Reflexology is no different. No matter how good your intent and how well you practice, you will always want to be prepared to cover yourself if someone decides to turn on you.

Sometimes you will work with very ill people. Sometimes when people are suffering they look for someone to blame. The proactive approach to avoiding this situation is to require a signed consent form for everyone you work on, before you work on them. Have a potential client sign a form releasing you from any liability. If the client is a minor, have the legal guardian sign *and* the minor, if they are old enough to write.

## Getting Consent

Another good rule if you are working with an elderly or sick person is to get family members to sign your form before you work on the person. If someone refuses to sign, this could indicate that you might have trouble in the future. If everyone is in agreement, then you are more likely to have the goodwill of everyone involved.

Following is a sample consent form. You can modify it as you wish and use it to inform your clients about reflexology and the cleansing reactions that may occur. You will also be disclosing that you are not a medical doctor. Remember, you are really not doing anything more to them than if they were to walk barefoot in the gravel! But the consent form is a necessary ingredient for our protection and the client's information.

**Tread Lightly**

Keep these words out of your vocabulary: **treat, diagnose, prescribe,** and **cure** when in practice. If you use them, you could be charged with practicing medicine without a license. Reflexologists do not do any of the above. Make it clear to your clients that you are not a medical doctor (unless you are, of course!).

# *Reflexology Consent Form*

Our services neither diagnose nor prescribe for disease conditions. All clients are encouraged to seek competent medical help when those services are deemed necessary. The client accepts total responsibility for his/her own health care and maintenance.

Nothing said, done, performed, typed, printed, or produced by us is intended or meant to diagnose, prescribe, treat a disease, or take the place of a licensed physician. This work is not medical treatment. It is a form of health maintenance utilizing the techniques and principles of reflexology.

I understand that there may be some physiological responses that are sometimes related to the self-healing process such as: nausea, dizziness, diarrhea, muscle soreness, or depression, all of which may occur naturally as part of a cleansing process due to reflexology treatments. I further understand that reflexology may be helpful in the alleviation of pain from any suspected ailment(s) I may have had before the session. However, alleviation of pain is not synonymous with "recovery" from any suspected dysfunction, and I will therefore refrain from any excessive activity that might cause further injury to myself during my healing process. By signing below, I acknowledge and fully agree with the above information.

_____

Client's Signature                                        Date

_____

Practitioner's Signature                                 Date

# Client Instructions

Please remove your jewelry.

Please remember to breathe. Holding your breath holds tension and pain, while exhaling tends to help release tension and pain.

Pain is not gain in reflexology. Pain will cause the body to tense automatically. Though deep pressure may be used in various techniques, please discuss any discomfort with me, so that techniques may be adjusted to your particular needs.

After the treatment: Everyone responds differently to this type of therapeutic treatment. Take a few moments to feel the effects of your treatment and please feel free to discuss with me any impressions you may have.

Drink lots of extra water. Typically, reflexology stimulates blood and lymph flow, releasing toxins from the body. Eight glasses of pure water per day will help the reflexology refresh your body completely.

CANCELLATION POLICY: So that I may better serve all my clients, 24-hour notice is required for cancellations. You will be charged for the full session with less than 24 hours notification.

I have read all of the above and understand and agree with it completely. I, therefore, consent of my own free will to this and any subsequent treatments, on this _____ day of _____ month, year _____.

_____
Print Client's Name

_____
Client's Signature

_____
Print Practitioner's Name

_____
Practitioner's Signature

# Information, Please

When setting up appointments over the phone, use caution in the words you use. Be sure to let people who are inquiring about your services know that you are not a medical doctor and that you do not treat diseases. What you can tell them is that you utilize a natural healing therapy (reflexology) that assists the body in healing and balancing itself. I always tell the person what my fees are, what forms of payment I accept, and how long the appointment will last when they make their appointment. I also suggest that they wear comfortable clothing, such as sweat pants or shorts, for their comfort.

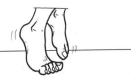

### Tip Toe

If you use a massage table in your practice, have a footstool next to the table to help your clients onto the table. I learned this lesson when working with a petite woman who had to "jump" up on my table in order to sit on it! This action caused the structure of my table to crack! Since then I have always provided a footstool to clients short and tall!

When you see a client for the first time, you will want to let them know what to expect up front. Make sure you have verbally addressed the information in the preceding "Client Instructions" sheet.

Have a shallow container nearby where they can place their jewelry and eyeglasses safely. And, if it's not obvious to them, ask them to remove their shoes and socks, too!

Make sure that the new client has read and signed your consent and instruction forms. Ask them if they have any broken bones or injuries on the feet or hands that you need to know about. Using a medical case history form is also a good idea. Having lots of information about the person will allow you to better help them and understand some of the conditions they are experiencing. For instance, if they have checked asthma on their medical history form, you might want to ask them if they have trouble breathing while lying on their back; if so, address that up front by propping some pillows under them, or simply work on them in a chair instead.

You can make your own medical history form, or use the one I have provided for you if you wish. The most important things I look for on the forms are:

➤ If the person bruises easily

➤ If there are any broken bones or other injuries on the hands or feet that I need to be aware of

➤ If the person has epilepsy or any other disorder that can come unexpectedly that I need to be aware of

➤ If the person is pregnant

The following form I provide is a little detailed because I practice more than one modality, and therefore the information I retrieve is more than what might be needed to give a reflexology session, but it never hurts to have this information on file.

# Medical History

Have you had or do you currently have any of the following on a regular basis?

Circle the item if you have the condition *presently*, "X" the item if you have had the condition in the *past*.

| Diagnosed Diseases | Ailments | Surgeries or Injuries |
| --- | --- | --- |
| \_\_\_\_ HIV/AIDS | \_\_\_\_ Fatigue | \_\_\_\_ Removal of *any* organs (hysterectomy, appendix, tonsils, gallbladder, etc.) |
| \_\_\_\_ Cancer—where? | \_\_\_\_ Stressful lifestyle Explain: \_\_\_\_\_ _____ _____ | \_\_\_\_ Broken bones—which? _____ _____ |
| \_\_\_\_ Lupus | \_\_\_\_ Depressed | \_\_\_\_ Hernia operation |
| \_\_\_\_ Fibromyalgia | \_\_\_\_ Cold sores | \_\_\_\_ Chemotherapy |
| \_\_\_\_ Manic depressive | \_\_\_\_ Moodiness | |
| \_\_\_\_ MS | \_\_\_\_ Bloating | |
| \_\_\_\_ Epilepsy | \_\_\_\_ Belching | |
| \_\_\_\_ Addictions—what? | \_\_\_\_ Gas (intestinal) | |
| \_\_\_\_ Ulcer—where? | \_\_\_\_ Mouth ulcers | |
| \_\_\_\_ IBS/Colitis | \_\_\_\_ Thin fingernails | |
| \_\_\_\_ Diverticulitis | \_\_\_\_ Irregular bowel movements | |
| \_\_\_\_ Hemorrhoids | \_\_\_\_ Rashes | |
| \_\_\_\_ High/low blood pressure | \_\_\_\_ Red blotches on face | |
| \_\_\_\_ Endometriosis | \_\_\_\_ Insomnia | |
| \_\_\_\_ Diabetes | \_\_\_\_ Oily skin/acne | |
| \_\_\_\_ Arthritis | \_\_\_\_ Irregular menstruation or difficulty | |
| \_\_\_\_ Asthma | \_\_\_\_ Short of breath | |
| \_\_\_\_ Kidney stones/ bladder infections | \_\_\_\_ Painful urination | |

Allergies: \_\_\_\_ foods \_\_\_\_ medicines \_\_\_\_ environmental \_\_\_\_ animals

*continues*

*continued*

---

Are you currently taking any medications? _____ yes _____ no

If yes, please list which drugs and what they are for:

_____ for _____

_____ for _____

_____ for _____

Are you pregnant? _____ yes _____ no

If yes, have you ever had trouble carrying before? _____ yes _____ no

Are you breast-feeding? _____ yes _____ no

Family physician name: _____

Address: _____

_____

Phone: _____

General complaints or is there anything I have not asked you that you feel I need to know?

_____

_____

_____

PLEASE MARK ANY AREAS OF PAIN OR TENSION ON MODEL BELOW:
(This is where I have an outline of a body, and a pair of feet too!)

---

While first observing your new client's feet and medical history form you should discover if they have any of the contraindications for reflexology (see Chapter 15, "How to Touch"). Ask if they have had reflexology before and if there is anything they would like to share about that. Also inquire if there is anything, especially physical complaints, that they want you to focus on for the therapy. These things should all be communicated between you and your client before you start.

# Certifiably Certifiable

Reflexology is not necessarily recognized by every state as a separate modality apart from massage therapy. Therefore, either there are no licensing laws governing the practice of reflexology, or there are laws that require you to be a licensed massage therapist to practice reflexology. Find out what the laws are in your state/country before you start on your path to becoming a reflexologist.

If you are in an area where reflexology is not regulated by the government, this does not mean that you will be safe from legislation at a later time. For example, some massage therapy groups wish to have local licensing laws for their practices. Depending on how they write these laws, if the laws get passed, this could make it illegal for you to practice reflexology unless you are a massage therapist! (Another reason why I don't care for this type of legislation.)

It is not that the massage therapists intend to put you out of business. If the wording in the bill says that in order for you to have a business where you touch another person (feet or otherwise) you have to be a licensed massage therapist, then you will not be able to practice reflexology!

## A Foot into the Future

Keep these tips in mind to stay ahead of any possible future government regulations that could put you out of practice:

➤ After reflexology training and certification by your private reflexology teacher/school/ program, begin preparing for national certification through an independent national certification board for the country you intend to practice in. See more on what these boards' goals are in Chapter 17, "Tools of the Trade."

➤ Find out the minimum number of hours or credits that a licensed massage therapist needs to practice legally in your hometown. Whatever that number is, make sure that you acquire the same amount of hours or credits in your area of specialty—foot, hand, and ear reflexology—even if it requires you to attend more than one school. Be creative.

**Tip Toe**

Once you are certified (nationally) by your own country's organization, they should be able to keep you informed of changing laws that may affect your practice. They should also work to protect your rights to practice reflexology locally. If not, seek out another organization that protects the rights of natural health practitioners in general to practice their modalities. One of these national organizations that has been especially helpful to me is:

Coalition for Natural Health
1200 L Street N.W., Suite 100–408
Washington, D.C. 20005
800-586-4264
E-mail: ttchh@naturalhealth.org
Web site: www.naturalhealth.org

➤ Stay on top of all local legislative laws that come into play as they relate to all holistic practitioners. Any laws affecting the broad natural health field could possibly affect you.

## Credit Where It's Due

Reflexologists owe a debt of gratitude to the massage therapists who have paved a path for other disciplines in making bodywork legitimate. They have also paved the way for us to work beside other health care professionals. And they have awakened the medical insurance companies to the preventative value in natural therapy so that reimbursement for our services is becoming a reality.

### Foot Note

I would always suggest to an aspiring reflexologist that they work toward their country's highest certification levels. If, in the future, reflexology stands alone as its own modality, then more than likely it will be your national, independent testing organizations who will set the standards for what qualifies a reflexologist to practice. See Appendix A, "Reflexology Schools, Teachers, and Associations," to find a reflexology organization that can teach you more.

Reflexology boards are working together to push for reflexology to become a separate modality from massage. If this happens, your training as a reflexologist will also be separate from the massage training. You will become a foot, lower-leg, and hand specialist. You will know the foot and the zones and the reflex points better than any massage therapist who doesn't have your specialized training.

You will also be able to talk intelligently with acupressure specialists and acupuncturists alike with your in-depth knowledge of the energy zones and pressure points on the feet, hands, and ears. So keep your ears and eyes open and never stop learning! Have a good time with it, add your own style, and you will have a long-lasting, rewarding career in reflexology.

### The Least You Need to Know

➤ Being sincere in your intent will help you gain repeat business and a practice built by word of mouth.

➤ Make your reflexology treatments an extension of your personality, and customize your atmosphere to reflect your unique style.

➤ You might want to choose a niche in reflexology. Use your passion or your successes to help you choose.

➤ Get certified in reflexology, then work to increase your skills.

➤ Set up a safe and comfortable work space, tell your clients what to expect, and always get a signed consent form.

# Part 5
# Reflexology in Action

*Even though reflexology does not claim to treat or cure diseases, many people have had their symptoms relieved and ailments reversed because of the use of reflexology. Anecdotal evidence lets us experience firsthand our clients' healing process. The next section will give you specific points to work on for some common ailments and will highlight some positive testimonials to the value of reflexology.*

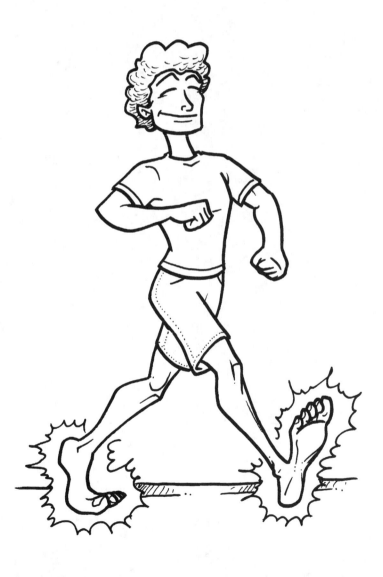

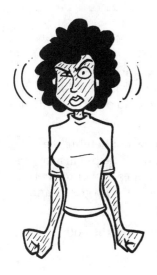

# Chapter 23

# Keeping Your Glands in Order

---

## In This Chapter

➤ Learn what specific reflexes to work on for PMS

➤ Find out how to help diabetics with reflexology

➤ Learn which reflexes best help balance hormones

➤ See how working on the thyroid reflexes can balance the glands

➤ Hear a few testimonials from folks helped by reflexology

---

I had a phone call from a man one day: "Is this Frankie, the reflexologist who just worked on my wife Karen this morning?" "Yes, how can I help you?" I asked, a little nervous about the seriousness I detected in his voice. "Do you sell gift certificates for your sessions?" he asked, still leaving me no clue what he was really after. "Yes," I replied. "Well, I would like to buy a year's worth for my wife," he said sternly. "What?" I asked, feeling bemused. "She came home after her treatment a new woman! I haven't seen her this relaxed and happy in years. I really don't want to know what you're doing to her," he said, "but I would like you to keep on doing it!"

The moral of this short story is that reflexology can make you feel very good, particularly when it comes ro relieving the tension associated with PMS and glandular imbalances. And it might even do wonders for your relationships!

# Are You Unbalanced?

Reflexology is not meant to diagnose or treat disease conditions. However, many of us suffer from imbalances of the body that medical doctors can offer no cure for or assistance with. I have seen these imbalances regain balance over and over, not only in my own health, but also in the lives of many of my clients.

**Tip Toe**

Many women (including myself) have used the herbal supplement evening primrose oil, which has hormone-like substances to eliminate the cramps associated with periods. Evening primrose oil seems to be most effective when you take three to six capsules daily for at least one week before menstruation.

Reflexology has the mysterious effect of helping the body do what it was designed to do. It helps balance the glands and stimulate the sluggish ones back into action. It seems to be able to wake up those sleepy glands and get them moving again.

Our glands control myriad functions in the body, including the following:

➤ Metabolism

➤ Growth

➤ Menstrual cycles

➤ Fertility

➤ Emotions

➤ Body temperature

➤ Weight regulation

If any one of these is not working properly, it can makes us feel slow or hyper, have irregular cycles, experience sterility, frigidity, or mood swings, or feel too hot or too cold! None of these imbalances are any fun, and any of them can be a real nuisance in our lives.

The preceding conditions are not always medical diseases, but they are things that we can deal with if we can incorporate natural healing therapies like reflexology into our lives. We will see how some people have been helped by reflexology and learn which reflexes to work on to help get you back in balance!

# How to Ride a Twenty-Eight-Day Cycle

Here's a story about one of my past reflexology students/clients and how her periods were regulated with the use of reflexology. For as long as she could remember, her periods were irregular. Sometimes they were 20 days apart, other times she went as long as 70 days! Not only did she never know when her periods were going to begin or end, but when they did come, they were excruciatingly painful! The pain was merciless and would usually last for four hours and usually made her sick.

**Foot Note**

A small percentage of all menstruating women experience **dysmenorrhea**, a period associated with pain, nausea, vomiting, and sometimes faintness. The cause may be related to fibroid cysts, endometriosis, pelvic inflammatory disease, or the presence of an IUD.

Even her OB-GYN was insensitive to this problem. So she sought another. Both told her that some women "just get cramps" and that she should take a "strong" pain medication like ibuprofen. "Well, let me tell you," she says, "I would have taken a truckload of ibuprofen if it would have even come close to helping me! Nothing that I took seemed to help my pain or regulate my periods."

## A Learning Experience

Then, she enrolled in her first reflexology class. The day after her first class she began her period. To her surprise, the cramps were not as severe after practicing in reflexology class as they had been before. They still lasted four hours, but the pain did not make her cry or throw up!

The reflex points that help regulate periods include:

➤ Ovary

➤ Uterus

➤ Fallopian tube

➤ Pituitary

"I never linked my lessened cramps or the start of my period to the reflexology treatments," she says, "at least not then. But as I continued with my monthly reflexology sessions and followed up at home on myself weekly, my cycle started to even out. I had three periods within three months of beginning to use reflexology! Coincidence or not, I was delighted."

She continued to come in for treatments. Being skeptical, she did not necessarily link her improvement with the reflexology sessions; however, it was the only significant change she had made to her life over the course of the time that she improved!

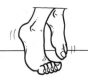

### Tip Toe

Zone therapy works for relieving the pain of menstrual cramps. For menstrual pain, press and hold the ovary and uterus reflex points until the pain subsides. The uterus and ovary reflexes are located on either side of the flat part of your heel. The fallopian tube reflex connects both of these points around the top side of the ankle joint.

## Coping with Cramps

I told her that when she experienced cramping, she should apply pressure to both her ovary and uterus reflex points and hold them until the pain subsided. (These reflexes are located on either side of the flat part of your heel.) This worked very well to help diminish the pain, especially during the first four hours of her most severe cramping.

"Now," she says, "if I do not get regular reflexology treatments and choose to neglect reflexology for my own feet, my period has a tendency to begin a day or two late. As soon as I become aware of this, I have my husband apply pressure on my ovary and uterus reflex points. The stimulation works almost immediately, and I will get my period usually within 12 hours."

*Menstrual trouble reflex points: Working these spots on both feet has helped many with balancing cycles and alleviating pain associated with menstrual cramps.*

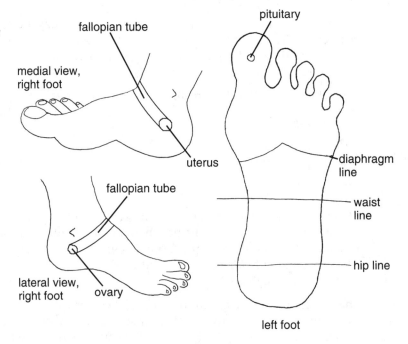

She was finally convinced that her sessions were the main reason for her improvement. By aiding her hormones and helping her glandular system through the use of reflexology, her body balanced itself. Although I have since moved away from this client's hometown, I do visit occasionally to see her and other clients in the area. She keeps in touch, and every time I see her she expresses her gratitude to me for introducing her to reflexology and says she has been on a regular cycle now for years. Not only that, but reflexology is a fulfilling career for her, too!

**Foot Note**

In addition to reflexology, herbs and supplements can be the finishing touch to a pain-free lifestyle! Look for my *The Complete Idiot's Guide to Herbal Remedies,* coming soon to a bookstore near you!

# Dealing with Diabetes

I have worked with a handful of clients who had adult onset diabetes. Coincidence or not, after working with these people, not only did they all feel better, but at least one of them was able to lower the amount of insulin that she was required to take. Another client was on two types of insulin and was able to eliminate one of them with regular reflexology sessions!

Of course, this was done under the direction of their physicians. Both these women felt that their improvement was a testimonial that natural therapies can help the body work better. This also shows how reflexology can not only be a preventative or an alternative therapy, but a complementary therapy to regular medical care.

Both of these diabetic women were on several medications during their treatments with me. The natural therapy, along with medical care, helped them recover and lessened their requirement for some medications.

**Tread Lightly**

Never take yourself off a medication without the assistance of your trusted physician. Also, as a reflexologist, NEVER tell your clients to take themselves off their medications, or to use reflexology IN PLACE OF their prescriptions! This can be dangerous to the person and can also get you in trouble. Always refer the client back to their physician for medical matters.

### The Sole Meaning

**Diabetes mellitus** is a disorder of carbohydrate metabolism in which sugars in the body are not oxidized to produce energy due to lack of pancreatic insulin. Symptoms of diabetes include excessive thirst, sugar in the urine, and poor digestion. Complications can include poor circulation leading to slow healing, poor eyesight, weight gain, and coma if insulin and diet are not regulated.

# How Sweet It Isn't

Let's take a closer look at what diabetes is all about. Diabetes occurs when the pancreas fails to secrete enough insulin. *Diabetes mellitus* is the medical term for what most of us commonly call diabetes. It is a disorder of carbohydrate metabolism in which sugars in the body are not oxidized to produce energy due to lack of the pancreatic hormone insulin or because of the body's resistance to insulin.

The accumulation of sugar leads to its appearance in the blood, or *hyperglycemia*, which literally means high blood sugar. Symptoms include thirst, weight gain or loss, and the excessive production of urine. The use of fats as an alternative source of energy leads to disturbances of the acid/alkaline balance in the body and can cause *ketosis*, which is the imbalance of fat metabolism. If left untreated, diabetes can eventually lead to convulsions and even diabetic coma.

## Triggers and Treatments

Although there appears to be an inherited tendency to diabetes, diabetes may also be triggered by various factors, including physical stress (affecting the adrenals). Diabetes that starts in childhood or adolescence is usually more severe than that beginning in middle or old age.

Treatment is based on a carefully controlled diet, with injections of insulin or drugs that are taken by mouth to lower blood sugar levels. Lack of balance in the diet or in the amount of insulin taken leads to *hypoglycemia* (over-production of insulin by the pancreas, which lowers blood sugar levels).

Long-term complications of diabetes include thickening of the arteries, which can affect the eyes. Other effects include circulation problems that can manifest as slow wound healing. This is probably due to the fact that blood supply to the wounded area is decreased due to a sluggish circulatory system.

This is another reason why reflexology can be such a great therapy for people who suffer with diabetes. Reflexology stimulates circulation, which is necessary in healing wounds and can help get the blood supply moving and help bring the blood to the extremities such as the hands and feet.

# Back in Circulation

Because of poor circulation associated with diabetes, several areas of the body are affected by the disease. The entire urinary system is affected, since the body is trying to rid itself of excess acid wastes. The eyes can also be troubled due to a lack of circulation. The adrenals are also affected, as well as the pancreas and the digestive system.

### Foot Note

Some diabetics are prone to fungus growth on the toenails. This is probably due to the fact that there is a lack of blood supply carrying oxygen to the extremities, making an ideal environment for fungus growth. If you are diabetic, you might want to try a natural remedy first before scheduling a toenail removal (as some doctors have ordered for this problem). Since your healing time is slower, the recovery time from such an operation can be agonizingly long. See the table in Chapter 20, "Podiatry Matters," for some natural therapies that have helped many get rid of athlete's foot and toenail fungus.

When working on someone who suffers from diabetes, work the areas that are most tender, as usual, but make sure you do not skip the following important areas:

➤ Eyes*

➤ Spleen

➤ Liver

➤ Pancreas*

➤ Stomach

➤ Adrenals

➤ Urinary system

➤ Kidneys*

The reflex areas marked with an asterisk (*) above are the three *most important* areas to work for diabetes. Reflexology will not necessarily lower blood sugar levels, but it can help balance the glands and increase circulation. Increasing the circulation of a diabetic can help their body speed up the healing process and help them get blood moving up to the head where it can nourish the eyes!

### Foot Note

A Danish study in 1984 showed a clear increase in blood flow in the subject's body following reflexology treatments. Pictures taken with infrared rays, which can show changes in heat loss, showed the increased blood flow. It is assumed that the improved circulation achieved through reflexology treatments increased the oxygen supply to the brain (blood carries nourishing oxygen).

# PMS: Calming the Beast Within

Since *premenstrual syndrome*, or *PMS*, is a common ailment in women around the world, it is natural for you to see many clients who experience PMS.

Some specific symptoms of PMS include the following:

➤ Mood swings

➤ Tension

➤ Irritability

➤ Bloating

➤ Headaches

### The Sole Meaning

**PMS** stands for **premenstrual syndrome**. It is called a syndrome because of its host of symptoms, which may include tension, irritability, emotional disturbance, headache, abdominal bloating, tender and swollen breasts, pimples, and water retention.

Usually, hormones are on a rampage, which can make a woman feel like she's out of control. Her spouse and children might think the same thing!

Since the pituitary gland (in the brain) is responsible for sending hormonal messages to the rest of the body, it would make sense to stimulate this point when suffering from PMS or to stimulate the point on someone else who is experiencing PMS symptoms. Talk about making your point!

## Too Tense

PMS seems to cause tension in the body. To ease tension, work all along the brain and spinal cord areas to help relax all the muscles in the body. Utilize the relaxation and stretching techniques you learned in this book. Of course you should always work the ovary and uterus areas when dealing with any type of female issues (see the figure earlier in this chapter).

Working the top of the foot (the opposite of the ball of the foot) can also prove useful for lessening tenderness in the breasts during PMS. To work the chest, you can squeeze the webbing between all the metatarsals in the feet and hands. Here's a summary of the points you can work on for PMS, so you can find them in a hurry:

➤ Pituitary (helps with water retention and regulating hormones)

➤ Brain (calms nerves, improves circulation)

➤ Spinal cord (calms nerves, brings out serotonin)

➤ Ovary (regulates hormones)

➤ Uterus (can ease contractions)

➤ Fallopian tube (relaxes pain in pelvic area)

➤ Chest area (opposite lymphatics on top of foot, work by squeezing webbing between metatarsals)

## PMS = Pre-Meditated Surgery Avoided!

Next is a great testimonial to the positive effects that reflexology can have on PMS sufferers. A young woman in her early 30s who I used to work with came to me as her last resort. Her PMS symptoms were so intolerable to herself and her family that her doctor had suggested that she have a hysterectomy. (Remember—removing the hysteria?)

Before such a radical treatment, she wanted to see if reflexology could help her. She told me that we had exactly six weeks before her scheduled surgery date and that if reflexology was going to help her, she had better see improvement before then. Talk about pressure!

**Tread Lightly**

Emergency medical treatment should not be foregone in favor of reflexology. However, reflexology used before an elective surgery or other medical treatments may help alleviate the need for the medical procedure. Give reflexology a try first, and if it doesn't help you completely, at least it can help you recover from your surgery.

Well, needless to say, her regular reflexology treatments proved to be her saving grace—and my saving face! Her symptoms disappeared, and she remained steady and tolerable to herself and her family each month. She made significant improvement after one month, which made her rethink her scheduled surgery. She could see steady improvement and also experienced more dramatic results after about three months of treatments three times per week. Her family was so impressed that they all came to have me work with them, too!

My client never opted to have her hysterectomy and was happy and grateful to have found reflexology as a natural alternative. In addition, she lost approximately 30 pounds of excess weight and told me that she felt she had a new lease on life!

### Foot Note

In 1991, an American study involving 52 women was conducted on the effectiveness of reflexology on premenstrual syndrome. A 46 percent reduction in symptoms was reported over a six-month period on those receiving regular reflexology sessions (information compliments of ARCB).

# Thyroid Be Done

For some reason, thyroid trouble seems to be getting more and more prevalent in younger people. Could it be radiation pollution in the air? Electromagnetic pollution? Something in the pesticides or fertilizers in the foods we eat? Or could it just be a general lack of iodine in our foods?

There are many things to consider when the thyroid is not working properly. Since medical tests will only show a problem with the thyroid's hormone production after the thyroid is already halfway shot, it is best to try and monitor yourself for thyroid troubles. Know what to look for and work preventatively to help yourself before your thyroid gives up on you!

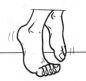

### Tip Toe

Here's a self-test designed by a physician if you suspect you have an underactive thyroid:

Keep a thermometer next to your bed for one week.

Each morning take your temperature under your armpit before getting out of bed, and chart the results.

If your body temperature is below 97.8 for a few days or more, make an appointment to discuss the possibility of low thyroid activity with your doctor.

## *What to Watch For*

Since your thyroid hormone regulates your metabolism, it will have an effect on your movements, your temperature, and even your body development and weight gain or loss. Red flags that something *could* be wrong with the thyroid are covered in Chapter 12, "Sexy Stuff: The Glandular System." Here are some general things to look for. Look for any extremes or significant changes in these areas:

➤ Extremes of body temperature

➤ Change in speech speed

➤ Unexpected changes in weight

➤ Change in sleep patterns

➤ Change in appearance of skin color or texture

➤ Change in hair texture or hair loss (especially women)

# *Working Together*

Since the thyroid works in conjunction with the ovaries and some of the other glands, it is a good idea to work with all the glands of the body if you suspect any problems with the thyroid. Reflexes to work on for thyroid trouble include the following:

➤ Thyroid area (along the ball of the foot under and around the neck of the large toe)

➤ Parathyroids

➤ Pineal gland

➤ Pituitary gland

➤ Ovaries

Since reflexology works on helping the body do what it is supposed to do naturally, stimulating the thyroid reflexes cannot damage the functioning of the organ. You will only help to achieve balance. So don't worry about overstimulating the thyroid with reflexology. Natural therapies do not cause this kind of reaction. It takes synthetics to force your body to do something unnatural.

Overall, you can see that reflexology has helped many to balance their glandular system by stimulating balance in the body. Since it is safe and effective, some lucky ducks have been able to use reflexology to avoid radical surgeries or have been able to reduce the amount of medication they were taking. And because of reflexology's amazing abilities to smooth hormonal ups and downs, marriage counselors may discover reflexology to be instrumental in helping save marriages, too!

---

### The Least You Need to Know

➤ Reflexology is a safe therapy to complement medical treatments.

➤ Never suggest that your client use reflexology in place of their medications. Medications need to be monitored between doctor and patient only. Steer clear of giving any medical advice!

➤ Reflexology cannot force the body to do anything unnatural. It will only stimulate natural healing and balancing.

➤ Refelxology can help diabetics because of its ability to increase circulation and help the glands to balance.

➤ Reflexology can help PMS sufferers by balancing glands and promoting the release of tension.

---

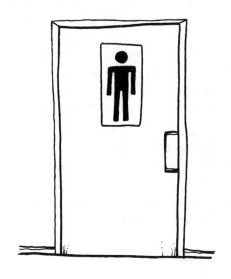

# Chapter 24

# Let's Get Things Moving

---

### In This Chapter

➤ Learn about the cleansing effects of reflexology

➤ Find out about colon transit time

➤ Discover how the nervous system affects our bowel

➤ Get personal with a few clogged-up friends

---

"What did you do to me?" a voice on the other side of the phone asked. "I'm not sure I understand. What's happening?" I politely asked the client I had just seen two days before. "After I left you the other day, I went home and used the bathroom, and it seems this has been my favorite place for the entire weekend!" "Doing some cleansing, eh?" I retorted, "I mentioned to you that this might happen."

"Yes," she said, "and I just wanted to thank you very much. I have never felt so light, so alive, and so relieved in literally what feels like years! I didn't believe you when you told me that I might be constipated, but now I understand!"

This client was chronically constipated but didn't believe that constipation was that big of a deal. In fact, her doctor told her that everyone has their personal regular cycle and that once a week was considered "normal" for her. In this chapter we will talk about what the "ideal" regular schedule should be for digestion and elimination so that you see how your elimination matches up. Then we can see how reflexology can help you catch up if you are slacking in this area. So now, let's get rolling!

# Reflexology: A Moving Experience

One of the first things you experience, especially after your first reflexology session, may be considerable cleansing of the lower bowel. Because reflexology relaxes the entire body, it is especially effective for cases of constipation related to stress or tension.

The bowel is a muscle, and it is closely linked to the nervous system. Reflexology treatments not only help to relieve stress and tension, but will relax all the muscles in the body, resulting in a "moving" experience.

The bowel-loosening effect does not necessarily happen right away, but is usually felt the day after the treatment. If you have a problem with constipation, you will really get "a run for your money" with a reflexologist!

**The Sole Meaning**

**Colon transit time** is a phrase used by holistic nutritionists to address how fast or sluggish your colon may be. It refers to the time it takes for a meal to be eaten and eliminated. A healthy colon's transit time should be between 16 and 18 hours.

**The Sole Meaning**

The **alimentary canal** is the scientific name for what I refer to in this book as the food tube. It is the canal or tube that begins at the mouth and ends at the rectum and processes food for absorption and elimination.

## Transit Time

There is a big difference between the ideal healthy bowel and what most of us have. (See Chapter 6, "A Lot to Swallow: The Digestive and Intestinal System," for more on the digestive and intestinal system.) Ideally, for a person who eats three meals daily, a person with a healthy bowel should evacuate once for every meal eaten.

There is a phrase used by holistic health practitioners referred to as *colon transit time*. Colon transit time is the length of time it takes the food you eat to be digested, absorbed, and the waste products from the digested meal to be evacuated. Entire colon transit time for a healthy bowel should be between 16 to 18 hours.

## The Food Tube

I have labeled the entire digestive and eliminatory system or the *alimentary canal* "the food tube" because the food goes in through the mouth (the top of the tube), to the stomach and intestines, and heads back out of the body as waste materials—all through the same "tube."

The digestive system functions best on regularity. This means that when we eat on a regular schedule, such as three meals a day, there will always be three meals being processed through our food tube. Let me demonstrate:

➤ Breakfast is meal number one. Let's say you are now reading this book at breakfast time, while enjoying a steamy cup of Starbucks latte and munching on a bagel. Just the process of chewing signals to your digestive system to get to work.

➤ At this time, meal number two, which was last night's dinner, is being assimilated and will be found about halfway or more through the food-tube's process.

➤ Meal number three is yesterday's lunch, which will be eliminated shortly after you eat today's breakfast.

➤ By lunchtime today, yesterday's dinner will be ready to be evacuated, and so on it goes with each meal eaten.

See the following illustration to digest the whole picture.

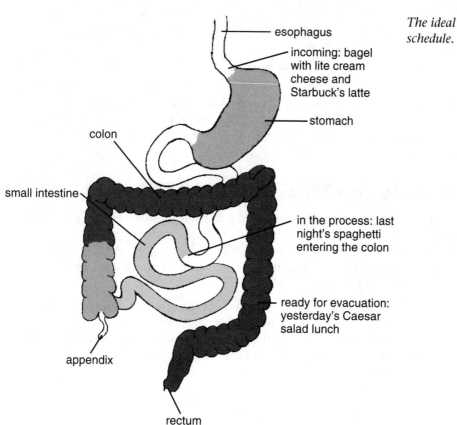

*The ideal food tube schedule.*

329

How can I discern which meal is the one being eliminated, you ask? An old nutritionist's trick is to eat some corn at one of your meals. Note which meal it was and write down the time that you ate it. Once the corn shows up for an encore, you have your colon transit time!

**Foot Note**

Ideally the bowel will be stimulated to eliminate within approximately 20 minutes to one hour after you eat a meal. The evacuation is usually the waste products from two meals ago. Fruit is the exception here because fruit has a much faster colon transit time and serves as a cleanser of the digestive tract and bowel. Some fruits can go through the system in less than four hours.

Anything more than 24 hours is too long. Increase your reflexology treatments, drink more water, eat more fiber and whole, raw foods, try taking two capsules of the herb cascara sagrada before bedtime each night, and go back to Chapter 6 to get more tips on strengthening your bowel.

# Constipation: When Things Are NOT Moving

It is not uncommon during reflexology treatments to hear the stomach and intestines begin to growl. The growling is actually a good sign, since it means you are moving energy. If shortly after beginning a treatment strange noises begin to emerge from beneath the blanket, you can guess that the digestive track is being stimulated into action and the bowel is preparing for elimination.

I have had success with helping people overcome constipation and also spastic bowel conditions using reflexology. In addition, nausea has subsided during the administration of reflexology. A backup of bowel toxins causes some headaches. Stimulating the bowel reflex points on the feet and hands can relieve a headache by allowing the bowel to evacuate promptly.

## A Stimulating Session

Constipation can be relieved with reflexology by stimulating the following reflexes:

➤ Ascending colon

➤ Transverse colon

➤ Descending colon

➤ Small intestine

➤ Liver

A headache or nausea caused by constipation will require the same reflex stimulation with the addition of the brain, neck, and head areas.

**Tread Lightly**

Although fiber is necessary for a smooth-running colon, if your body is not used to the fiber, you may experience intestinal gas or some abdominal bloating for the first few days of adding a fiber supplement (such as psyllium hulls) or extra fruits and vegetables to your diet. This should subside as digestion improves.

## Not By the Zit on My Chinny, Chin, Chin

Another frequent complaint that can be related to constipation is adult acne. More women than men seem to experience this annoying ailment. The first question that should come to mind when faced with this problem is "How often do you frequent the bathroom?"

If the answer is once per day or less, consider focusing on the bowel reflex points. The skin is as clean as the blood is, and the blood is as clean as the bowel. Therefore, cleansing the bowel should get at the root cause of the adult acne problem.

Other than constipation, adult acne can be caused by a hormone imbalance. Daily reflexology self-treatments along with weekly or biweekly treatments administered by a practitioner until the problem subsides may be required to completely balance the glands. For adult acne, especially in women, work the following reflexes:

➤ Bowel

➤ Pituitary

➤ Ovaries

➤ Liver (responsible for filtering excess hormones from the blood)

Once the bowel is cleansed, any related symptoms and ailments clear up. This is the beauty of reflexology; it gets to the source of the problem and helps the body correct itself.

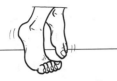

**Tip Toe**

Eat flour-based products less frequently if you suffer from constipation. Such foods as bread, crackers, pastries, and pastas can slow digestion and clog up the colon.

# Joe's Story

My friend Joe is truly an amazing man. His energy is only exceeded by a 170 mph wind mixed with a lightening storm with a bit of swirling hail thrown in. Before his wife Val introduced me to him she exclaimed, "You'll know Joe, he's the one bouncing off walls!"

I thought that was an exaggeration until I met him. After our meeting, I was struck by Val's restraint in describing her husband. In fact, I thought that if Joe ever needed work he could volunteer himself as the methamphetamine poster child.

With Joe's extremely high energy, it is no wonder he has high arches. He moves like lightning and is always on the go. As an electrician, Joe epitomizes the phrase "be one with your work."

## Fixing the Electrician's Shorts

In holistic reflexology we might assume that a person with such high energy tends toward one extreme or another in their bodily functions. We can discern this just observing Joe's personality and energy levels. When Joe does sleep, he sleeps like he is in a coma, but when he is up and running, he is really running!

When working with a high-strung personality, it is important to start out by getting them to relax. Be sure to include the following:

➤ Stretches

➤ Rotations

➤ Central nervous system reflexes

**Tread Lightly**

Drinking prune juice will stimulate things to get moving quickly! However, prune juice should only be used as a home remedy for constipation occasionally and not relied on as a regular "treatment" or replacement for a balanced diet, water, exercise, and reflexology.

About 20 minutes into his first reflexology treatment with me, Joe was fast asleep. Joe never seemed to have any complaints except that he had a hard time gaining weight and that he occasionally experienced constipation. Both of these symptoms are very understandable knowing Joe's fast metabolism and high-strung nature.

## Corn? When Did We Have Corn?

The day following his treatment, Joe called me and asked what I had done to him. He reported that he had to run to the bathroom nearly every hour during the day and was wondering when this might subside! Joe enthusiastically commented that he identified whole pieces of yellow corn in the toilet, but couldn't remember the last time he had eaten corn!

This just goes to show that the bowel can hold onto lots of materials for long periods of time. Our nervous systems can affect the bowel in negative ways by tightening it and hindering its eliminative abilities. By using deep pressure on the bowel reflex points on the feet and hands, the nervous system relaxes and the bowel has the opportunity to release its built-up toxins.

Having energy is not a bad thing, but being high-strung also brings with it the possibility of having "stuck" energies. Don't be surprised if after a treatment you, too, discover yourself releasing components of meals past.

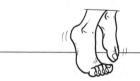

**Tip Toe**

Nervous stress or tension can cause constipation. Use reflexology points for the brain and nervous system along with the food-tube reflexes to encourage the body to eliminate.

# Branden the Constipated

Another client of mine we will talk about here is another overachieving personality. Branden is a beautiful young girl in her early 20s. She is a perfectionist, at least with her expectations of herself. Branden is a top-notch downhill skier who races in National Championships and is a straight-A college student.

Branden was voted high school prom queen, participated in student council, and is a general favorite of her classmates—at least the boys! One of the most noticeable things about Branden, once you get past her fabulous outward beauty, is her speech. Branden speaks so fast that sometimes you cannot understand a word she says! This was the first clue that she might have an uptight colon.

**Foot Note**

Many high-strung types have high-strung colons that can cause constipation or spastic colon conditions. Fast-paced speech is another clue that a person may be high-strung. What do I mean by fast-paced? For instance, at a dinner party, if someone tries to ask you if you ate yet, and instead of hearing "Did you eat?" it sounds like the person said "Jeet?" then you are probably dealing with a high-strung personality type.

# All Stuffed Up and Not Going Anywhere

Branden seems to have clogged-up sinuses that makes her sound nasal, as if she were crying. When talking to Branden, you might notice that she always seems to have a slight sniffle and will sniff periodically throughout your conversation. This constant sniffling is a sign to me that not only are her sinuses clogged up, but that she probably has a sluggish elimination system overall.

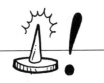

**Tread Lightly**

Keep yourself from getting constipated by eating whole, raw foods on a regular schedule, drinking pure water, and getting exercise and regular reflexology treatments!

When the elimination system is sluggish, symptoms may include:

➤ Constipation

➤ Sinus and respiratory congestion

➤ Rashes or other skin ailments such as pimples

➤ Headaches

➤ Appendicitis

➤ Urinary tract problems

Branden had her appendix removed at the age of 16. Her complaints included breakouts of the skin, frequent head colds, bouts of anger, and not surprisingly, constipation! Branden's constipation seems to run in the family. She was not breastfed as a baby, her eating habits were irregular and did not consist of 80 percent whole, raw foods, nor was her daily water intake adequate. All these factors put together paint a picture for a chronically constipated body!

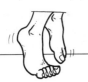

**Tip Toe**

When an organ has been surgically removed, its corresponding reflex needs to be stimulated regularly to keep energy balanced throughout the body.

In Branden's case, the bowel has obviously been under-active since childhood. First of all, most of us who have not been breast-fed lack the proper bacteria in the intestines that help us absorb nutrients and assist proper digestive processes. An acidophilus or bifidophilus supplement can restore the proper reserves to our digestive tract.

Since Branden's diet was not consistent, her digestive system was not able to get into a consistent pattern of digestion and elimination. And since her diet lacked whole, raw, organic foods and proper water intake, the bowel lacked sufficient materials to operate properly. The appendicitis at the age of 16 only enhanced the picture that this girl was a clogged-up cookie!

# Toxic Wasteland

The pimples Branden was experiencing were just her body's way of trying to eliminate the backed-up toxins through her skin. These toxins were originating from a toxic bowel. This was the obvious source of the problem, and this is what we focused on for her reflexology treatments.

When I first began working on Branden's feet, the most notable part of her treatment was the sonic effect that it created across the room. Breaking up the hardened crunchies in her feet was so loud that we could actually hear an echo as the sound bounced off the walls!

It was all I could do to hold Branden down the first time I worked on her. I barely used any pressure at all, but the toxic buildup in her feet was so great that it was impossible to work deeply on her. After the first few minutes of the first treatment, Branden had to sit up and blow her nose. Toxins were being released almost immediately from her sinuses.

We noticed that the bladder area on her foot was swollen and red. I asked her if she had had any problems with her urinary tract. She replied that she had been repeatedly fighting off severe bladder infections for years. The bladder reflex spot was very tender for her, but I believe the work helped to prevent a potential bladder infection.

# Eliminate the Negative

To get effective results, Branden required more treatments than she was able to commit to; however, after her first treatment, she eliminated several times the following day and did not experience another bladder infection for at least another month.

Because of distance and Branden's hectic lifestyle, she became an infrequent client of mine, but nevertheless came whenever she could for treatments. The treatments she did have resulted in almost immediate effects. She nicknamed them her "poop treatments" and would come to see me when her constipation became a problem for her.

Frequent reflexology treatments for Branden would have served her well to stimulate her eliminative channels and keep her from experiencing excess mucus and frequent bladder infections. Both of these symptoms are the result of a sluggish bowel that is unable to eliminate the toxic waste materials effectively. The other eliminative organs such as the skin and urinary tract and even the respiratory system try to make up for this sluggishness and therefore experience the negative side effects of a toxic overload.

### Foot Note

For constipated small children, fruit on an empty stomach makes a wonderful home remedy to use to correct the condition. Applesauce can work wonders. If not, a drop of liquid senna, cascara sagrada, or turkey rhubarb in a baby's drink will get results right away. For infants, first try rubbing a few drops of the liquid herb on the lower abdomen before giving internally. Remember that reflexology should not be overdone in babies, and a total of 10 minutes for the hands and feet should be sufficient.

# Cliff—Not Your Regular Baby

Visiting my friends in Durango, Colorado, one year, I had the privilege of getting to know their three-year-old son Cliff. I first met Cliff when he was an infant, but I was sincerely blown away with his clear focus, his adamant personality, and the expressive mature attitude he possessed at the ripe old age of three!

Cliff was a strong little boy with blond, fine, straight hair and large blue eyes. Because he was a very bright child, I had the opportunity to ask him straightforward questions and actually get straightforward answers.

Cliff told me he enjoyed the outdoors, animals, and dried fruit that his mom dehydrated from their garden. Cliff had been breast-fed for almost a year and appeared quite healthy and balanced. Cliff also demonstrated an entertaining sense of humor. I could discern from Cliff's personality that he had a special mission to accomplish on this earth, and he definitely had the personality to carry it out.

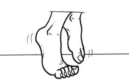

### Tip Toe

Reflexology is a self-help therapy that you can take anywhere you go! If you normally get constipated when you travel, be sure to utilize reflexology to help stimulate your colon, relax your body, and help it adjust to the different schedule.

## Cute Little Stinker

Since Cliff was out of diapers, his mom was not necessarily as colon-conscious as I was at the time. However, she complained that Cliff was experiencing some intestinal gas and wondered if my reflexology treatments could do anything for the little stinker.

Well, being the personable flirt Cliff was, he expressed his eagerness for me to practice reflexology on his feet and hands by immediately removing his socks and lifting his foot into my lap. Cliff watched me intently as I worked gently on each of his little feet. His facial expressions changed, his eyes squinted, and his eyebrows formed odd patterns as I worked on the "crunchy" spots I found on his bowel reflex areas on the soles of his feet. By the time I finished working on his feet and hands, Cliff was heavy lidded and asked his mom to put him to bed. The next day the proof of the effectiveness of the therapy was in the pudding, so to speak.

## Again?

Cliff's mom reported to me the next evening that she and Cliff ran errands the whole day after his treatment. At each store and office they visited, Cliff politely asked to be taken to the bathroom. One of their errands was at a construction site where no bathroom was available. But the need was so great that mom had to accompany little Cliff to the woods!

Cliff's energy was higher than normal that day, and he appeared to be very cheerful. He had a total of six bowel movements in one day! Quite a feat for a little three-year-old body! After this cleansing, Cliff's bowel movements returned to normal, and his mom has not complained about his gas since.

**Tread Lightly**

Be prepared by planning on having access to a bathroom the day after a reflexology treatment. Especially if it is one of your first treatments, you may experience cleansing through frequent bowel elimination.

The only complaint my friend did have was that if she knew that reflexology was going to be so effective she would have arranged to have me work on Cliff on a day that they were planning to stay home!

## Stop and Smell the Roses

The moral of the story is that reflexology can be an effective treatment for constipation, especially during the initial treatments. Because of its effectiveness in this area, one should be aware of this and not schedule a treatment immediately before an important event where frequent trips to the bathroom may not be possible.

Notice that in all these cases, the clients were overachieving, energetic, on-the-go type people. I believe that sometimes these energetic folks just do not take the time to relax or slow down enough to give the bowel a chance to relax and eliminate naturally. These people are more likely to eat faster than a lower-energy person and therefore create extra work for the digestive system.

Performing reflexology on this personality type may help them relax and facilitate a release of body toxins through the bowel. If you are practicing on one of these types of people, you should let them know what they can look forward to the following day.

## The Least You Need to Know

➤ Problems with the elimination system can be the base cause of a host of symptoms, from adult acne to headaches and urinary tract infections.

➤ A healthy colon transit time should be approximately 16 to 18 hours.

➤ Reflexology sessions can help the body to relieve constipation.

➤ High-strung personalities may have high-strung colons, leading them to extremes of constipation and/or spastic bowel conditions.

➤ Although each body responds in different times and degrees, you might experience a cleansing reaction after your first reflexology treatment, and you may want to plan on taking time to cleanse.

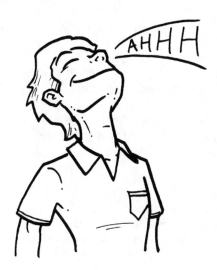

# Chapter 25

# Reflexology Helps You Breathe

## In This Chapter

➤ Discover how reflexology can help relieve bronchitis symptoms

➤ Learn to differentiate between an illness and a healing crisis

➤ Find the specific points to work on for sinus congestion

➤ Learn how a doctor used reflexology to help asthma

Another great use for reflexology is for ailments of the respiratory system—the lungs, sinuses, and bronchials. It is not understood how this works, except, of course, for the improved circulation, normalization of the glands, and relaxation of the muscles.

Relaxing the muscles can help ease conditions such as a spastic cough. How does it work to relieve asthma symptoms, bronchitis, and clogged-up sinuses? I don't know, but I do know that reflexology has helped me and many others to relieve a clogged-up head or kick out a chest cold!

In this chapter we are going to take a look at some respiratory ailments and then see how reflexology can help. I will then give you some pointers on which areas to work on if you are experiencing any of these symptoms. Isn't that a breath of fresh air?

# Take a Deep Breath

If you've ever had bronchitis, you probably would be willing to do anything to avoid this irritating illness again! *Bronchitis* literally means inflammation of the *bronchi* (pronounced *bronk-eye*), the air passageways of the lungs. How did they come up with a name like that? It was probably named after some guy from the Bronx. "Hey, how's that bronchi? He had some type of lung condition didn't he?"

Viruses and bacteria cause bronchitis. Symptoms that characterize bronchitis include a persistent, phlegmy, hacking cough with copious amounts of mucus. (Yes, that was the medical definition.) When one suffers with bronchitis the bronchial tubes narrow in spasmodic contractions.

Some causes of bronchitis include smoking and air pollution. Air pollutants, smoke, and tar are toxins that clog up the small passageways of the respiratory system and make it more difficult for the body to filter out airborne viruses and bacteria.

**The Sole Meaning**

**Bronchitis** means inflammation of the **bronchi**. It is an illness characterized by coughing, a constriction of the bronchi due to spasms, and the production of copious amounts of mucus from the bronchi. Culprits are smoking, air pollution, and generally dirty or underactive lungs!

## Can You Get Bronchitis from Living in the Bronx?

Weakened or filthy lungs will make you more vulnerable to bronchitis. However, bronchitis is your body's way of trying to protect you from viruses and bacteria entering deeper into your body. Your body makes mucus to surround the offending toxins, and then puts constriction on your bronchials, forcing you to cough, and hopefully rid yourself of these invaders!

A bout with bronchitis should not be suppressed. You should help your body rid itself of the lung toxins. Reflexology is a therapy that will assist your body in detoxifying and will support you in fighting off illness.

## Work Those Reflexes

Points to work on to help your body relax its spasmodic contractions and boost your immune system include the following:

➤ Lungs

➤ Chest

➤ Upper lymphs

➤ Bronchus

➤ Throat

➤ Sinus

➤ Thymus

Sometimes reflexology will "stir up" old catarrh and mucus that have been sitting in the lungs for a long time. This can bring on what seem like symptoms of bronchitis, but may actually be a cleansing process of the lungs.

# Don't Call 911 for a Healing Crisis

You can tell a cleansing process from an illness by its length and severity. This process is known as a *healing crisis* and is the result of your body becoming strong enough to eliminate old poisons or toxins that have settled in the tissues.

A healing crisis is characterized by a short duration (usually counted in threes: three hours, three days) of isolated symptoms, and afterward the person will feel much better than they did before the crisis—as long as they let it run its course.

For example, one of my clients who comes regularly for reflexology treatments has had bronchitis many times. This person does not smoke, nor is she a city dweller, so her air pollution factor is lower than most.

During her first reflexology session, there was much tenderness in her lungs and upper respiratory system reflexes. We broke up a large number of crunchies during the hour-long treatment. Since her chest and lung areas were where we discovered the most crunchies, I worked these areas most frequently.

## *Feeling Much Better*

Later that afternoon she called me and her voice was hoarse! She was coughing, and said she had "come down with bronchitis"! I wondered if this wasn't a healing crisis, so I asked her what other symptoms she was experiencing. She reported that although she had had bronchitis in the past, this was different.

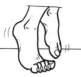

**Tip Toe**

Reflexology can help stimulate the body to heal naturally by speeding up the healing process. If you take medications that suppress your respiratory symptoms, this can cause the irritants to stay in your body and settle back down into the tissues. Try to bear through the natural healing if possible, and refer to Chapter 9, "Remember to Breathe! The Respiratory System," for more tips on keeping your respiratory system healthy.

**Tread Lightly**

Usually a healing crisis comes when a person has made significant changes in their lifestyle, including the intake of supplements and herbs, healthy diet, and exercise, along with reflexology.

She was coughing up mucus; however, she did not have the weak, achey feeling that she always had before with bronchitis. She did not have a fever, and her energy was high. As she described how isolated her symptom was, she began to realize that this was probably a reaction to the reflexology treatment.

Because this was the only symptom she experienced, I concluded that the pseudo-bronchitis was caused by a cleansing process and not by a new viral infection. She waited to see how she would feel later, and in less than three full days her condition was gone and she felt even better than before she had the coughing attack!

## Healing Crisis or Illness?

This is a good example of how reflexology can bring on a healing crisis disguised as an illness. How will you know if you have a full-blown illness or if you could possibly have stirred up a cleansing? Note the differences in the following table.

### Healing Crisis and Illness Contrasted

| Healing Crisis | Illness |
| --- | --- |
| Usually only one isolated symptom | Usually a host of symptoms |
| Person retains energy | Loss of energy and fatigue |
| Acute symptoms | A slow building of symptoms |
| Symptoms are short-lived, usually in threes: three hours, three days | Symptoms last longer |
| Symptoms appear after a natural health therapy was begun | Symptoms appear at any time |
| Symptoms get progressively better | Symptoms get progressively worse |

**The Sole Meaning**

**Asthma** is a respiratory condition characterized by bronchiolespasms causing difficulty in breathing. Asthma is brought on by an array of stimuli, including exposure to allergens, exertion, emotions, and infections.

## Attacking Asthma

*Asthma* is a condition characterized by attacks of bronchiolespasms causing difficulty in breathing. Asthma is brought on by an array of stimuli, including exposure to allergens, exertion, emotions, and infections.

Reflexology can play a role in helping asthmatics because of the relaxation it can bring to the bronchial tubes and entire nervous system. If emotions are a factor in bringing on an attack, a caring reflexology treatment may help a person let go of their worries—at least temporarily.

## Working It Out

Hardened mucus, or what some refer to as "mucus plugs," in the lungs can only make us more vulnerable to all sorts of lung and upper-respiratory conditions; therefore reflexology can help by stimulating the body to cleanse itself of excess mucus. Reflex points and areas to work if you have asthma include:

➤ Bronchials

➤ Lungs

➤ Upper lymphs

➤ Chest

➤ Adrenals

➤ Heart

➤ Diaphragm

➤ Colon

Another consideration when working with folks with asthma is that some people with severe asthma are not able to lie flat on their backs because of breathing difficulty. Therefore, a reclining chair is best for working on these people. If this is not available, try to make them comfortable in a chair while you sit on a pillow or cushion on the floor below them.

## The Boy Who Loved Animals

The following story about one of my asthmatic clients illustrates how effective reflexology can be for helping asthma and allergies.

A young mother with a six-year-old, red-headed, blue-eyed boy came in to see me for reflexology. He was fair-skinned, and the skin around his eyes appeared pink and swollen. He had a runny nose and appeared to be a mouth breather. There was a horizontal crease across the bridge of his nose giving me more clues that this boy was suffering from allergies. The mother appeared exhausted.

"Eric just started having allergies about a year ago, and now it's worked its way into asthma," she complained. "It tears my heart out to see him so uncomfortable. He loves animals, but they trigger his asthma and he is not even able to look at one without a problem. He wants to play with the neighbors' pets, but the last time he petted a cat we almost had to rush him to the emergency room! His wheezing makes us very uneasy, and I find myself up at night checking in on him to make

**Tip Toe**

Experiments at the Kiev Research Institute of Pulmonary Disorders showed that 89 percent of asthmatic patients were helped through the use of reflexology alone.

sure he is still breathing. He cannot run and play like he wants to either. I heard about reflexology being good for this sort of thing. Do you think you can help?"

I explained to the mom how reflexology works and that we were not treating disease, just helping the body help itself. I agreed to work on the little boy once per week, and had her follow up with mini sessions at home. My sessions with the boy only lasted about 20 minutes each time. I concentrated on his sinus, lung, bronchus, adrenal, immune system, and bowel reflexes.

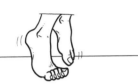

**Tip Toe**

Reflexology not only works to stimulate the body into action, but helps boost the other organs of elimination (bowel, kidneys, skin) to help the upper respiratory system in its detoxification process.

After the sessions with me, the mother reported that the boy would run and play and not experience any signs of asthma for a day or two. Mom followed with her home sessions on her boy once or twice per week before tucking him into bed.

We used this routine for about three months, and the boy responded very well. His chronic runny nose cleared up and overall he seemed more "at ease" and relaxed, although still full of little boy energy!

The last time I saw the mom, she brought the boy in and was beaming herself. The boy's nose was clear, the inflammation around his eyes was gone, and he was smiling as she sat him on her lap to talk to me. "I am so grateful; thank you so much for helping Eric! Guess what we did yesterday? We took Eric to ride a pony! He loved it, and did not have one sign of allergies or asthma!"

How wonderful that reflexology can be instrumental in the healing process and help a little boy enjoy the things little boys can! Just keep in mind that asthma is a complicated disease and should be handled with a holistic approach that analyzes the sufferer nutritionally and emotionally, as well as medically.

**Foot Note**

I am a living testimonial to the efficacy of the holistic approach to asthma. A holistic program of reflexology, herbal supplements, and balancing my blood sugar levels has left me without a trace of asthma. For years my only relief from asthma attacks and shortness of breath was the use of aerosol inhalers and sometimes bronchodilator medication. I haven't had to use an inhaler for years, not even when cross-country skiing!

# Oh, Stop Your Sniffling!

Do you experience any of the following?

➤ When you talk on the phone do people ask you if you are cutting an onion?

➤ Do you sound like you've been crying all the time?

➤ Do some suspect you might be sniffing something other than air?

➤ Do clerks give you funny looks around Mother's Day when you ask them to help you find a card for your "Bomb"?

If you can answer yes to any of these questions, you may be suffering from chronic sinusitis!

## Sinusitis Is Not an Allergy to Signs

Allergies are the main cause of *sinusitis*. What exactly is sinusitis? You guessed it, inflammation of the sinus cavities! Okay, let's get a little more technical. Sinusitis is an inflammation of one or more of the mucus-lined air spaces in the facial bones that communicate with the nose. (Hello nose!)

It is often caused by infections spreading from the nose. Symptoms include headache and tenderness over the affected sinus, which may become filled with a purulent material that is discharged through the nose. In persistent cases, treatment may require the affected sinus to be washed out or drained by a surgical operation. How's that for technical?

The fingers and the toes all correlate to the zones and reflexes for the sinuses. Squeezing these when you have a sinus infection or sinus congestion may help you relieve the pain and pressure. Reflexology is not a substitute for fighting infection, but it can help you with the discomfort and help boost the immune system to help you fight infection. And don't forget, when you are suffering from infection or your body is discharging mucus, make sure you keep up your fluid intake.

**The Sole Meaning**

**Sinusitis** is an inflammation of one or more of the mucus-lined air spaces in the facial bones that communicate with the nose. It is often caused by infections spreading from the nose. Symptoms include headache and tenderness over the affected sinus, which may become filled with a purulent material that is discharged through the nose.

## Footbaths for Sinus Congestion

To help break up congestion you also may want to try a footbath. My husband occasionally will get sinus infections, especially during ragweed season and when the ranch below us cuts their hay. This is a time of great suffering for him, so we will always employ the use of footbaths and reflexology treatments to help him feel better.

For sinus congestion, we have used the following with success:

➤ Find a container that will hold water, is large enough to allow your foot to be submerged in it, and deep enough so that the water can come up to your ankle.

➤ Fill the container with cold water, just enough to cover your ankles.

➤ Now fill up the bathtub with enough water to cover the ankles. Make the water as hot as you can tolerate, and add a few drops of the essential oil of oregano, peppermint, horseradish, or other stimulating aromatic to the hot water.

➤ Place the container of cold water in the bath water, or next to the tub, if you prefer.

➤ Sit on the side of the tub, and place one foot in the hot water and one foot in the cold water. The hot water draws blood to the foot, while the cold water pushes blood away from the foot. This whole process moves circulation quite nicely and many times will offer almost instant relief to one side of the head! And when you are suffering with a clogged nose, one opened air passageway is better than none!

You can try switching feet once you get relief from the first footbath, but my husband usually is satisfied with one airway and will be able to sleep because of having at least one passageway open.

You can also work the tips of the fingers and toes by squeezing them and holding each one individually until you notice the pain subsiding in your sinuses. If you are at home, you may want to put clamps on the toes or fingers to help alleviate the pain of a sinus infection. Just don't leave them on too long. Five minutes at a time is plenty!

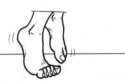

**Tip Toe**

You can make your own clamps to use on your fingers or toes to stimulate the sinus reflex points. Find some spring-loaded clothes pins. Remove the wire and replace with a rubber band, and voilà, instant clips! Put one on each toe or finger when you have allergies or sinus troubles.

## Allergies No More

For the chronically stuffed-up head, reflexology has worked instantaneous wonders in my experience. Along with asthma, I used to be one of those who pronounced my "Ms" like "Ebbs." If you can't relate, hold your nose and say the letter "M"—see what I bean?

If you are stuffed up with a clogged head from allergies, but do not have an infection, reflexology can help relieve the congestion. Points to help relieve head congestion include:

➤ Eyes

➤ Ears

➤ Inner ear

➤ Sinuses

I frequently see folks with sinus congestion from a head cold or allergies. Many times sinus congestion is released immediately after I begin working on them. This release has been described as a popping sensation followed by a relief of congestion. Working primarily on the padding of the foot just below the toes has helped in these conditions.

Allergies and asthma, bronchitis, and all ailments of the respiratory tract limit us in taking a full breath of life! It is wonderful to know that reflexology can be useful in changing these problems. Reflexology is safer than asthma and allergy medications, and has no ill side effects. Reflexology used at home is as free as the air we breathe, and may make a huge difference in how we feel!

---

### The Least You Need to Know

➤ Reflexology can facilitate a cleansing process in the lungs and bronchials that can cause a person to cough up excess mucus after a treatment.

➤ If you think you are ill after a reflexology treatment, investigate whether it is a healing crisis rather than an illness.

➤ Reflexology can play a role in helping asthmatics because of the relaxation it can bring to the bronchial tubes and entire nervous system.

➤ Squeezing the padding of the fingers and toes can lessen the pain of a sinus infection.

➤ Working the eye, ear, and sinus reflex points can instantaneously relieve sinus congestion.

---

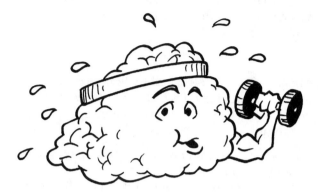

# Chapter 26

# A Nervous-System and Psychological Workout

---

## In This Chapter

➤ Discover the ways reflexology can help the nervous system

➤ See how reflexology helps with insomnia

➤ Learn which reflexes may be helpful to work for psychological and nervous-system disorders

➤ Find out how reflexology can calm nausea

➤ Discover the top 10 ways to tell you're a reflexologist

---

When I first met Linda, an attractive 28-year-old, she appeared slight in stature, although she was not petite. It was her lack of energy and the way she carried herself that made her appear smaller. Linda spoke to me softly with lowered eyes and in a nervous voice. "I can't believe I made it here to see you," she whispered hurriedly. "I am getting more and more panicky about leaving the house. I have been suffering from almost daily panic attacks, and I'm at my wits end with it!"

Linda and I worked together on a holistic program that included reflexology sessions every other week for six months. Her husband came in a few times to watch my techniques so that he could follow up with some general reflexology on her at home.

After six months, Linda's attacks were becoming less frequent. She was improving. Was this because reflexology was working to balance her glands? Working on the nervous system? Or was it the psychological factors of being taken care of and having her husband work on her at home that cured her mind and soul? We will never know, but the main thing is that she is living a more productive and settled life and if reflexology can help Linda, it may be able to help others with similar conditions. Let's take a look at some of the ways reflexology works on the mind and brain.

# Central Processing

The nervous system encompasses the brain and spinal cord, and we tend to associate the mind with the brain and thinking. However, the mind is really something that we don't know much about. Although ailments of the nervous system can be linked to the mind, they are not necessarily the same thing.

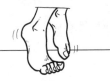

**Tip Toe**

Maybe I'm just lucky, but the people who come to me for guidance and truly believe in themselves do heal. That's why I have these wonderful stories to share with you that can give you inspiration to do the same!

**The Sole Meaning**

**Multiple sclerosis** is a chronic nervous-system disease in which the myelin sheaths surrounding the nerves and spinal cord are damaged, affecting the function of the nerves involved. Symptoms vary but may include an unsteady gait, shaky limbs, and involuntary movements of the eyes.

In Linda's case, I wasn't sure whether her problems were coming from her mind or her body, and it did not matter to me. I knew that my good intentions, her dedication to sessions, and her intent to be well would come together and help her balance.

The central nervous system is the highway that carries all the messages for all of the body processes and functions. As long as we are not under anesthesia, the nervous system is aware of everything that goes on in the body. Reflexology is great for relaxing the nerves and balancing glandular secretions and can help with disorders of the nervous system.

In this chapter I have included both nervous-system disorders and psychological disorders. These may include:

➤ Manic-depressive disorder (now called bipolar disorder)

➤ Severe stress-related conditions

➤ Parkinson's disease

➤ Multiple sclerosis

➤ Some addictions

➤ Insomnia

➤ ADD

This chapter will highlight a few imbalances that are directly related to excessive stress or worry and will show you how to help yourself or others with reflexology sessions. We will specifically discuss insomnia, bipolar disorder, nausea from nervous tension, and Attention Deficit Disorder, commonly referred to as ADD. You will see how others have been helped with these problems through reflexology.

# Rock a Bye Baby

When we discussed the nervous system way back in Chapter 8, "What Nerve: The Nervous System," we discussed the pineal gland and its production of melatonin, a hormone nicknamed "the sleep hormone" or the "anti-aging hormone."

Melatonin is the chemical messenger our body manufactures to make us feel tired and help us go to sleep. As we age, our pineal gland produces less and less of this hormone. Other things may interfere with melatonin production, such as hormone therapy and the ingestion of alcohol and some drugs.

*Insomnia* can occur when there is not enough melatonin being produced by the pineal gland. Insomnia has many other causes, including worry or high stress, blood sugar imbalances, thyroid imbalance, and side effects of drugs or prescription medications or the use of legal or illegal stimulants.

**The Sole Meaning**

**Insomnia** is the inability to fall asleep or to remain asleep for an adequate length of time.

# When Counting Sheep Doesn't Work

Insomnia is the inability to fall asleep or to remain asleep for an adequate length of time, resulting in constant exhaustion. Reflexology can be very useful in helping those with insomnia. It is best that someone with insomnia have another person work on them to help with this problem. Working to put yourself to sleep can be difficult.

If you create the right atmosphere for your insomniac subject, making sure they are comfortable and feel secure, then they may just fall asleep while you work on them! This has happened to me several times and is a great compliment to the reflexologist.

The main reflexes to work on an insomniac are:

➤ Pineal

➤ Brain

➤ Adrenals

➤ Solar plexus

➤ Thyroid and parathyroid

Start with the pineal gland reflex point, located on each large toe and thumb. This gland may be sleeping itself and not producing enough of the invaluable melatonin hormone! Stimulate this point three times on each large toe and also on each thumb.

**Tip Toe**

Sipping a nice warm cup or two of chamomile tea before bedtime helps many relax and may help you get a good night's sleep. Chamomile is soothing to the nervous system, tastes good, and is a safe herb to take.

You will know when you stimulate the point by the feeling of electric shock that your partner will feel when you find it (see Chapter 8 for details). Ask your partner for feedback when you are trying to find this point. Most people will jump when the point is correctly stimulated, although not everyone responds so outwardly.

Also make sure that you work the entire brain area (all along the tops of each toe and fingertip) when a person complains of insomnia. In addition, all the relaxation techniques, such as the stretching and rotating techniques, will help the body to relax.

The adrenals may be weakened because of stress, and therefore they should also be reflexed. Be sure to also work the thyroid and parathyroids, since an imbalance of these glands affects metabolism and can be the cause of insomnia. The solar plexus is a new area we haven't covered yet, but it is key in relaxing the body, nerves, and mind, so we will talk about it in more detail next.

# A Bundle of Nerves

Since many people who have insomnia are worriers, you should be sure to work the solar plexus reflex in the feet and hands. The *solar plexus* is found right in the middle of the upper half of the trunk of the body, where the rib cage comes together about at the stomach level in front of the diaphragm. See the tear card chart in the front of this book to find the reflex location for the solar plexus. You will see that it is centered in the middle of the diaphragm line on both the hands and feet. The solar plexus is a great network of nerves that goes out to all parts of the abdominal cavity and has sometimes been called the abdominal brain. It is affected by stress, especially worry.

**The Sole Meaning**

The **solar plexus** is found right in the middle where the rib cage comes together about at the stomach level in front of the diaphragm. It is a great network of nerves that goes out to all parts of the abdominal cavity.

The fine network of nerves extends from the part of the aorta (the main artery of the body) below the diaphragm and includes the front of the abdominal aorta as well as the adrenal glands. The solar plexus helps to regulate the sympathetic nervous system.

When a person is worried or stressed, stimulating the solar plexus reflex can make them jump off your table! You will need to warn a person before you stimulate their solar plexus, especially if they are worriers or have insomnia. Then follow these steps:

➤ Grip the foot as shown in the following photo. Or you can work on two feet at the same time if you prefer, for an all-over rush!

➤ Find the indentation in the middle of the base of the ball of the foot (feet) just under the diaphragm (see the tear card).

➤ Ask the person to take a deep breath. If you like, you can take a deep breath with them to guide them. Press in and slightly upward with your thumb for three seconds while your partner holds their breath.

➤ Have your partner exhale while you slowly release pressure on the spot and pull the feet (foot) toward you. Do not remove your thumb(s) from contact with the spot, just relax the pressure.

➤ Repeat the stimulation of this point a total of three times.

**Tip Toe**

A variation on the solar plexus technique described in the text is done using both hands, one on each foot at the same time. Try both ways and choose the one that is most effective for you.

You can go deeper each time you work this reflex according to the tolerance of your partner. Afterward, they should feel invigorated and relaxed. See the following photo to help you refine your technique.

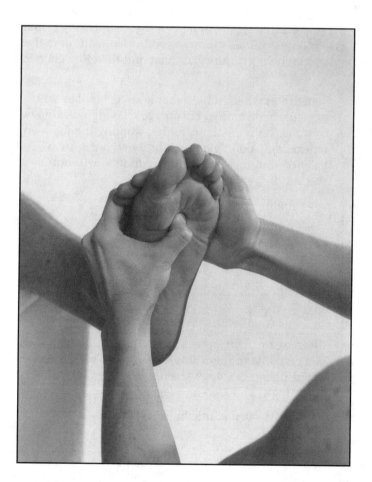

*Stimulating the solar plexus on one foot, using one hand. A variation includes stimulating each solar plexus reflex simultaneously.*

353

# Leveling Out the Highs and Lows

"What do you call a bear with depression?"

"A bipolar bear!"

*Manic-depressive psychosis*, or as it is now called, *bipolar disorder*, is a severe mental illness usually caused by a chemical imbalance. The severity of this disorder varies, but its main characteristics are severe depression and then mania (excitability). The episodes can be precipitated by emotionally upsetting events, but the reactions are often out of proportion to the causes.

The disease can be genetically inherited, but the full expression can be altered by environmental factors. I have seen many bipolar people come to a manageable balance with the help of a holistic approach such as reflexology, nutritional supplementation, and psychotherapy. I have been amazed and encouraged at the progress I have seen my clients experience. Reflexology has played a role in helping these people facilitate balance in their lives.

The people who want to have a hand in their own healing are the ones who always do the best. The folks I work with who are afflicted with bipolar disorder usually respond quickly to sessions. Such a serious illness should always be addressed with more than reflexology; however, reflexology can help with the glandular and therefore chemical imbalance of the brain.

Sometimes when in their manic state, bipolars will experience insomnia. Encourage relaxing reflexology sessions. With bipolar disorder, working the following reflexes will aid in glandular and nervous-system balance, and the relaxation techniques will soothe the mind:

➤ Brain

➤ Spinal column

➤ Adrenals

➤ Solar plexus

➤ Pineal

➤ Pituitary

### The Sole Meaning

**Manic-depressive psychosis,** or **bipolar disorder,** as it is now called, is a severe mental illness characterized by severe depression followed by bouts of mania. Mania takes the form of obsession, compulsion, or an exaggerated feeling of euphoria.

I have seen clients relax when they are in a manic state as a response to reflexology. I have also seen these people lift from their depression during a reflexology session. With regular sessions these people begin to level out their highs and lows and regain a sense of stability.

That is all we can ask for as reflexologists—just a little bit of balance.

**Foot Note**

Although bipolar disorder is a chemical imbalance, I have seen a difference in those who have been brave enough to face the illness, actively take part in their recovery, and choose to be more conscious of their behaviors. I have seen some people make startling progress with natural therapies to supplement their traditional psychotherapy or other counseling sessions. Responsibility is empowering and will help anyone in their progress toward good health.

# What Do You Mean I'm Hyper? A Look at ADD

Many children are now known to suffer from a recently recognized disorder commonly referred to as *ADD*, or *Attention Deficit Disorder*. The problems associated with ADD include an inability to focus attention on routine activities. Some will have high frustration and choose to express themselves in violent outbursts. Others seem to not be able to sit still.

The adult suffering from this disorder may not necessarily show it outwardly as "misbehavior." In fact, these people often make great business entrepreneurs, as their overactive mental states can help breed creativity. Not only that, but adult sufferers of ADD usually will have the drive to work ridiculous hours to make their businesses successful. The danger in this type of behavior is that the adult's ADD-induced energy will eventually burn out.

**Foot Note**

An ADD adult may run his/her body into the ground and neglect family or friendships. Based on this behavior, many make too many promises that are impossible to follow through with. Needless to say, life works best for us in balance. Entrepreneurs with ADD may have great start-up businesses, but if they don't get their disorder under control, they might be better off selling their businesses before employees or the businesses suffer any damage.

## Cause and Effect

While some blame this disorder on a pure lack of parental discipline, many children diagnosed with ADD could have an underlying physical problem aggravating or possibly causing the hyperactivity. Some theories held about an underlying physical irritation can include the following:

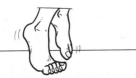

**Tip Toe**

Refined sugar is digested quickly and causes a "spike" in blood sugar, since sugar gives energy to the body. This burst of energy created by sugary snacks may aggravate a child afflicted with nervous or behavioral problems. Replace sugars with protein snacks instead.

➤ Food allergies

➤ Hyperglycemia

➤ Essential fatty acid deficiency

➤ Environmental allergies

The problem is that other than a major psychotropic medication, doctors have not been able to come up with a cure-all for this disorder. No matter, reflexology has its place in working with the hyperactive, children or adults.

## Working It Out

Specific reflex points to work on for those who suffer from problems concentrating or who feel or appear hyper include the following:

➤ Brain

➤ Adrenals

➤ Central nervous system (spine and brain)

➤ Pineal gland

➤ Pancreas

Since many children with food allergies or blood sugar imbalances suffer with ADD, these possibilities should be investigated. In the meantime, working the reflex points to help the glands involved will not hurt, and more than likely will prove useful.

# Calming Things Down

We can feel nauseated because of psychological or nervous-system disorders. The brain plays a key role in making us feel sick or well, whether it is because of real or perceived threats that make us tense. When we relax the nerves, other symptoms that are caused by nerves, like nausea, can be alleviated.

Reflexology makes a great therapy for children who are fussy, but are too young to tell you what is wrong. I have seen car sickness alleviated with the use of reflexology. If you have someone in the car with you who can work on the child, ask them to press some reflexology buttons on the child's hands. If a car-sick child is old enough, you can instruct them how to perform reflexology on themselves.

## Push My Nausea Button

Dizziness is what usually causes nausea. Dizziness, or the sense of losing balance, comes from sensations in our inner ear. Therefore, the inner ear reflex points are excellent areas to work for children (or adults) experiencing car, air, or sea sickness, or anything that involves a continuous rocking motion.

You can also work the stomach reflex in the hand, which will aid a sick stomach. And finally, you can try the renowned foot, hand, and *body reflexologist* and author Mildred Carter's button for nausea. Mildred says this "nausea button" is located on the inside of the wrist, between the two large tendons, found about three fingers from the wrist.

It may take a constant pressure for up to 20 minutes on this spot before relief is experienced. You may have seen bracelets claiming to relieve motion sickness; these bracelets are nothing more than elastic bands with a small "pea" that is placed on this reflex point.

**The Sole Meaning**

**Body reflexology** is similar to foot and hand reflexology, but the reflexes are found over the entire body, not just the feet and hands.

Reflexology points helpful for nausea include:

➤ Inner ear

➤ Stomach

➤ Nausea button

➤ Spine

If car sickness is a common problem, one of the best herbal remedies for this is ginger root. Ginger can be taken in capsules or eaten raw or candied. Just a little goes a long way, and you can take a little just before your car ride. Ginger is safe for pregnant women, too, and has been used to alleviate morning sickness.

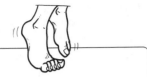

## Go to Sleep My Little Baby

Car sickness, or just plain old car grouchiness, can be cured with reflexology fairly quickly, as this story about a nine-month-old baby reveals:

Some years ago while visiting some friends and clients in Georgia, I had the privilege of sitting in the backseat next to my friend's nine-month-old baby boy for a three-hour car trip.

Being a bit road weary myself and not knowing how to deal with children, I was not particularly delighted with the situation, especially since the boy had just discovered how to make long, loud noises with his throat and was fascinated with his ability to sound like a lawn mower running out of gas!

**Tip Toe**

The relaxing benefits of reflexology often will put a baby or young child to sleep in the car, which makes them unconscious of their nausea!

After he got bored with his verbal experimentation, he decided he was grouchy. He began fussing and squirming in his car seat and began to whine quite loudly. In a desperate attempt to save my own sanity, I took his little hand in mine and began working his reflexes. In less than three minutes (and let me tell you I was counting) the little bugger had his eyes closed and was quickly falling asleep.

The funniest thing about it was that as I finished up working one finger, he would stretch out the next finger as if to say, "Okay, now do this one!" The next two and a half hours were peaceful bliss for both of us! Reflexology to the rescue once again.

## Care with Compassion

As you have learned, although reflexology can be used as a self-help technique, when administered by another person, reflexology can be a mind, body, and soul healing experience. Psychological disorders are complicated illnesses, but reflexology works by sharing compassion, too. It not only balances the glands, but may facilitate emotional release for folks dealing with emotional trauma or pain.

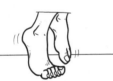

**Tip Toe**

No action is without consequence. When we decide to make a conscious effort to help ourselves, the consequences are commitment, dedication, patience, discipline, and consistency. These are also the key ingredients to earn anything that has any value in our lives.

They say that making up your mind is 90 percent of anything you do. Maybe some psychological or chemical disorders and even nervous-system disorders cannot be "cured," but they can certainly be managed to make them easier to live with. Sometimes just making the conscious decision to incorporate a natural healing therapy, such as regular reflexology treatments, into your life is a positive affirmation toward better management of your illnesses.

I hope you will become dedicated in your commitment to healing yourself, your family and friends, and maybe others through the wonderful therapy of reflexology.

# The Reflexology Top Ten

Now that you are briefed—to say the least—in some basic reflexology techniques, concepts and theories, and know what you can look forward to when using this therapy, I hope you will consider incorporating it into your life. Or maybe you have been inspired through my stories to seek training and become a reflexologist yourself. In either case, working with feet and the people attached to those feet is more than rewarding, and by now you should be able to understand my list of ways you can tell if you are a reflexologist.

**Top Ten Ways to Tell You're a Reflexologist**

1. Frequently, people bare their soles to you and say "heel me."

2. You have a foothold on the competition.

3. You knead your clients and they need you.

4. You always have what you need for your work at your fingertips.

5. You no longer think of corn as just a vegetable.

6. You're all thumbs.

7. You see where your clients stand.

8. You put a lot of pressure on your clients to heal.

9. You look forward to working on your feet all day long.

10. You are known for your "healing feats."

I hope *The Complete Idiot's Guide to Reflexology* has been as fun for you to read as it was for me to write. Please don't skip the appendices in the back, since they will give you some companies, schools, and organizations to contact to obtain everything you need for your career in the natural health field (including my Web site address!).

I look forward to meeting up with you again in my next book, *The Complete Idiot's Guide to Herbal Remedies*. Until then, maybe you will come visit my healing spa for some reflexology so you can bare your sole(s) to me! I wish happiness and balance for you with every footstep in your life journey.

**Tip Toe**

Learning without thought is labor lost; thought without learning is perilous.

—Confucius (K'ung Fu-tzu; 551–479 B.C.), Chinese philosopher, *Analects*

If a little knowledge is dangerous, where is the man who has so much as to be out of danger?

—T. H. Huxley (1825–1895), British biologist, *On Elementary Instruction in Physiology*

## The Least You Need to Know

➤ The solar plexus reflex on both hands and feet is the best reflex to work on when under a great deal of stress or worry.

➤ The pineal gland manufactures the hormone melatonin. It may be helpful to stimulate the pineal gland reflex if you have insomnia.

➤ Work the inner ear and stomach reflexes if you are experiencing nausea or car sickness.

➤ Fussy babies can quickly be relaxed with the use of reflexology.

➤ Reflexology facilitates relaxation for the body, mind, and soul, making it an excellent remedy for nervous-system and psychological disorders.

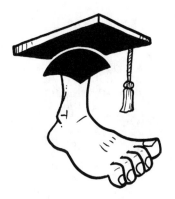

# Reflexology Schools, Teachers, and Associations

## Where to Find a Reflexologist

There are many ways to find a reflexologist. If you have not heard about a good one by word of mouth in your area, contact your country's national organizations to find a local member. If there are none in your area, try some of the following suggestions:

➤ Personally recommended reflexologists in the U.S. and Canada are listed on my Web site: http://www.healingfeats.com/reviewof.htm.

➤ Check your local phone book under reflexologist, holistic health practitioners, or bodyworkers.

➤ Call any local reflexology school for a list of their graduates. Read on for some schools you might want to call. Remember that many schools teach students from all over the world.

➤ See your local holistic practitioner publication/guide book.

➤ Check with your local health food store. Many times they will have a bulletin board or area where practitioners leave their cards, brochures, and flyers.

# Reflexology Organizations

## *Canada*

**The Reflexology Association of Canada**
English Administration (RAC Head Office)
Box #110
541 Turnberry Street
Brussels, Ontario
N0G 1H0
Telephone: 519-887-9991
Fax: 519-887-9792
Toll-free orders only: 877-RAC-FEET (722-3338)
E-mail: reflexca@reflexologycanada.com
Web site: www.reflexologycanada.com

**The Reflexology Association of Canada**
French Administration
305 St. Henri
Drummondville, Quebec
Telephone: 819-474-3351

## *China*

**China Reflexology Association**
P.O. Box 2002
Beijing, 100026
Fax: 861-5068309

## *Ireland*

**National Register of Reflexologists**
c/o The Registrar
Gerald du Bois, Unit 13
The Mall, Terryland Retail Park
Headford Road,
Galway
Ireland
Telephone: +353 91 56 8844
E-mail: footman@tinet.ie
Web site: http://homepage.tinet.ie/~footman/

Note: This organization is not currently online, but you can contact Anthony Larkin, co-founder of the organization, at the above Web site or e-mail addresses for more information. Anthony claims to have the largest collection of reflexology books in the world. This one is his 100th!

## South Africa

South African Reflexology Society
P.O. Box 201858
Durban North 4016

## United Kingdom

**Association of Reflexologists**
27 Old Gloucester Street
London WC1N 3XX
Telephone: 0990 673320
E-mail: aor@reflexology.org
Web site: www.reflexology.org/aor

Note: You can request a catalog of their practitioners along with "friends" or associate members in other countries.

## United States

**American Reflexology Certification Board (ARCB)**
P.O. Box 620627
Littleton, Colorado 80162
Telephone: 303-933-6921
Fax: 303-904-0460

Note: This organization will provide you with a list of members in your area or a contact for an organization near you.

## International Organizations

**International Council of Reflexologists (ICR)**
P.O. Box 621963
Littleton, Colorado 80162 USA
Phone: 303-627-4052

# Reflexology Schools

The following list of schools is organized by home country. However, many of these schools offer classes that come to your area. Check them all out before you decide!

# Australia

**Victorian School of Reflexology and Herbal Studies**
19 Dickson Street
Sunshine, Victoria 3020
Telephone: 61 03 312 5573
Fax: 61 03311 3501

# Canada

**Shanti D. Parakh**
6980 Coach Drive
Niagara Falls, Ontario L2G2J1
Telephone: 905-374-3067

Note: Workshops and lectures on reflexology and related health modalities are offered. Shanti is from India. He offers extremely intuitive and effective reflexology sessions. Shanti visits Rochester, New York, frequently, so I have also added him under the U.S. heading as well.

**Touchpoint**
Yvette Eastman
3186 Bedwell Bay Road
Belcarra, B.C. V3H 4S1
Telephone: 604-936-3227
Toll-free: 800-211-3533
E-mail: touchpnt@npsnet.com
Web site: www.Touchpoint-Institute.com

Note: Certificate courses in reflexology via home study, videos, and Internet make this unique. Instructor will arrange to come to your area! Call for details.

# Ireland

**Larkin School of Reflexology**
Anthony Larkin, Founder
41 Parkfield
New Ross, Co. Wexford
Ireland
Telephone: +353 51 422209
E-mail: footman@tinet.ie
Web site: http://homepage.tinet.ie/~footman

Note: Visit Larkin's Web site for the most comprehensive book list on reflexology anywhere!

# United Kingdom

**Association of Reflexologists**
27 Old Gloucester Street
London WC1N 3XX
Telephone: 0807 5673320
E-mail: UKaor@aol.com
Web site: www.reflexology.org/aor

Note: There are many schools all over the UK. A full listing of Association of Reflexology accredited schools in the UK is listed on their Web site, or you can write and request a catalog.

# United States

**Academy of Natural Healing**
Isabelle Hutton, R.N.
5114 South Emporia Way
Greenwood Village, Colorado 80111
Telephone: 303-779-1094
E-mail: ISHutton@aol.com
Web site: No Web site at this time, but you can see Isabelle listed on my Web site at www.healingfeats.com/reviewof.htm.

Note: Isabelle certifies students and prepares them to pass the national certification exam.

**Colorado School of Healing Arts**
7655 West Mississippi Suite 100
Lakewood, Colorado 80226
Telephone: 303-986-2320
Toll-free: 800-233-7114
Fax: 303-986-6594

Note: Reflexology certificate programs offered.

**Idaho School of Massage Therapy**
5353 Franklin Road
Boise, Idaho 83705
Telephone: 208-343-1847
Fax: 208-363-0938
E-mail: idschmassage@rmci

Note: This massage school currently offers a 140-hour reflexology module technician certificate.

**International Institute of Reflexology**
P.O. Box 12642
St. Petersburg, Florida 33733-2642
Telephone: 727-343-4811
Fax: 727-381-2807

Note: A private International Certification certificate is offered. This school teaches the Ingham Method of Reflexology.

**Modern Institute of Reflexology**
7063 West Colfax Avenue
Denver, Colorado 80215
Telephone: 303-237-1562
Toll-free: 800-533-1837
Fax: 303-237-1606
E-mail: footdocs@ix.netcom.com
Web site: www.reflexologyinstitute.com

Note: This reflexology school offers a 350-hour certification for reflexologists. They also offer correspondence courses and a hands-on finishing school. Fully bonded and licensed by the Colorado Department of Higher Education. Worldwide student body. This school teaches Full Spectrum Reflexology and the use of instruments.

**Shanti D. Parakh**
6980 Coach Drive
Niagara Falls, Ontario L2G2J1
(Also practices in upstate New York)
Telephone: 905-374-3067

Note: Workshops and lectures on reflexology and related health modalities are offered. Shanti is from India. He offers extremely intuitive and healing reflexology treatments. Shanti visits Rochester, New York, frequently, so I have also added him under the U.S. heading. Call him to find out more about classes.

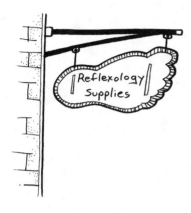

# Supplies and Where to Find Them

## Tables, Chairs, Charts, Tools, and Machines

Call and request a catalog or flyer on these great products that can be used at home for self-help with reflexology.

## *Reflexology Charts*

**Academy of Natural Healing**
Isabelle Hutton, R.N.
5114 South Emporia Way
Greenwood Village, Colorado 80111
Telephone: 303-779-1094
E-mail: ISHutton@aol.com

Note: Beautiful foot and hand charts suitable for framing, also companion muscle charts corresponding to organ/meridian flows. See order form in back of this book.

**Stirling Enterprises**, listed under "Hand Tools," also carries charts.

**Modern Institute of Reflexology**, listed under "Reflexology Schools" in Appendix A.

**International Institute of Reflexology**, listed under "Reflexology Schools" in Appendix A.

# Reflexology Chairs

**Modern Institute of Reflexology**
7043 West Colfax Avenue
Denver, Colorado 80215
Telephone: 303-237-1562
Toll-free: 800-533-1837
Fax: 303-237-1606
E-mail: footdocs@ix.netcom.com
Web site: www.reflexologyinstitute.com

Note: LaFuma collapsible chairs, handmade in France.

# Massage Tables

**Living Earth Crafts**
Don Payne, CEO
600 East Todd Road
Santa Rosa, California 95407
Telephone: 888-380-9044
International: 707-584-4443
E-mail: sales@livingearthcrafts.com
Web site: www.livingearthcrafts.com

Note: Offers environmentally friendly quality massage tables and equipment.

**Ultra Light Corporation**
3140 Roy Messer Highway
White Pine, Tennessee 37890
Telephone: 800-999-1971
International: 423-674-8111
Fax: 423-674-8004

Note: Call for a catalog.

# Hand Tools

**Modern Institute of Reflexology**
7043 West Colfax Avenue
Denver, Colorado 80215
Telephone: 303-237-1562
Toll-free: 800-533-1837
Fax: 303-237-1606
E-mail: footdocs@ix.netcom.com
Web site: www.reflexologyinstitute.com

Note: Dr. Richard Long, retired chiropractor and current reflexologist, handcrafts wooden probes to your specifications. Several different tools and charts are available.

**Stirling Enterprises**
Mildred Carter
P.O. Box 216
Cottage Grove, Oregon 97424
Telephone: 800-766-FOOT (3668)
Fax: 541-942-1046

Note: Wooden probes, plastic clips, and other products and books by Ms. Carter. This is also a source for reflexology charts.

# Complementary/Electronic Machines

**Academy of Natural Healing**
Isabelle Hutton, R.N.
5114 South Emporia Way
Greenwood Village, Colorado 80111
Telephone: 303-779-1094
E-mail: ISHutton@aol.com

Note: Offers the "Chi Machine," a self-help roller-type machine designed to increase life-force energy and oxygenate the body.

**International School of Reflexology and Meridian Therapy**
P.O. Box 68283
Bryanston
Johannesburg 2021
South Africa
Principal: Inge Dougans
Telephone/Fax: +27 11 706-4206
E-mail: vacuflex@iafrica.com

Note: The school has branches worldwide and holds the patent rights for the Vacuflex Reflexology System. Inge gives seminars throughout the world.

**Modern Institute of Reflexology**
7043 West Colfax Avenue
Denver, Colorado 80215
Telephone: 303-237-1562
Toll-free: 800-533-1837
Fax: 303-237-1606
E-mail: footdocs@ix.netcom.com
Web site: www.reflexologyinstitute.com

Note: Foot rollers, Percuss-O-Matic, and several different plug-in tools available.

# Mind Machines and Technology

**Tools for Exploration**
47 Paul Drive
San Rafael, California 94903-2118
Telephone: 888-74-TOOLS (888-748-6657)
International orders: 415-499-9050
Fax: 415-499-9047
E-mail: toolsforexploration@yahoo.com
Web site: www.tools4explore.com

Note: Large, colorful catalog specializing in mind technology, biofeedback, music, and much more.

# Holistic Health Supplies

## Bulk Herbs/Teas

**Pool Ridge Herbals**
Donna Burch, President
P.O. Box 526
Guerneville, California 95446
Telephone: 707-632-6003
Toll-free: 888-422-0320, PIN 6003
Fax: 707-632-6003
E-mail: Poolridg@wco.com
Web site: www.poolridge.com

Note: Pool Ridge Herbals—"Wellness Tonic Teas"—home to 16 varieties of highest quality whole-leaf organic/wild-crafted blends designed for system support and wellness. Beautifully packaged with detailed directions for use on each package.

**Nature Sunshine Products, Inc.**, listed below, also carries some bulk teas and herbs.

## Herbs/Herbal Combinations/Capsules and Tablets

**Nature's Sunshine Products, Inc.**
P.O. Box 19005
Provo, Utah 84605-9005
Telephone: 801-342-4500
Toll-free customer service: 800-223-8225
Fax: 800-472-9328
Web site: www.nsponline.com

Note: This is a quality source for many herbs mentioned in the book. Call customer service for a local supplier in your area.

# Nutraceuticals

**Mannatech, Inc.**
600 South Royal Lane, Suite 200
Coppell, Texas 75019
Telephone: 972-471-8111
Toll-free information line: 800-832-0797
Fax: 800-825-6584
E-mail: jmcfarla@mail.mannatech-inc.com
Web site: www.mannatech-inc.com

Note: Offers a line of nutraceuticals. Nutraceuticals are natural products that have scientific studies that prove their effectiveness.

# Supplements/Vitamins

**Nature's Sunshine Products, Inc.**
P.O. Box 19005
Provo, Utah 84605-9005
Telephone: 801-342-4500
Toll-free customer service: 800-223-8225
Toll-free Spanish: 800-321-4652
In the U.K.: 44 95 267 1600
In Canada: 905-458-6100
Fax: 800-472-9328
Web site: www.nsponline.com

Note: This is a source for high-quality supplements mentioned in the book, including liquid chlorophyll, colloidal silver, colloidal minerals, and zinc. (NSP has offices in several countries. Visit their Web site for more information.)

**Mannatech, Inc.**
600 South Royal Lane, Suite 200
Coppell, Texas 75019
Telephone: 972-471-8111
Toll-free information line: 800-832-0797
Fax: 800-825-6584
E-mail: jmcfarla@mail.mannatech-inc.com
Web site: www.mannatech-inc.com

Note: Offers food-based vitamins and metabolic typing profiles to choose your formulas. Call to find a local distributor in your area.

# Essential Oils/Aromatherapy/Diffusers

**Young Living Essential Oils**
250 South Main Street
Payson, Utah 84651
Telephone: 801-263-6200
Fax: 801-465-5424
Web site: www.youngliving.com

Note: This company manufactures essential oils they say are grade A. Call for more clarification or a local distributor.

**Nature's Sunshine Products, Inc.**
P.O. Box 19005
Provo, Utah 84605-9005
Telephone: 801-342-4500
Toll-free customer service: 800-223-8225
Toll-free Spanish: 800-321-4652
In the U.K.: 44 95 267 1600
In Canada: 905-458-6100
Fax: 800-472-9328
Web site: www.nsponline.com

Note: Nature's Sunshine carries a line of grade A essential oils.

# Flower Essences

**Pegasus Products, Inc.**
P.O. Box 228
Boulder, Colorado 80306-0228
Telephone: 970-667-3019
Toll-free: 800-527-6104
Fax: 970-667-3624
E-mail: STARVIBE@indra.com
Web site: www.pegasusproducts.com

Note: Offers a great line of flower and gem essences.

# Ear Cones

**Coning Works**
Irene McFee
c/o 2370 West Highway 89A Suite 11-144
Sedona, Arizona 86336
Telephone: 520-282-7812

Note: Irene manufactures a whole line of ear cones utilizing different herbs for specific uses. Call for a full listing of her cone choices.

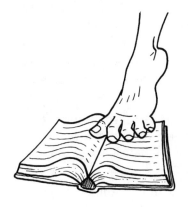

# What Does It All Mean? A Brief Glossary

**Acupressure**   A traditional Chinese therapeutic technique whereby pressure is applied to acupuncture points. Acupuncture and acupressure use the same points; the difference is that acupuncture utilizes sterile needles, and acupressure does not penetrate the skin.

**Alimentary canal**   The scientific name for what I refer to in this book as the food tube. It is the canal or tube that begins at the mouth and ends at the rectum and processes food for absorption and elimination.

**Alveoli**   Small pockets that stick out along the walls of alveolar sacs in the lung. This is where carbon dioxide leaves the blood and the blood takes in oxygen.

**Anaerobic**   The inability of the body to utilize molecular oxygen for proper cellular respiration.

**Anemia**   A reduction of the amount of hemoglobin being carried in the blood. A spleen not doing its job efficiently can cause anemia. Symptoms of anemia include fatigue, pallor, lowered immune response, and exhaustion. Next time you're thinking "anemia boost of energy," work your spleen reflex.

**Antibodies**   Substances made in the lymphoid tissue and released into the bloodstream to attack antigens and render them harmless.

**Antigens**   Any type of substances foreign to the body that are potentially dangerous. When antigens are discovered in the body, antibodies are created in response.

**Aromatherapy**   The therapeutic use of aroma or smells to gain a positive, desired effect.

**Arteriosclerosis** A chronic disease where the arteries become thick, hard, and lose their elasticity, which results in impaired blood circulation. Symptoms may include cold hands and feet, blurred vision, high blood pressure, and difficulty in thinking and breathing. Causes have been linked to too much saturated fat in the diet, lack of aerobic exercise, and too much caffeine, salt, or alcohol in the diet.

**Asthma** A condition characterized by attacks of bronchiolespasms causing difficulty in breathing. Asthma is brought on by an array of stimuli including allergens, exertion, emotions, and infections.

**Athlete's foot** A fungal condition that is actually ringworm. The medical name for this infection is *Tinea Pedis*. This fungus is contagious. Athlete's foot was so named because it has been a common condition among athletes who share locker rooms (barefoot) and showers.

**Autonomic nervous system** The part of your nervous system that is in control of the bodily functions like digestion, heartbeat, perspiration, and so on, that we do not consciously direct.

**Autopsy** A medical term used to describe the dissection and examination of a dead body to determine the cause of death or the presence of the disease process.

**Ayurveda** The ancient Indian form of healing medicine. Ayurvedic colleges are equivalent to Western medical schools. Ayurveda is based on the principal that illness is caused by toxin buildup in the body and/or nutritional deficiencies.

**Bedside manner** A term used to describe how a doctor behaves in front of or toward his patient. Reflexologists also need to develop a good bedside manner for the recipient to feel comfortable, at ease, relaxed, and well cared for.

**Blood-brain barrier** A protective mechanism made of a semi-permeable membrane that keeps solid particles and large molecules from entering the brain cells.

**Body reflexology** Similar to foot and hand reflexology but the reflexes are found over the entire body, not just on the feet and hands.

**Bronchiole** A small airway of the breathing system from the bronchi to the lobes of the lung. The bronchioles allow the exchange of air and waste gases between the alveolar ducts and the bronchi.

**Bronchitis** Inflammation of the bronchi. It is an illness characterized by coughing, a constriction of the bronchi due to spasms, and the production of copious amounts of mucus from the bronchi. Culprits are smoking, air pollution, and generally dirty or underactive lungs.

**Catarrh** Rhymes with guitar and is the excessive secretion of thick phlegm or mucus by the mucus membranes of the nose or nasal cavities. The term is not used in a scientific context, but is used as a general term and usually will be referred to as mucus that has been dried up or hardened in the sinus passages.

**Central nervous system**   Includes the brain and spinal cord and controls conscious thoughts and actions like movement and talking.

**Colon transit time**   A phrase used by holistic health practitioners to address how fast or sluggish your colon may be. It refers to the time it takes for a meal to be eaten and eliminated. A healthy colon transit time should be between 16 and 18 hours.

**Contraindication**   A term meaning any factor in a condition that makes it unwise to pursue a certain line of treatment. For a light example, you would not give a massage to a person with a severe sunburn!

**Dehydration**   The lack of water in body tissues. Lack of efficient water intake, vomiting, diarrhea, and sweating can all be causes of dehydration. Symptoms may include great thirst, nausea, and exhaustion. If drinking plenty of water does not immediately correct the problem, sometimes water and salts need to administered intravenously at an emergency room.

**Diabetes mellitus**   A disorder of carbohydrate metabolism in which sugars in the body are not oxidized to produce energy due to lack of the pancreatic hormone insulin or to resistance to insulin. The accumulation of sugar leads to its appearance in the blood (hyperglycemia), then in the urine; symptoms include thirst, loss of weight, and the excessive production of urine. Complications can include poor circulation leading to slow healing, poor eyesight, weight gain, and coma if insulin and diet are not regulated. *See also* Hyperglycemia.

**Diverticulitis**   A disease of the bowel where compacted fecal matter causes pressure in the bowel that produces small pouches or bowel pockets along the intestinal walls. These sacs can fester and swell, causing severe discomfort. These infected pockets can be dangerous or deadly if they burst.

**Emphysema**   A disease characterized by breathlessness. Victims of this disease usually require oxygen tanks to assist their breathing capacity. The disease occurs because the area of the lungs that is responsible for exchanging oxygen and carbon dioxide is damaged. There is really no known cure for emphysema, therefore prevention is best.

**Endorphins**   Substances in the nervous system released by the pituitary gland that affect the central nervous system by reducing pain. Their effect on the body is similar to the effects of using pain-killing medications such as morphine.

**Entrainment**   The phenomenon of self-regulated synchronization of the pulsing of two objects. For instance, clocks put together in a room and left alone will eventually synchronize and beat at the same pulse. Some researchers think that our heart entrains with the beat of the earth.

**Fallen arches**   Can happen with prolonged standing or excessive weight, tearing, or weakening of the muscles of the arch of the feet, causing flat feet.

**Femur, tibia** and **fibula,** and **patella**   All bones of the leg. The patella is the kneecap, the femur is the largest leg bone, and the tibia and fibula make up the shins.

**Footbath**   The use of water and sometimes essential oils applied to the feet and lower legs to change the condition of or circulation in the body.

**Four-element model**   Used as a tool to teach a philosophical way of seeing the elements (air, fire, water, and earth) in everything we do.

**Gallstone**   A hard stone-like mass made up of cholesterol (blood fat), bile pigments, and calcium salts. Gallstones can cause trouble when and if they get stuck in a bile duct, where they can cause jaundice.

**Glandular system**   A general term used to describe all the glands of the body. The glandular system is divided into two categories, the endocrine glands (without ducts) and exocrine glands (with ducts). Glands are considered to be an organ or group of cells that make and secrete fluids, such as hormones.

**Goiter**   An enlargement of the thyroid gland. Goiter is usually caused by a lack of iodine. The thyroid is actually working hard to attract the nutrient iodine (its main source of food) and enlarges in the process.

**Grounded**   A term used commonly to refer to being focused and connected to the earth or physical reality. It is used interchangeably with the phrase "having both feet on the ground." Being grounded can be used to describe a practical, down-to-earth, goal-oriented person.

**Hallux valgus**   A deviation of the large toe at its metatarsophalangeal joint. This deviation causes what is known as a bunion. *Hallux* is Latin for "great toe," and *valgus* means "an overt positional deformity, turning away from the midline of the body."

**Hammer toe**   A deformity of the toe. Most often this occurs in the second toe (the wealth toe!) and is caused by fixed flexion of the first joint. In other words, the joint of the toe gets permanently fixed in a bent position.

**Hering's Law of Cure**   A standard philosophy for healing naturally. It states: "All healing starts from the head down, from the inside out, and in reverse order that the symptoms have been acquired."

**Hertz frequency**   A measurement of vibrational frequency and energy levels. Everything is composed of energy and therefore has a certain vibration.

**Hiatal hernia**   A condition of the stomach where the stomach is pushed up into the esophagus, causing pain, indigestion, heartburn especially when lying down, a feeling of a lump in the throat, inability to gain or lose weight, anxiety attacks, and can have many other symptoms. Some symptoms even resemble those of a heart attack.

**Holistic**   A term used to describe a way of living, practicing, or thinking that takes into account all factors of life. In holistic health, a practitioner will consider the physical, mental, emotional, and spiritual aspects of the person to help them back to balance.

**Homeostasis**   The medical term used for the body's internal balancing act. It means that our unconscious body functions, such as body temperature and glandular secretions, are working for us to keep us alive and functioning. Life truly is a balancing act.

**Hydrangea**   The leaves and root of the hydrangea plant have been used by herbalists and nutritionists for years as a solvent for calculus stones and other gravel deposits in the body. It has been used to relieve backaches due to kidney and rheumatic problems, prevent the formation of gravel deposits, gallstones, kidney stones, enlarged prostate gland, and help relieve the pain from each!

**Hyperglycemia**   Also known as diabetes, which is a disease relating to the pancreas and its insufficient production of insulin to keep the blood sugar level balanced. Diabetes, in effect, is high blood sugar. *See also* Diabetes mellitus.

**Hyperthyroid**   An overactive thyroid leading to symptoms such as nervous irritability, excitability, ferocious appetite, inability to gain weight, a racing heart, and popping eyes.

**Hypoglycemia**   A condition that is related to the over-production of insulin by the pancreas, which lowers blood sugar levels. Low blood sugar levels can affect brain function. If not controlled, low blood sugar can be a precursor to diabetes.

**Hypothyroid**   A thyroid that is worn out and underactive. It usually is too weak to produce the correct thyroid hormones. Symptoms of hypothyroidism are a general slowing down of the metabolism, causing coldness, slowed speech, slower movements, lethargy, and trouble staying asleep.

**Hysterectomy**   The removal of a woman's uterus. Sometimes a full utero-ovarian hysterectomy will be performed, which also removes one or both of the ovaries.

**Insomnia**   The inability to fall asleep or to remain asleep for an adequate length of time.

**Kegel exercises**   Commonly referred to as Kegels. Exercises for women that involve tightening the lower pelvis muscles, simulating the same feeling as stopping urine flow. Contractions should be held for 6 to 10 seconds, followed by complete muscle relaxation. This should be done four or five times in a series three to four times a day.

**Keratosis**   Any horny growth of the skin. Most commonly seen as warts or corns.

**Lecithin**   A substance produced by the liver if the diet is adequate. It is needed by every cell in the body and largely makes up cell membranes; without it they would harden. Lecithin protects cells from oxidation, protects the brain, and is a fat emulsifier. Supplements are usually derived from soybeans, which contain a fair amount of lecithin.

**Manic-depressive psychosis** or **bipolar disorder**   A severe mental illness characterized by severe depression followed by bouts of mania. Mania takes the form of obsession, compulsion, or an exaggerated feeling of euphoria.

**Menopause**   When a woman's ovaries stop producing eggs. The ovaries discontinue their hormone production, which sometimes leads to dry skin, emotional instability, hot flashes, and heart palpitations.

**Meridians**   Invisible lines of energy that run longitudinally along the body. The mapping of these meridian lines along the body is known as zone therapy, which many say is just another name for reflexology.

**Moroseness**   Feeling ill-humored and depressed. Can be caused by an improper functioning of the pituitary gland located in the midbrain. Stimulating this gland with reflexology just might be key to alleviating depression and can lift your spirits!

**Mouse shoulder**   A spasm of the muscles behind the shoulder blade that can pull the vertebrae in the upper neck and back out of alignment. This situation is usually found on the side of the body that is used to operate a computer mouse and can cause pain and stiffness or even numbness in the arm and hand on that side. Mouse shoulder will give you something to squeak about.

**Multiple sclerosis**   A chronic nervous system disease in which the myelin sheaths surrounding the nerves and spinal cord are damaged, affecting the function of the nerves involved. Symptoms vary but may include an unsteady gait, shaky limbs, and involuntary movements of the eyes.

**Orthotic inserts**   Special prescription shoe inserts designed to support or supplement weakened joints or limbs.

**Ovulation**   Occurs in females and is a term used to describe the time in a woman's menstrual cycle when the ovaries produce an egg and deliver the egg to the uterus to be (sometimes) fertilized. This process is controlled by the hormones secreted by the pituitary gland.

**Papovavirus hominis**   A virus that causes painful plantar warts. Footbaths may help in killing the virus.

**PMS**   Stands for **premenstrual syndrome**. Because of its host of symptoms, this ailment is known as a syndrome. PMS symptoms may include: tension, irritability, emotional disturbance, headache, abdominal bloating, tender and swollen breasts, pimples, and water retention.

**Podiatry**   The health profession that cares for the human foot. The doctor of podiatric medicine is called a **podiatrist** and examines, diagnoses, and treats diseases, injuries, and defects of the foot.

**Pretense**   A false action or appearance or intention to deceive. In some belief systems, hurting your pinky finger means that you are trying to be someone you are not or are "trying too hard" to make something appear different than it is. In Jin Shin Jyutsu, the pinky fingers are associated with the emotion "to try, trying to, or pretense."

**Pronate** *(verb)* or **pronation**   The lowering of the inner edge of the foot by turning it.

**Psychoneuroimmunology**   The study of how our thoughts affect our health. Broken down to its components, *psycho* means "the mind," *neuro* means "the nerves," *immun* stands for "the immune system," and *ology* means "the study of." The word literally means mind + nerves + immune + the study of.

**Phytochemicals**   Natural plant substances such as hormones, bioflavonoids, or carotenoids (and thousands of others) that make up a plant and are considered nutrients for our body.

**Reflexology**   The term literally means the study of how one part reflects or relates to another part of the body. Reflexology is a holistic therapy used for health management and maintenance and can also be used as a health and personality analysis tool.

**Rosacea**   A skin disease on the face in which the blood vessels on the cheeks and nose enlarge, causing the face to appear bright red or flushed. The cause is uncertain, but it is believed that extremes in temperature, food irritants, and too much alcohol can all play a part in aggravating the condition.

**Schizophrenia**   A severe mental disorder characterized by delusions, hallucinations, and the belief that his/her thoughts and actions are shared by or controlled by others.

**Sciatica**   A pain felt down the back and outer side of the thigh, leg, and foot, even radiating into the heel. It is sometimes caused by a degeneration of an intervertebral disk that compresses a spinal nerve root. The onset may be suddenly brought on by awkward twisting or lifting movements.

**Seasonal Affective Disorder**   Otherwise known as SAD. A syndrome characterized by severe depression during certain times of the year. This disorder brings on a desire to overeat, especially carbohydrates. Most notably the depression is experienced during times when there is a lack of sunshine. Stimulating the pineal gland may help SAD people.

**Sinusitis**   An inflammation of one or more of the mucus-lined air spaces in the facial bones that communicate with the nose. It is often caused by infections spreading from the nose. Symptoms include headache and tenderness over the affected sinus, which may become filled with a purulent material that is discharged through the nose.

**Solar plexus**   Found right in the middle of where the rib cage comes together about at the stomach level in front of the diaphragm. It is a great network of nerves that goes out to all parts of the abdominal cavity.

**Subluxation**   The fancy word for any joint being out of alignment. If you visit a chiropractor, you will usually find that she will diagnose you with one or more subluxations along your spinal column. Reflexology can help chiropractic adjustments last longer by keeping the muscles relaxed.

**Supination**   A condition in which the foot is turned inward so that the medial (outer) margin is elevated.

**Symbology** or **symbolism**   Describes how a symbol can represent something else. For instance, each country has a flag that symbolizes the particular country. Everyone has their own personalized set of symbolic meanings based on their life experiences. This is why you can be the best interpreter of your own dream details.

**Tinnitus**   A condition characterized by any noise, buzzing, or ringing in the ear. Causes of tinnitus may be excess ear wax, damage to the eardrum, Meniere's disease, or thinning blood due to overuse of aspirin or other drugs. Dr. Bernard Jensen also links tinnitus to a lack of magnesium.

**Torque**   A turning or twisting force. In reflexology treatments, you need to be careful not to torque the knee, since the knee is only designed to bend one way.

**Zone therapy**   Used interchangeably with reflexology. Zone therapy was coined by a medical doctor in the late 1800s and is used to describe the theory of energy zones that run longitudinally along the body.

# Index

# C

**389**

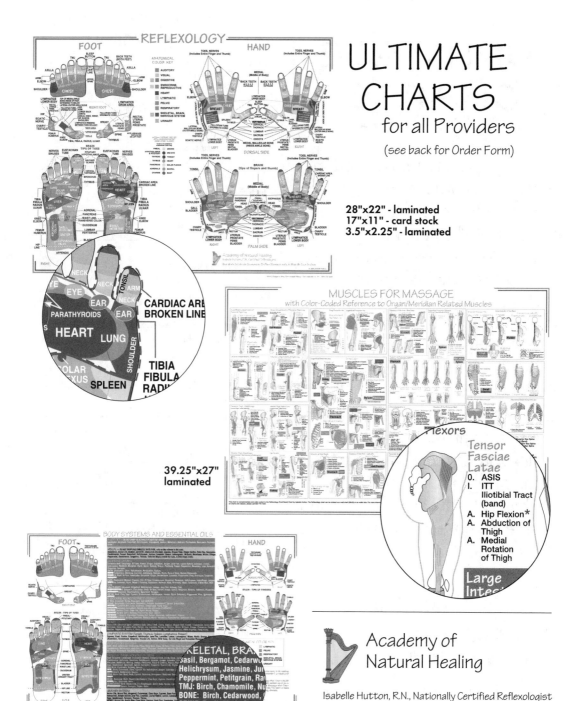

# ULTIMATE CHARTS
## for all Providers
(see back for Order Form)

**REFLEXOLOGY**
FOOT — HAND

28"x22" - laminated
17"x11" - card stock
3.5"x2.25" - laminated

39.25"x27"
laminated

MUSCLES FOR MASSAGE
with Color-Coded Reference to Organ/Meridian Related Muscles

Flexors

Tensor
Fasciae
Latae

0. ASIS
I. ITT
Iliotibial Tract (band)
A. Hip Flexion*
A. Abduction of Thigh
A. Medial Rotation of Thigh

Large Intes...

CARDIAC AREA
BROKEN LINE

HEART LUNG

TIBIA
FIBULA
RADIUS

SPLEEN

BODY SYSTEMS AND ESSENTIAL OILS
FOOT — HAND

17"x11" - card stock

Basil, Bergamot, Cedarwood...
Helichrysum, Jasmine, Ju...
Peppermint, Petitgrain, Ra...
TMJ: Birch, Chamomile, Nu...
BONE: Birch, Cedarwood, ...
SPINE: Basil, Birch, Cypre...
BRAIN: Bergamot, Birch...
...TIC NERVE: Birch...

## Academy of Natural Healing

Isabelle Hutton, R.N., Nationally Certified Reflexologist
5114 S. Emporia Way • Greenwood Village, CO 80111
303-779-1094 • Email: ISHutton@aol.com

**393**

# ULTIMATE CHARTS
## for all Providers

At a glance, the color-coded charts show where and what to work on for the feet/hands/muscles of the body. Topical application of essential oils may be an added enhancement.

Color-coding is consistent on all three charts. The muscles are color-coded to relate to the organs/reflexes/meridians and oils for each body system. The "Body Systems & Essential Oils" chart is complimentary to the Reflexology and Muscle charts or it can stand alone.

These charts are an excellent source of knowledge for all healing modalities.

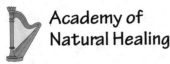

## Academy of Natural Healing

Isabelle Hutton, R.N., Nationally Certified Reflexologist
5114 S. Emporia Way • Greenwood Village, CO 80111
303-779-1094 • Email: ISHutton@aol.com

## ORDER FORM

**Reflexology Wall Chart**
**28"x22" - Laminated**

|  | | Qty. | Total |
|---|---|---|---|
| $35.00 | x | _____ | = _____ |

**Reflexology Chart**
**17"x11" - Card Stock**
$25.00     x _____ = _____

**Individual Hand and Foot**
**3.5"x2.25" - Laminated**
$3.00 (Hand)     x _____ = _____
$3.00 (Foot)     x _____ = _____

**Muscle Wall Chart**
**39.25"x27" - Laminated**
$45.00     x _____ = _____

**Body Systems and Essential Oils**
**17"x11" - Card Stock**
$15.00     x _____ = _____

SHIPPING & HANDLING          _____
(see below)
TAX (3.8% CO Residents)          _____
                    **TOTAL**  _____

### Shipping & Handling
Wall Charts (Reflexology & Muscle)
$8 for 1-5 charts, $1 for each additional chart

17x11 Charts (Reflexology & Essential Oil)
$5 for 1-5 charts, 50¢ for each additional chart

Individual Hand and Foot Mini Charts
$1 for 1-10 charts, 50¢ for each additional 10 charts

Name _____

Address _____

City/State/Zip _____

Telephone _____

E-Mail _____

Send order form with check to:
Isabelle Hutton
Academy of Natural Healing
5114 S. Emporia Way
Greenwood Village, CO 80111